Clinical Neuroscience

AN ILLUSTRATED COLOUR TEXT

Content Strategist: Jeremy Bowes
Content Development Specialist: Fiona Conn
Project Manager: Umarani Natarajan
Designer/Design Direction: Miles Hitchen
Illustration Manager: Jennifer Rose
Illustrator: Graeme Chambers

Clinical Neuroscience

AN ILLUSTRATED COLOUR TEXT

Paul Johns BSc BM MSc FRCPath
Consultant Neuropathologist and Senior Lecturer in Neuroanatomy
St George's Healthcare NHS Trust and St George's University of London
London, UK

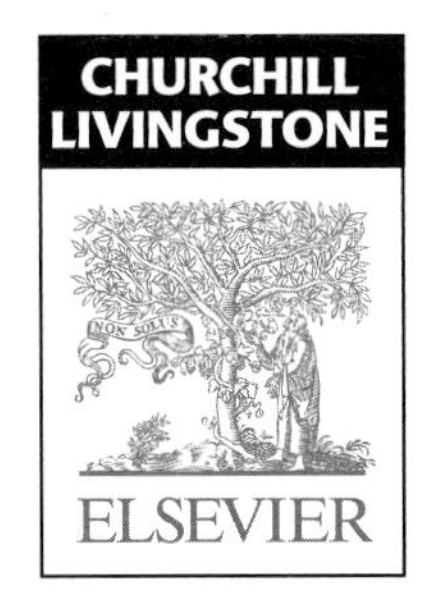

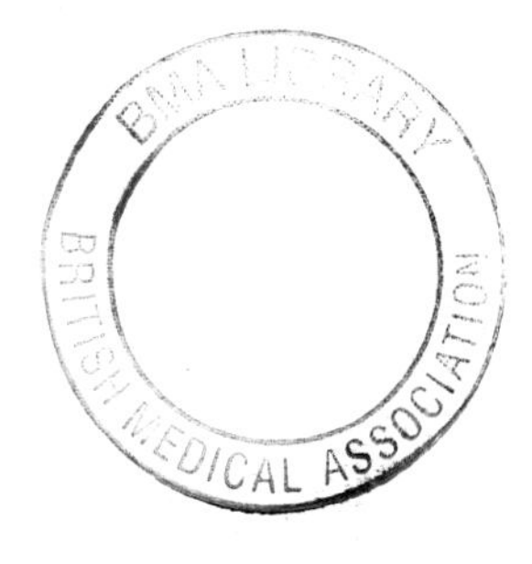

EDINBURGH LONDON NEW YORK OXFORD PHILADELPHIA ST LOUIS SYDNEY TORONTO 2014

CHURCHILL
LIVINGSTONE
ELSEVIER

ISBN 978-0-443-10321-6
ebook ISBN 978-1-4557-4212-7

British Library Cataloguing in Publication Data
A catalogue record for this book is available from the British Library

Library of Congress Cataloging in Publication Data
A catalog record for this book is available from the Library of Congress

Printed in China

The publisher's policy is to use **paper manufactured from sustainable forests**

For Iris,

Born on the 5th of December, 2013

Preface

This new addition to the *Illustrated Colour Text* (*ICT*) series provides a short, readable introduction to basic and clinical neuroscience. It is intended to contain 'all you need to know' to get a good understanding of the nervous system and its most important disorders. There are two main aims:

- Explain the core principles of cellular and molecular neuroscience, emphasising aspects that are important for understanding common brain diseases
- Provide an integrated, up-to-date description of the most important neurological disorders (such as stroke, epilepsy and dementia) and their scientific basis.

This text should be an ideal companion to the very popular *Neuroanatomy ICT* by Crossman and Neary and has been written in the same chapter-based format. Although the book is not divided into sections, the second half is more clinically-orientated than the first.

The earlier chapters introduce a number of core neuroscience topics, including the development, anatomy and cellular constituents of the nervous system. Some fundamental (and potentially confusing) concepts are explained, including the electrical properties of neurons and the principles of synaptic transmission. Before moving on to discuss specific neurological conditions in detail, there is an introductory chapter on the cellular mechanisms of neurological disease, which provides an overview of basic pathological processes (such as inflammation, gliosis, cell death and neurodegeneration).

The second half of the book focuses on the most common and important neurological disorders, with separate chapters on head injury, stroke, epilepsy, dementia, Parkinson's disease and multiple sclerosis. These provide a comprehensive and integrated introduction to each main disease, together with a number of associated and related conditions. Each chapter begins with the key clinical features (e.g., symptoms, signs and main imaging findings) before describing how each disorder is diagnosed and treated. Sections on aetiology and pathogenesis draw on relevant aspects of anatomy, pathology, physiology and pharmacology. In addition, numerous 'clinical boxes' (with a blue stethoscope icon) are scattered throughout the text, highlighting a wide range of neurological diseases, investigations and treatments.

Neuroscience is a challenging subject that is easier (and more interesting) to learn when it is understood rather than memorised; for this reason, emphasis has been placed on comprehension rather than rote learning. For instance, when new terms are introduced the word origins are usually given in brackets (at least when they seem to make sense!) and some of the more difficult-to-pronounce words have been spelled out phonetically. To summarise and reinforce the most important information (and to facilitate exam preparation) succinct 'key points' boxes are provided throughout.

The text has been prepared with the needs of medical students in mind and should be suitable for the majority of undergraduate medical courses; in addition, the integrated style should fit well with case-based and problem-based curricula. The content should be suitable not only for the earlier, more theoretical years of medical school (when exam preparation and revision are often foremost in the mind) but also in the later, more clinically-orientated years when the priority shifts towards survival during ward rounds and outpatient clinics! It should also be useful as an update and refresher for junior doctors embarking on potentially-daunting 'neuro' rotations – or for those entering specialist training in neurology-related disciplines.

Although it will be of particular interest to medical students and junior doctors, the book is suitable for anyone interested in the nervous system and its disorders, including undergraduate and postgraduate students in neuroscience, psychology and the biomedical sciences. The content is also relevant to a wide range of healthcare professions allied to medicine which require a basic knowledge of the nervous system and its disorders. To help make it more accessible to non-medical readers, a brief appendix of anatomical terminology has been included.

Much of this book was written during my specialist training in neuropathology at the National Hospital for Neurology and Neurosurgery (Queen Square, London) and was completed after I had taken up my present post as a consultant neuropathologist at St George's Hospital in Tooting (South London). Although it has certainly been extremely hard work at times, the process has also been very enjoyable – and I sincerely hope that this new volume in the *Illustrated Colour Text* series will prove to be a useful and worthwhile contribution.

Paul Johns
London, 2014

Acknowledgements

I am indebted to Professor Nick Fox, Professor Steve Gentleman, Dr Andrew MacKinnon, Dr Gemma Northam, Dr Gil Rabinovici, Professor László Seress and Professor Roy Weller for kindly providing various scans, micrographs and other images (in some cases more than one).

Thank you also to the following expert reviewers for their invaluable comments and suggestions on the stroke, epilepsy, dementia and Parkinson's disease chapters: Dr John Bamford, Professor Paul Bolam, Dr Peter Garrard, Professor Steve Gentleman, Professor David Mann, Dr Barry Moynihan, Dr Andrew Nicolson, Dr Dominic Paviour, Dr Maria Thom, Professor Michael Trimble and Professor Matthew Walker. I would also like to thank Dr James Thomas for the many hours of discussion, feedback and encouragement, particularly during the earlier stages of the project.

I am grateful to numerous individuals at Elsevier who have helped in various ways to bring this project to fruition, including Jeremy Bowes, Fiona Conn, Uma Natarajan and Andrew Riley. I would particularly like to thank Timothy Horne, who gave me the opportunity to write the book in the first place – and Graeme Chambers, who has managed to convert my many pages of hand-drawn pictures and scribbled explanatory notes into a superb collection of illustrations and diagrams.

Finally, I would like to thank Gemma (whose brain features in Figs 3.6c and A.5-7!), not only for helping me in many different ways with the book, but also for continuing to put up with all of my many faults – and most of all, for agreeing to be my wife.

Paul Johns
London, 2014

Contents

Chapter 1
Overview of the nervous system

CHAPTER CONTENTS

This chapter provides an overview of the main structural and functional components of the nervous system and introduces the topographical anatomy of the brain and its protective coverings. Many of the concepts introduced here will be discussed in more detail in subsequent chapters.

Parts of the nervous system

Central and peripheral nervous systems

The nervous system is divided into central and peripheral parts (Fig. 1.1). The **central nervous system (CNS)** is made up of the brain and spinal cord, encased within the bones of the skull and vertebral column. The CNS represents the main integrating and decision-making centre of the nervous system. The **peripheral nervous system (PNS)** includes 31 pairs of **spinal nerves** which emerge between the vertebrae (Fig. 1.2) and 12 pairs of **cranial nerves** which arise from the base of the brain (Fig. 1.3). At the roots of the upper and lower limbs, sensory and motor fibres are redistributed in the **brachial** and **lumbosacral plexuses** to enter a number of named **peripheral nerves** (Figs 1.4 and 1.5). The function of the PNS is to transmit nerve impulses to and from the brain and spinal cord.

The motor component of the peripheral nervous system is further subdivided into **somatic** and **autonomic** parts. The **somatic nervous system** innervates the skeletal musculature and is responsible for 'voluntary' (consciously initiated) actions. The **autonomic nervous system** supplies the internal organs and other visceral structures and operates at an automatic (mainly unconscious) level.

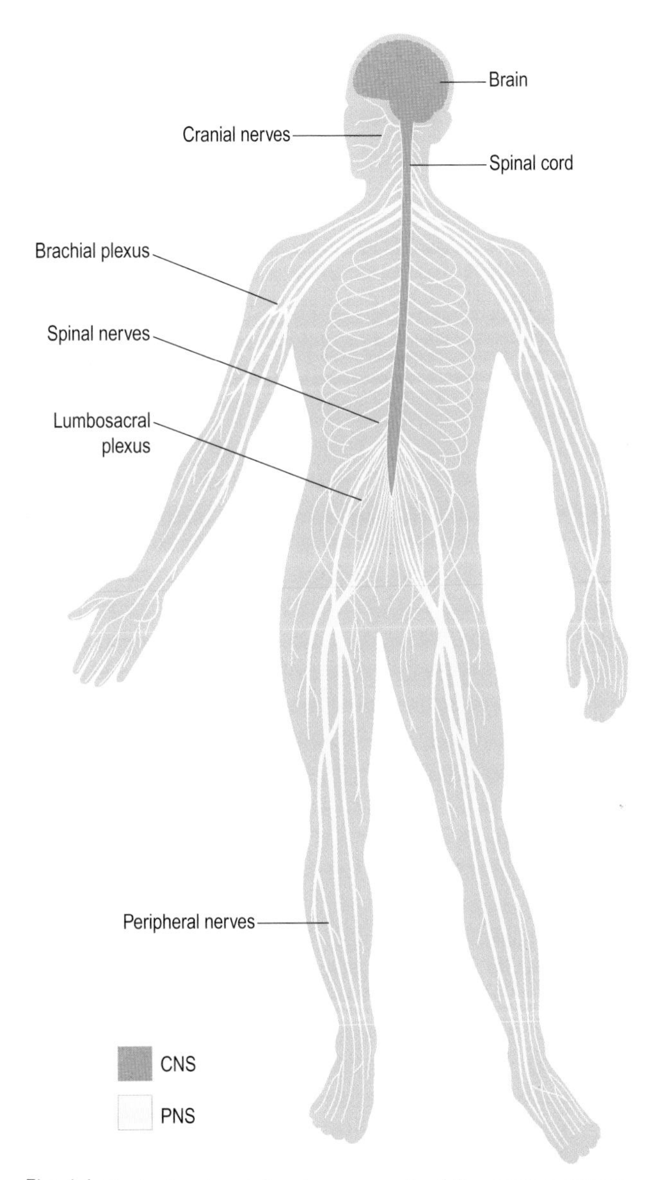

Fig. 1.1 **Central and peripheral components of the nervous system.** The central nervous system (CNS) includes the brain and spinal cord. The peripheral nervous system (PNS) is made up of sensory and motor fibres passing to and from the CNS.

Autonomic nervous system

The autonomic nervous system (ANS) or **visceromotor system** regulates the activities of the cardiovascular, respiratory, digestive and urogenital systems. It operates autonomously (Greek: autos, self; nomos, governed by law). The ANS depends upon a constant stream of sensory information from the internal organs and blood vessels which it uses to regulate the contraction of cardiac and smooth muscle and the secretory activity of glands. Ultimate control of the autonomic nervous system resides in the **hypothalamus**, a tiny region at the centre of the brain that is sometimes referred to as the 'head ganglion' of the ANS (described later; see also Ch. 3).

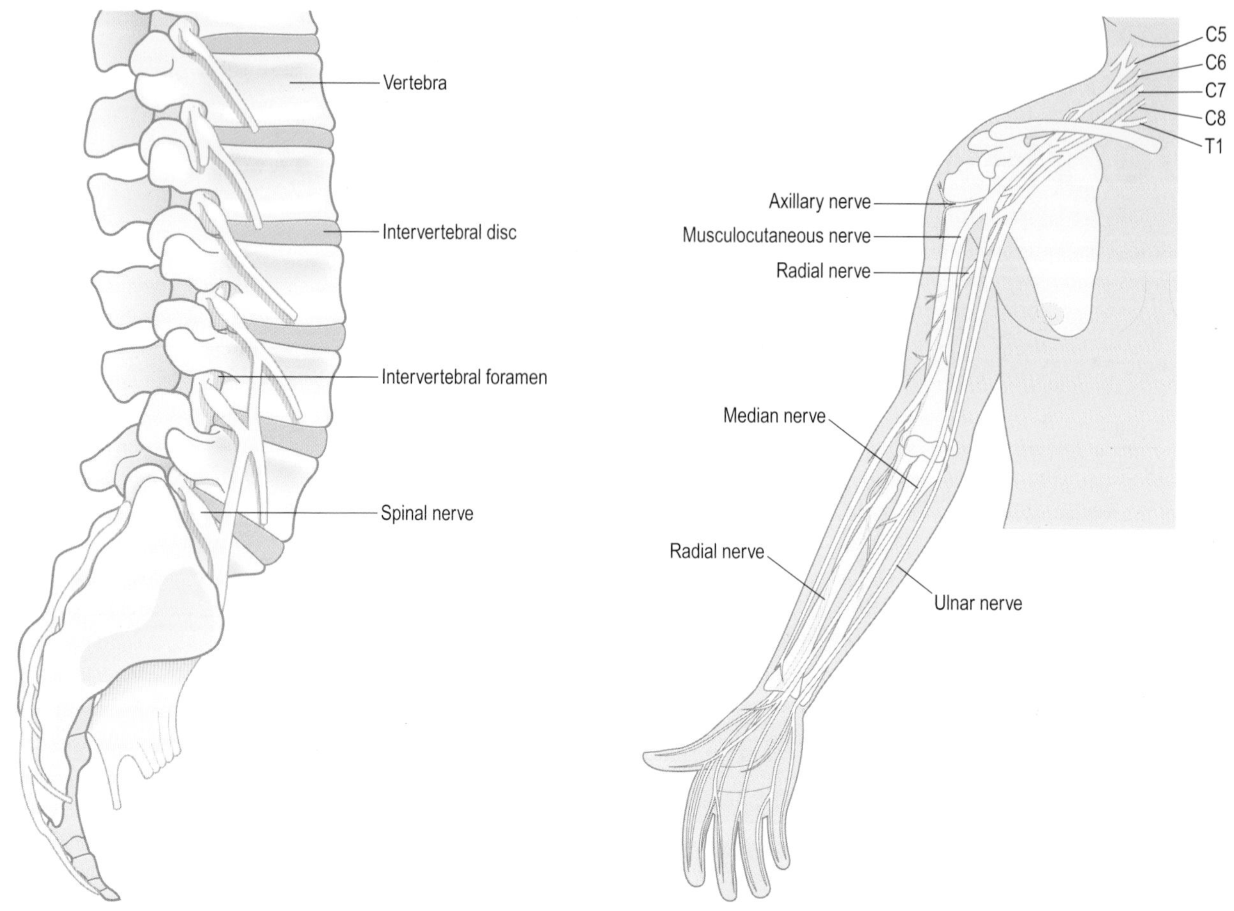

Fig. 1.2 **Lateral view of the vertebral column in the lumbosacral region.** The mixed spinal nerves can be seen emerging from the intervertebral foramina.

Fig. 1.4 **The brachial plexus giving rise to the main named peripheral nerves of the upper limb.**

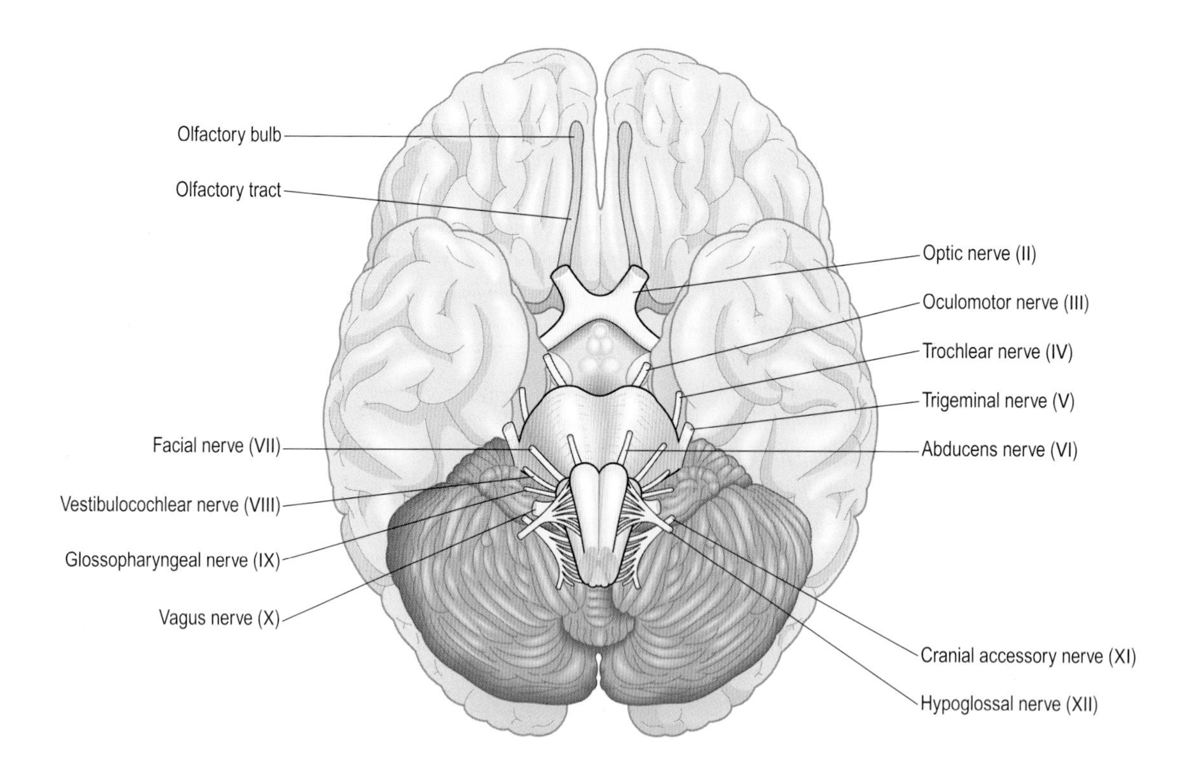

Fig. 1.3 **Ventral aspect of the brain illustrating the cranial nerves, which are conventionally labelled using Roman numerals.** The olfactory nerve (cranial nerve I) is not seen here; it consists of millions of filaments that arise from the nasal cavity and synapse in the olfactory bulb.

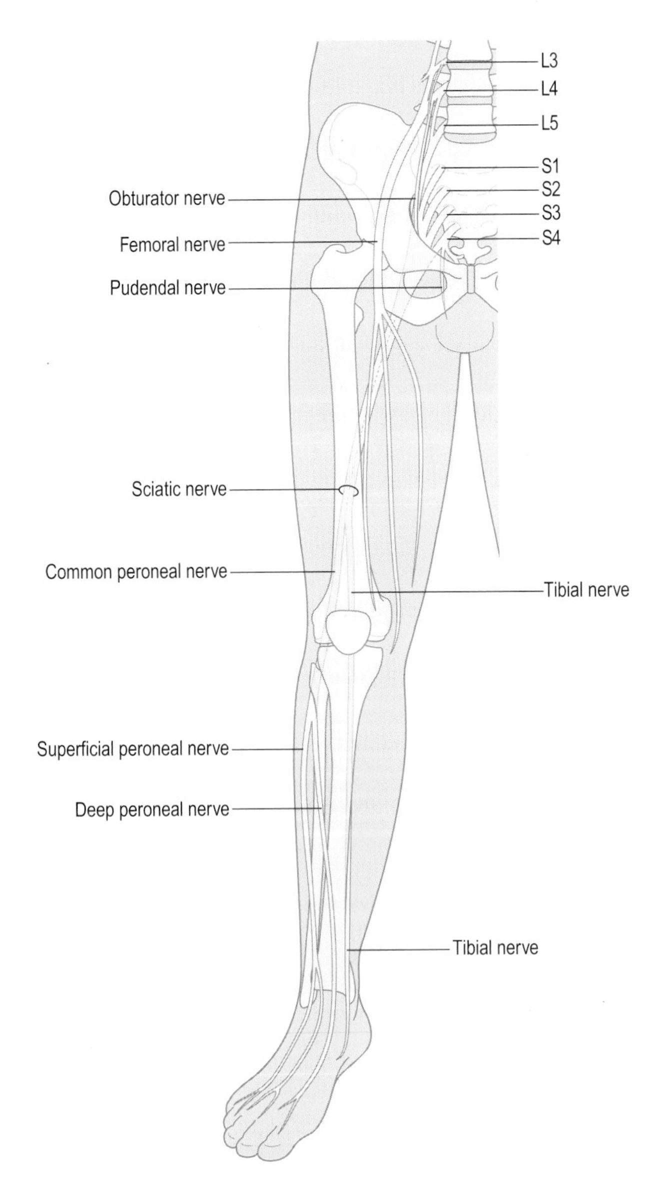

Fig. 1.5 **The lumbosacral plexus giving rise to the main named peripheral nerves of the lower limb.**

Sympathetic	Parasympathetic
Dilated pupils	Constricted pupils
Dry mouth	Salivation
Increased heart rate	Decreased heart rate
Dilated airways	Constricted airways
Inhibited digestion	Stimulated digestion
Retention of urine	Voiding of urine
Ejaculation	Erection

Fig. 1.6 **Comparison of the sympathetic and parasympathetic divisions of the autonomic nervous system.** The two limbs of the ANS tend to have opposing or complimentary effects on their target structures.

Divisions of the ANS

The autonomic nervous system has two divisions that widely innervate the body and tend to have opposing effects on their target structures (Fig. 1.6):

- The **sympathetic nervous system** is most active during highly stressful situations that provoke intense fear or rage, typified by the 'fight or flight' response: e.g. dilated pupils, dry mouth, racing pulse. It is said to act 'in sympathy' with the emotions.
- The **parasympathetic nervous system** generally has an antagonistic or complimentary effect on a given organ or tissue and is more associated with vegetative activities ('resting and digesting').

It is important to note that most structures are innervated by both divisions of the ANS and can be controlled independently (e.g. it is possible to dilate the pupils without increasing the heart rate); but the 'fight or flight' response is a useful way to remember the effects of the sympathetic division.

The two divisions of the ANS have distinct anatomical origins. Sympathetic fibres originate in the thoracic and upper lumbar segments of the spinal cord (T1–L2/3) as the **thoracolumbar outflow** (Fig. 1.7). This feeds into the **sympathetic chain**, on either side of the vertebral column, which provides sympathetic innervation to the entire body.

The parasympathetic fibres originate in cranial nerves III, VII, IX and X and the sacral spinal cord (S2–4). This constitutes the **craniosacral outflow** (Fig. 1.8). The vagus nerve (cranial nerve X) has a wide territory of distribution that includes most of the thoracic and abdominal viscera (Latin: vagus, wandering).

The term **enteric nervous system** refers to an extensive network of neurons within the wall of the gastrointestinal tract (Greek: enteron, intestine). This regulates the activity of digestive glands and coordinates the waves of peristalsis that propel food through the bowel lumen. Although it is a component of the ANS, it is sometimes regarded as a separate system since it is capable of coordinated activity, independent of the brain and spinal cord.

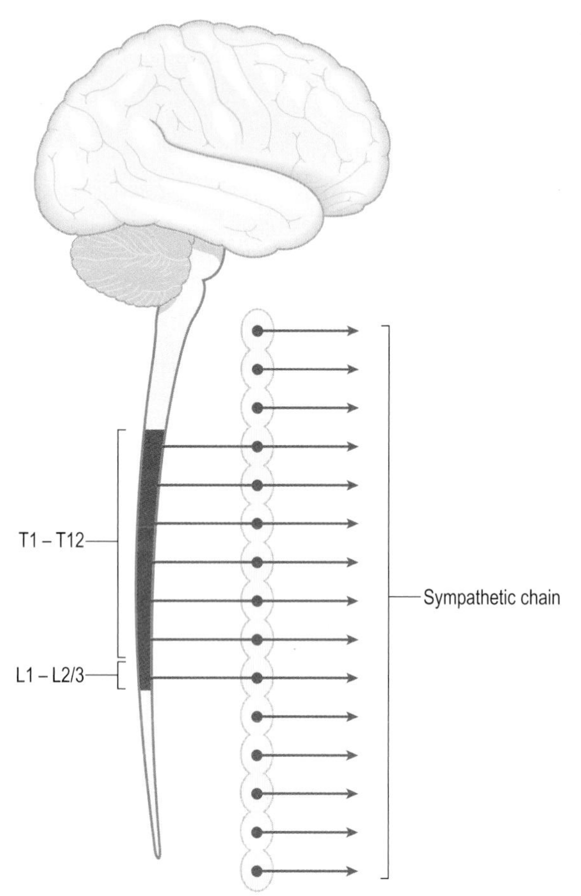

Fig. 1.7 **The thoracolumbar outflow gives rise to the sympathetic division of the autonomic nervous system.** Sympathetic fibres from the thoracic and upper lumbar spinal cord (T1–L2/3) innervate the sympathetic chain, which is located on either side of the vertebral column. Superior and inferior extensions of the sympathetic chain provide sympathetic innervation to the entire body.

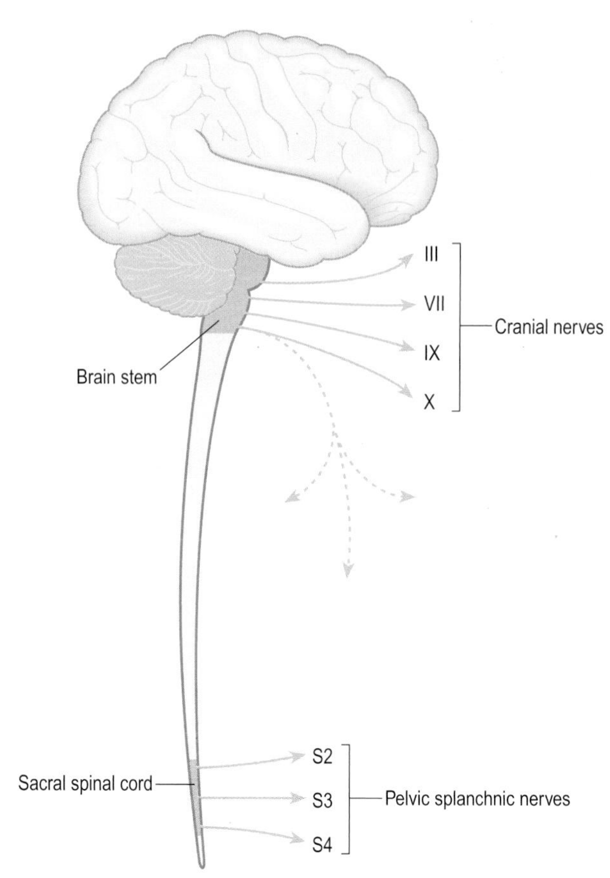

Fig. 1.8 **The craniosacral outflow corresponds to the parasympathetic division of the autonomic nervous system.** The craniosacral outflow includes contributions from cranial nerves III, VII, IX and X and the pelvic splanchnic nerves which arise from segments S2–S4 of the sacral spinal cord. Note that the vagus nerve arises in the brain stem but descends in the neck (dashed blue line) to supply most of the thoracic and abdominal organs.

Key Points

- The central nervous system (CNS) is composed of the brain and spinal cord, encased within the bones of the skull and vertebral column.
- The peripheral nervous system (PNS) includes 12 pairs of cranial nerves and 31 pairs of spinal nerves which carry sensory and motor fibres to and from the CNS.
- At the roots of the upper and lower limbs, sensory and motor fibres are redistributed in the brachial and lumbosacral plexuses to form a large number of mixed peripheral nerves.
- The motor component of the peripheral nervous system can be separated into somatic (somatomotor) and autonomic (visceromotor) divisions.
- The somatic nervous system innervates the voluntary (skeletal) musculature.
- The autonomic nervous system (ANS) innervates smooth muscle, cardiac muscle and glands within the internal organs (viscera) and blood vessels. It is controlled by the hypothalamus.
- The physiological actions of the sympathetic division of the ANS (originating from the thoracolumbar outflow) are typified by the 'fight or flight' response.
- The parasympathetic division of the ANS (represented by the craniosacral outflow) generally has an opposing action on a given organ or tissue.

Cells of the nervous system

Neural tissue contains two specialized cell types: **neurons** and **glia**. These will be introduced here and discussed further in Chapter 5.

Nerve cells (neurons)

The basic structural and functional unit of the nervous system is the **neuron** or nerve cell. Neurons are electrically excitable cells that are highly specialized for the receipt, integration and transmission of information via rapid electrochemical impulses. A typical neuron is illustrated in Fig. 1.9.

The **cell body** ranges from 5–120 μm in diameter and contains the nuclear DNA and the biological machinery for protein synthesis and other housekeeping functions. Two types of process (or **neurite**) arise from the cell body. A profusely branching 'tree' of **dendrites** (Greek: dendron, tree) is specialized to receive and integrate information and may receive projections from many thousands of other neurons.

Nerve impulses are triggered in the cell body and transmitted away from the neuron along the slender **nerve fibre** or **axon**. A typical nerve cell has a single axon which may be up to two metres long in humans. Axons make contact with their target cells (and may branch to influence more than one target cell) at swellings called **axon terminals**. Axons often give rise to branches (or **collaterals**) which typically arise at right angles to the long axis of the nerve fibre.

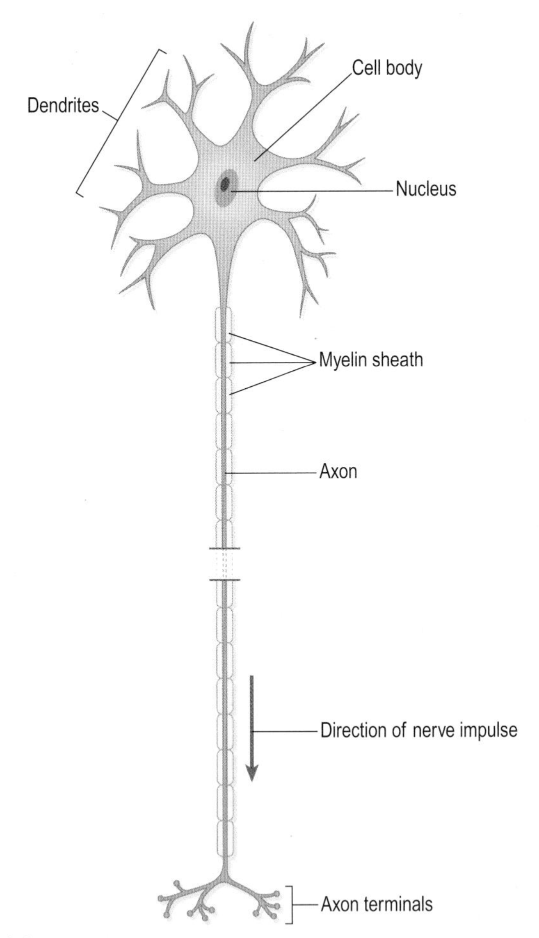

Fig. 1.9 **A typical neuron.**

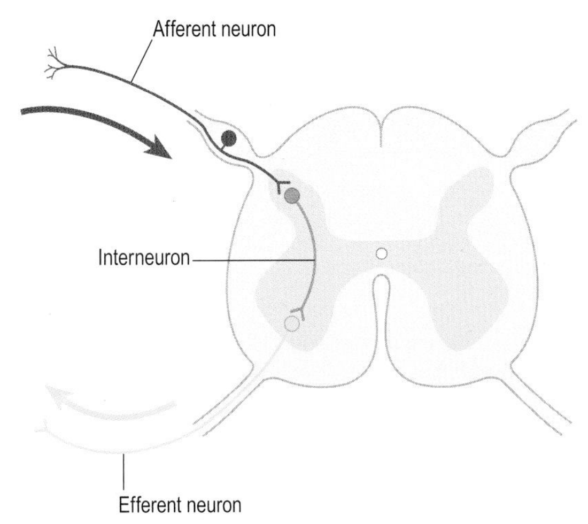

Fig. 1.10 **Afferent neurons, interneurons and efferent neurons.** The vast majority of nerve cells in the central nervous system are interneurons (association neurons).

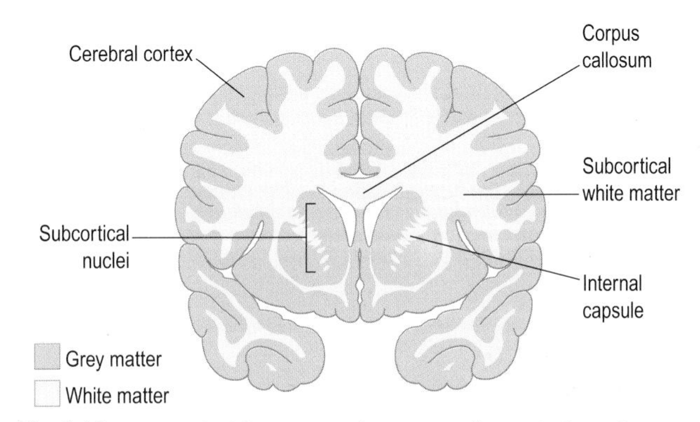

Fig. 1.11 **Grey and white matter.** The corpus callosum is the main commissural bundle linking the left and right cerebral hemispheres; the internal capsule is the major projection system, consisting of fibres passing to and from the cerebral cortex.

The point of contact between two neurons is called a **synapse** (Greek: sunapsis, point of contact). Neurons influence effector structures such as muscle fibres and glandular tissue at **neuroeffector junctions**. The specific junction between a somatic motor neuron and a skeletal muscle fibre is the **neuromuscular junction** (**NMJ**) (see Ch. 4). The electrical activity of the target cell is influenced by **neurotransmitters**, chemical mediators that are released at the axon terminal in response to the arrival of a nerve impulse. Neurotransmitters are stored in membrane-bound organelles within the axon terminal called **synaptic vesicles** (see Ch. 7).

Neurons can be classified into three functional types (Fig. 1.10):

- **Afferent neurons** carry nerve impulses towards the central nervous system. The term afferent fibre (or simply 'afferent') is also used to refer to any nerve process carrying impulses towards a particular structure. For example, 'cortical afferents' are fibres carrying impulses to the cerebral cortex. The term **sensory neuron** is usually reserved for afferent neurons conveying information that is to be consciously perceived.
- **Efferent neurons** carry nerve impulses away from the central nervous system. Again, the term efferent fibre (or 'efferent') can be used to refer to any process carrying impulses away from a particular structure. The term **motor neuron** is best reserved for efferent neurons that are involved in pathways concerned with voluntary movement.
- **Association neurons** (or **interneurons**) make up the vast network of interconnections within the brain and spinal cord. They have an integrative function, transforming sensory inputs into appropriate motor responses. The majority of neurons therefore fall into this category.

Neurons can also be classified by the number of processes that they have. The example shown in Fig. 1.9 is a **multipolar** neuron because it has several processes. Neurons with one or two processes are termed **unipolar** and **bipolar** respectively. The vast majority of neurons in the CNS are multipolar.

Grey and white matter

CNS tissue can be divided into grey and white matter (Fig. 1.11). **Grey matter** is composed mainly of neuronal cell bodies, dendrites and synapses. It is sharply demarcated from the adjacent **white matter**, which is made up of nerve fibres travelling to other parts of the nervous system. The pale colour of white matter is due to the lipid-rich **myelin sheath** that surrounds axons and enhances their conduction velocity (see Fig. 1.9; see also Chs 5 & 6). Discrete groups of neurons within the central nervous system are referred to as **nuclei** (singular: nucleus). In the peripheral nervous system, collections of neuronal cell bodies form aggregates that resemble knots on a piece of string. These are referred to as **ganglia** (singular: ganglion).

Neuroglial cells

In addition to neurons, the nervous system contains a variety of support cells that are known collectively as **glia**. These cells were originally thought to offer mainly physical support, literally holding nervous tissue together (Greek: glia, glue) but they are now known to carry out a wide range of important functions. The four main types of glial cell (discussed further in Chapter 5) are:

- **Astrocytes**, which provide structural and metabolic support to neurons and help to regulate the exchange of molecules between the bloodstream and the brain.
- **Oligodendrocytes**, which invest axons with a myelin sheath in the brain and spinal cord.
- **Schwann cells**, the peripheral counterparts of oligodendrocytes.
- **Microglia**, the resident phagocytic and immunocompetent cells of the central nervous system.

Although glial cells are relatively small, with an average diameter of around 4–8 μm, they outnumber neurons in a ratio of 10:1 and make up approximately 50% of the total volume of the CNS. Glial cells are able to undergo cell division (unlike neurons, which are **post-mitotic** cells).

Key Points

- The neuron is the basic structural and functional unit of the nervous system. The main types are afferent (sensory), efferent (motor) and association (interneurons).
- The dendritic tree is the afferent portion of the nerve cell, which may receive synaptic contacts from thousands of other neurons. Nerve impulses are generated in the cell body and transmitted to other nerve cells via the axon.
- Neurons communicate with other nerve cells, muscle fibres and glands at synapses. The arrival of a nerve impulse at the axon terminal triggers the release of a chemical neurotransmitter which influences the target cell.
- Grey matter is composed mainly of neuronal cell bodies, whereas white matter is made up of myelinated axons. Collections of nerve cells form nuclei in the CNS and ganglia in the PNS.
- Astrocytes are the main type of support (glial) cell. They perform important metabolic functions and help to regulate the passage of molecules between the CNS and the bloodstream.
- Axons are wrapped in a lipid-rich myelin sheath by central oligodendrocytes and peripheral Schwann cells. Myelin increases axonal conduction velocity.

Basic cerebral topography

The human brain is a pale pink organ with a mean mass of around 1.3 kg and a very soft, gelatinous consistency. It can be separated into three major parts – the **cerebrum**, **cerebellum** and **brain stem** (Fig. 1.12). The brain stem is further subdivided into the midbrain, pons and medulla oblongata.

Cerebrum

The cerebrum is dominated by the paired **cerebral hemispheres** which are responsible for cognition, language, memory, emotion and behaviour. The surface of the cerebral hemispheres is composed of a thin shell of grey matter, the **cerebral cortex** (Latin: cortex, bark) which is 2–4 mm thick. The cortex is thrown into numerous convolutions or **gyri** separated by furrows called **sulci** (singular: gyrus and sulcus) (Fig. 1.13). Cortical folding allows the maximum surface area of grey matter to be compressed into the limited confines of the skull, with two-thirds of the cortex hidden within the depths of sulci.

The cerebral hemispheres are divided by a deep cleft termed the **longitudinal fissure** and separated from the underlying cerebellum by the **transverse fissure**. Two prominent sulci on the cerebral convexity, the **lateral sulcus** and the **central sulcus**, help to divide the hemispheres into frontal, parietal, occipital and temporal lobes (Fig. 1.14; see also Ch. 3).

Crossing of sensory and motor pathways

A general principle of CNS organization is that sensory and motor pathways cross the midline at some point on their way to and from the cerebral hemispheres. The process of crossing over is termed **decussation** (Latin: decussis, the Roman numeral X) and means that each cerebral hemisphere is concerned with sensations and actions of the opposite (**contralateral**) side of the body. The reason for this is not known, but may reflect an escape response in our marine ancestors that is present in modern fish (the **C-start escape reflex**). This requires a sensory stimulus on one side of the body to trigger rapid contraction of the contralateral flank muscles (causing the fish to make a rapid U-turn).

Lateralization of function

The cerebral hemisphere in control of the preferred hand is said to be **dominant**. In most cases this is the left cerebral hemisphere because 90% of people are right-handed. Many of the remainder show mixed hand preference rather than being exclusively left-handed. The cerebral hemispheres are also specialized to carry out particular cognitive functions, which are said to be **lateralized**. The best example is language, which is also controlled by the left cerebral hemisphere in most people, regardless of hand preference.

Internal anatomy

Slicing the cerebrum reveals a number of grey matter structures including the **corpus striatum**, **amygdala** and **thalamus** (discussed further below) (Fig. 1.15). These subcortical structures are closely related to a collection of fluid-filled cavities and channels inside the brain, called the **ventricular system**.

The corpus striatum is the largest component of the **basal ganglia**. These are a collection of nuclei (the term 'ganglia' is a misnomer) that are involved in movement control and are affected in **Parkinson's disease** (Ch. 13). They also contribute to cognition, emotion and behaviour. The amygdala is concerned with emotional responses (especially anxiety and fear). It has close links to the **limbic lobe**, part of the brain that is particularly concerned with emotion and memory.

The thalamus and hypothalamus belong to the **diencephalon**. This region lies at the centre of the brain, surrounding the cavity of the third ventricle and is normally hidden from view between the cerebral hemispheres (Greek: dia-, between; enkephalos, brain) (Fig. 1.16). The thalamus is known as the 'gateway' to the cerebral cortex, since most ascending sensory pathways relay in one of its nuclei in order to reach their cortical targets. The **hypothalamus** controls the ANS and endocrine system and is involved in the maintenance of homeostasis.

Pituitary gland

The **pituitary gland** is just beneath the hypothalamus, connected to it by the **pituitary stalk**. It is separated into

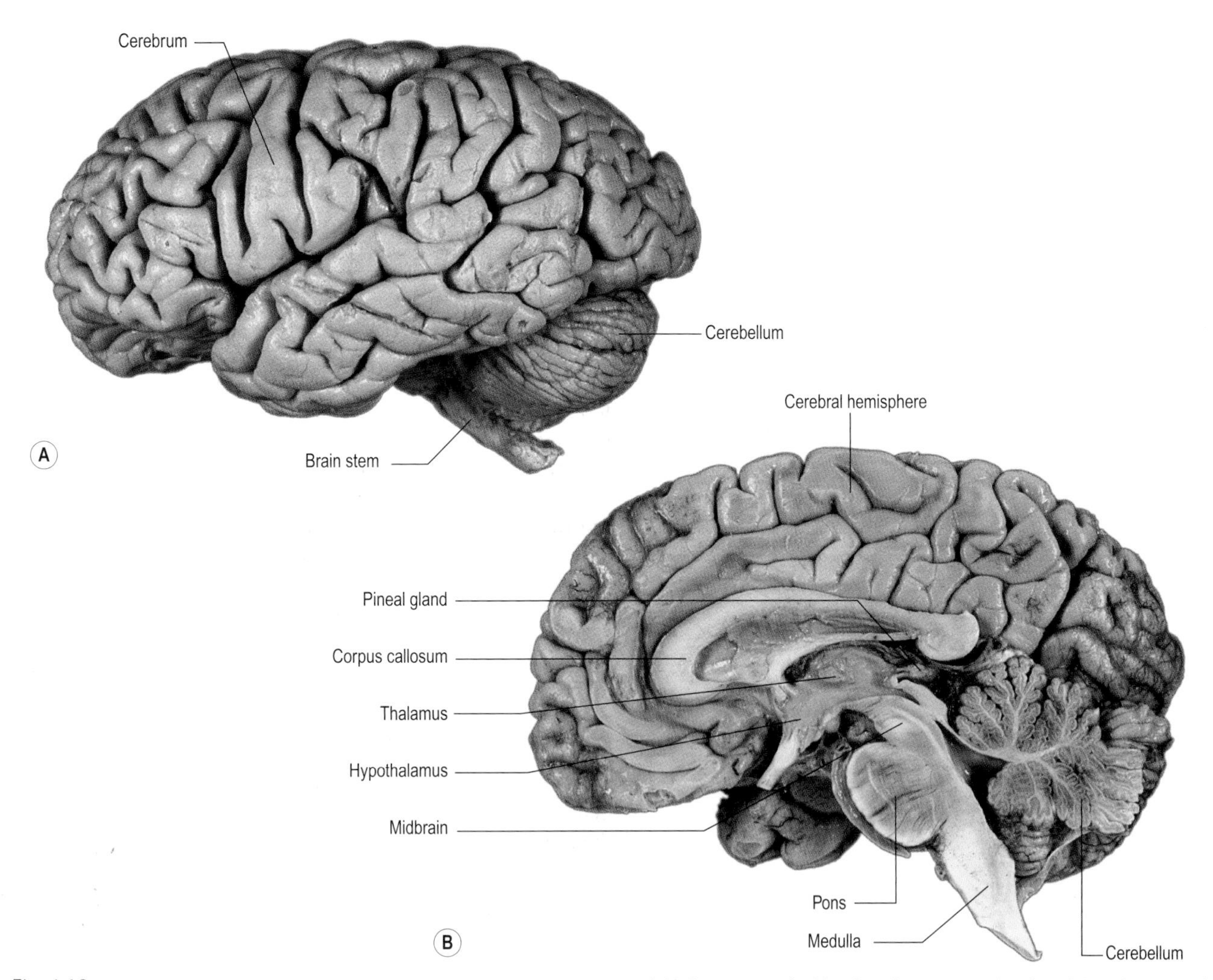

Fig. 1.12 **The human brain, illustrating the major subdivisions and some of the key anatomical landmarks. (A)** Lateral surface; **(B)** Median sagittal section. From Crossman: Neuroanatomy ICT 4e (Churchill Livingstone 2010) with permission.

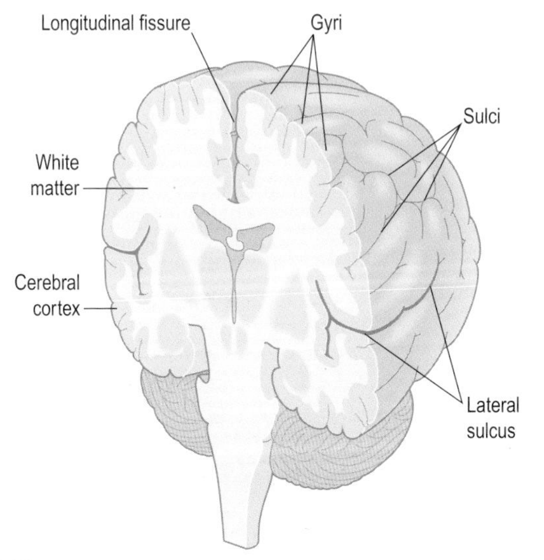

Fig. 1.13 **The folding of the cerebral cortex to form gyri and sulci.** In the cerebral hemispheres, all furrows that are lined by cortical grey matter are referred to as sulci; compare the lateral sulcus (which is lined by a continuous ribbon of grey matter) to the longitudinal fissure (which is not).

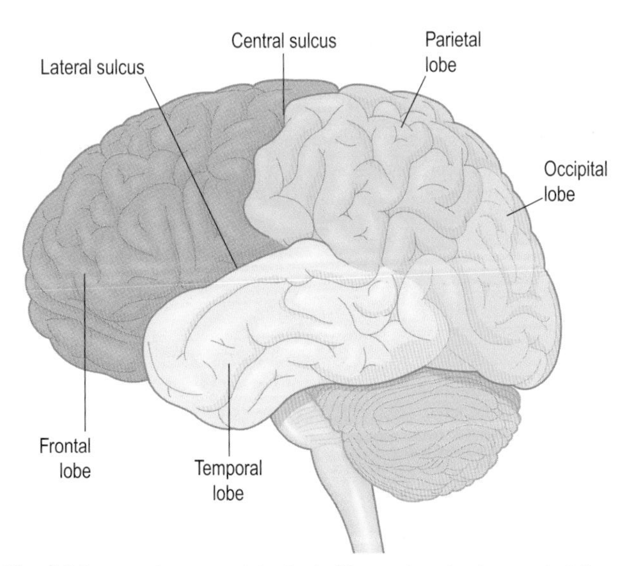

Fig. 1.14 **Lateral aspect of the brain illustrating the four main lobes of the cerebral hemispheres.** Note: there are no consistent sulci on the lateral surface of the hemisphere that clearly delineate the posterior lobar boundaries.

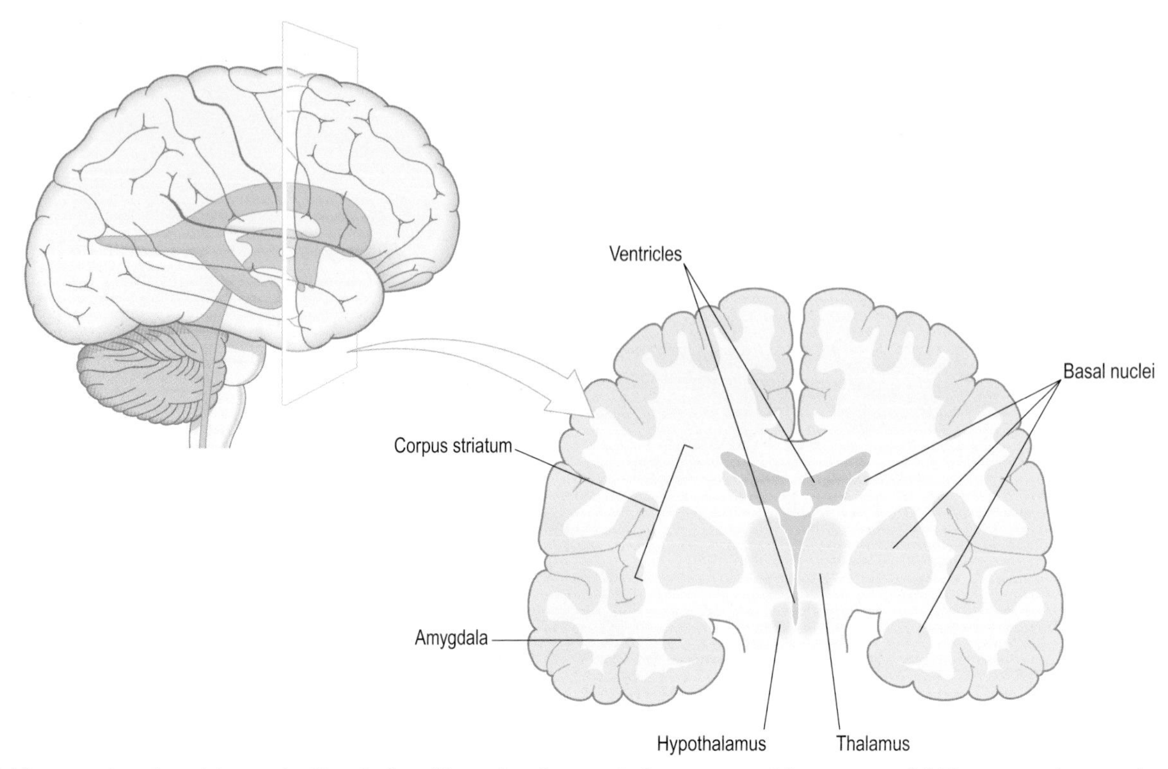

Fig. 1.15 **Coronal section of the cerebral hemisphere illustrating the ventricular system and deep grey nuclei.** The corpus striatum and amygdala are referred to as basal nuclei (grey matter in the base of the cerebral hemisphere). The thalamus and hypothalamus are not basal nuclei, but are instead part of the diencephalon, a central part of the cerebrum surrounding the cavity of the third ventricle.

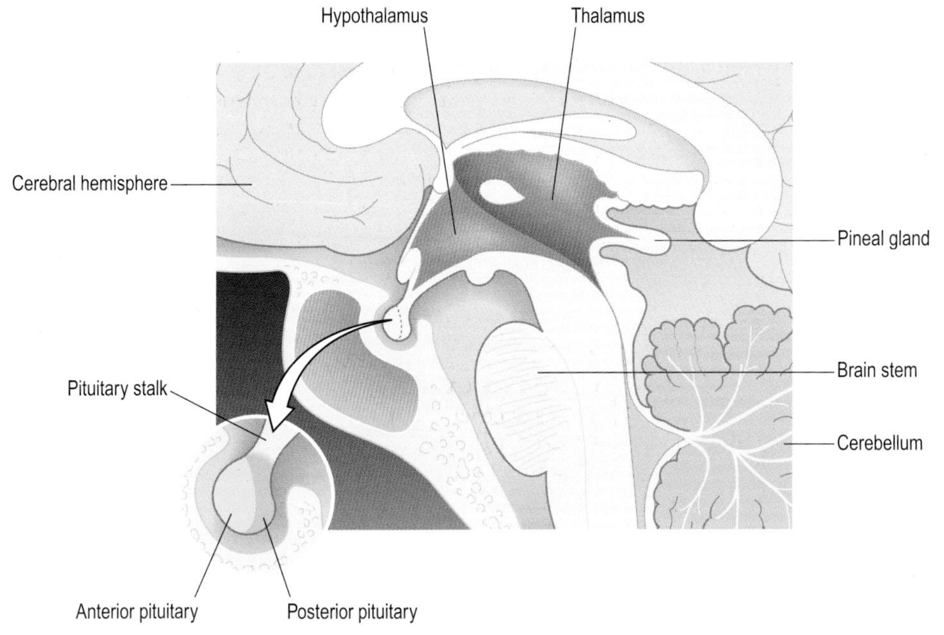

Fig. 1.16 **Median sagittal section of the brain illustrating the diencephalon (thalamic region) and pituitary gland.** The main components of the diencephalon are the thalamus and hypothalamus which form the side wall and floor of the third ventricle (coloured red). Although not part of the diencephalon, the pituitary gland is attached to the floor of the third ventricle and has links with the hypothalamus.

anterior (glandular) and posterior (neural) portions. The pituitary gland is an endocrine structure which releases **hormones** that control growth, metabolism and sexual function. It mainly regulates other glands (rather than having a direct physiological effect) and is therefore referred to as the 'master gland' of the endocrine system. Its activity is controlled in turn by soluble mediators released by the hypothalamus. These reach the anterior lobe of the pituitary gland via a capillary network called the **hypothalamo-pituitary portal system**. The hypothalamus communicates with the posterior lobe more directly via a bundle of nerve fibres termed the **hypothalamo-hypophyseal tract**.

Hemispheric white matter

The subcortical white matter is composed of numerous interlacing **tracts**, which are groups of axons with a common origin, destination and function. Two or more tracts running in company make up a bundle or **fasciculus** (plural: fasciculi). There are three main types of white matter bundle in the cerebrum, illustrated in Figs 1.17–1.19:

- **Association fibres** interconnect parts of the same hemisphere. **Short association fibres** (subcortical 'U-fibres') loop between neighbouring gyri. **Long association fibres** link more distant areas within a particular hemisphere.
- **Commissural fibres** cross the midline to connect with matching areas of the opposite hemisphere (Latin: commissūra, a joining together). The largest commissure is the **corpus callosum**, composed of some 200–300 million myelinated axons. The anterior and medial temporal lobes are linked by the much smaller **anterior commissure** (see Ch. 3, Fig. 3.25).
- **Projection fibres** pass to and from the cerebral cortex. The **internal capsule** is a massive white matter system composed of 20 million projection fibres that pass through the corpus striatum.

The internal capsule contains the **pyramidal tract** (primary voluntary motor pathway). This originates in the motor areas of the frontal lobe and projects to the brain stem and spinal cord.

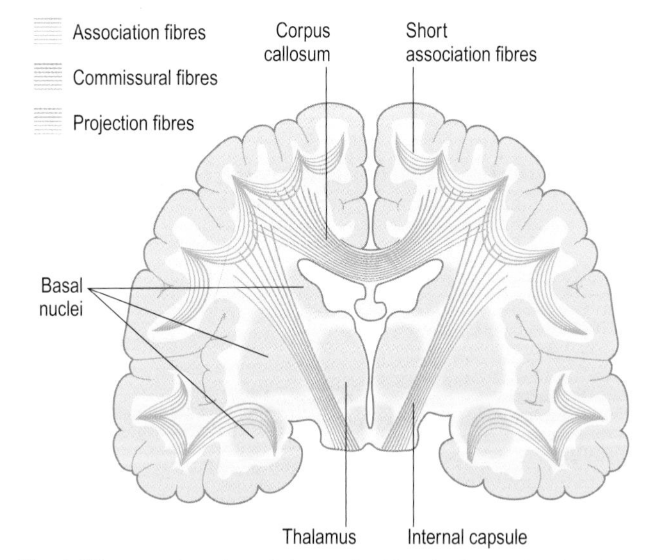

Fig. 1.17 **Coronal section of the cerebral hemispheres showing the main association, commissural and projection fibres in the subcortical white matter.** The corpus callosum is the main white matter connection between the cerebral hemispheres; the internal capsule is a massive white matter bundle consisting of fibres passing to and from the cerebral cortex.

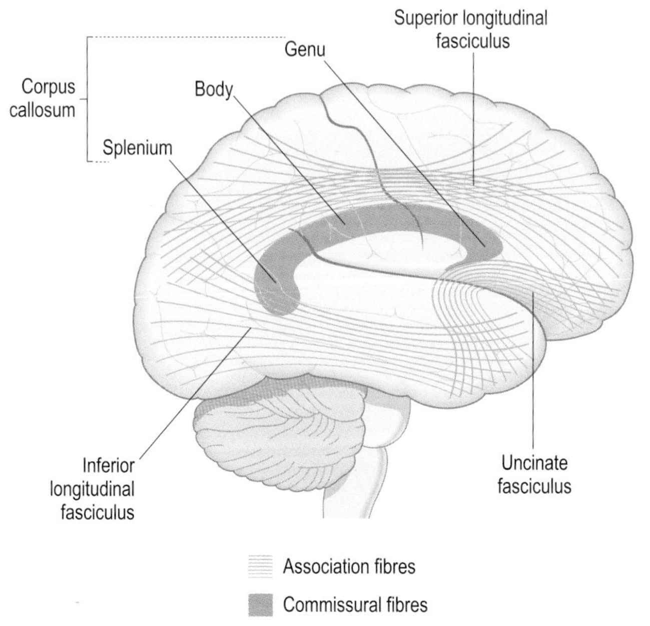

Fig. 1.18 **Lateral view of the cerebral hemisphere, illustrating white matter pathways.** Some of the major long association fibres are shown projected on to the surface of the cerebral hemisphere. The approximate position of the corpus callosum appears in transverse section; notice the genu and splenium, which give rise to fibres interconnecting the frontal lobes and the posterior parts of the cerebral hemispheres respectively.

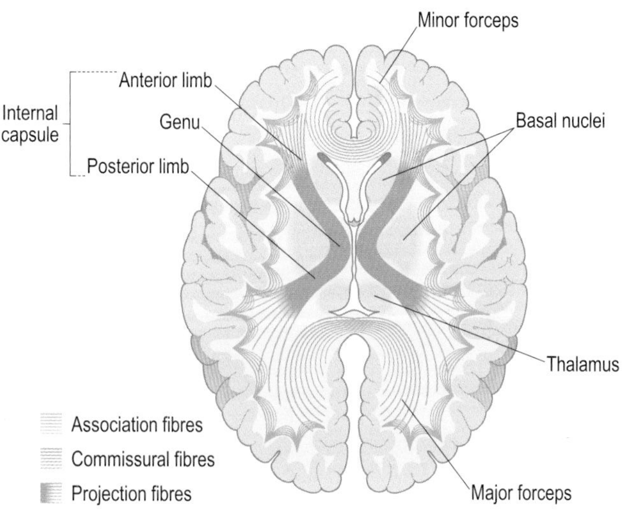

Fig. 1.19 **Axial (horizontal) section of the cerebral hemispheres showing the anterior and posterior limbs of the internal capsule passing through the deep grey matter.** The internal capsule (blue) is seen in transverse section and consists of ascending and descending axons passing to and from the cerebral cortex [to understand the orientation of the fibres, compare with Fig. 1.17]. The minor and major forceps are also seen in this view, which represent commissural fibres crossing the midline in the genu and splenium of the corpus callosum [compare with Fig. 1.18].

Key Points

- The brain consists of the cerebrum, cerebellum and brain stem.
- The cerebrum is dominated by the paired cerebral hemispheres which are responsible for personality, behaviour, language, intellect and emotion.
- The cerebral cortex is folded to form convolutions (gyri) separated by furrows (sulci). The central and lateral sulci help to demarcate the frontal, parietal, temporal and occipital lobes.
- The nuclei in the base of the cerebral hemisphere (basal nuclei) include the corpus striatum and amygdala. The corpus striatum is part of the basal ganglia and is involved in voluntary movement, cognition and emotion. The amygdala is concerned with emotional responses.
- The diencephalon is hidden between the cerebral hemispheres, surrounding the third ventricle. It includes the thalamus ('gateway to the cerebral cortex') and hypothalamus.
- The subcortical white matter contains: (i) short and long association fibres, linking cortical areas within a hemisphere; (ii) commissural fibres, which cross the midline to enter the opposite hemisphere; and (iii) projection fibres, passing to and from the cerebral cortex.

Cerebellum

The cerebellum (Latin: diminutive of cerebrum; cf. pig and piglet) is disproportionately large and well-developed in humans compared to other mammals. It clasps the brain stem from behind, forming the roof of the **fourth ventricle.** The cerebellum is involved in balance, muscle tone and coordination.

The cerebellum is composed of two large **cerebellar hemispheres** connected in the midline by the narrow **vermis** (which is said to resemble a segmented garden worm; Latin: vermis, worm) (Fig. 1.20A). The hemispheres and vermis are further subdivided into anterior and posterior lobes by the **primary fissure**. The cerebellum also contains a much smaller **flocculonodular lobe** that is composed of the paired **flocculi** (Latin: flocculus, tuft of wool) and the **nodule** of the vermis (see Chs 2 and 3).

Like the cerebrum, the cerebellum also has a folded outer layer of grey matter overlying a central core of white matter. However, the cortex of the cerebellum is arranged in parallel ridges called **folia** (separated by creases called **fissures**) and has a comparatively simple three-layered structure. Slicing the cerebellar hemisphere reveals the **dentate nucleus** embedded in the subcortical white matter (Fig. 1.20B). This is the principal efferent (outflow) nucleus of the cerebellum.

Cerebellar peduncles

The cerebellum is attached to the brain stem (on each side) via three white matter bundles (Fig. 1.21):

- The **superior cerebellar peduncles** are attached to the midbrain and contain a major projection from the dentate nucleus to the opposite thalamus and frontal lobe.
- The **middle cerebellar peduncles** arise from the pons and represent the principal afferent supply to the cerebellar hemispheres, which mainly originates from the opposite frontal lobe (see below).
- The **inferior cerebellar peduncles** are connected to the medulla and transmit afferent sensory information from the spinal cord.

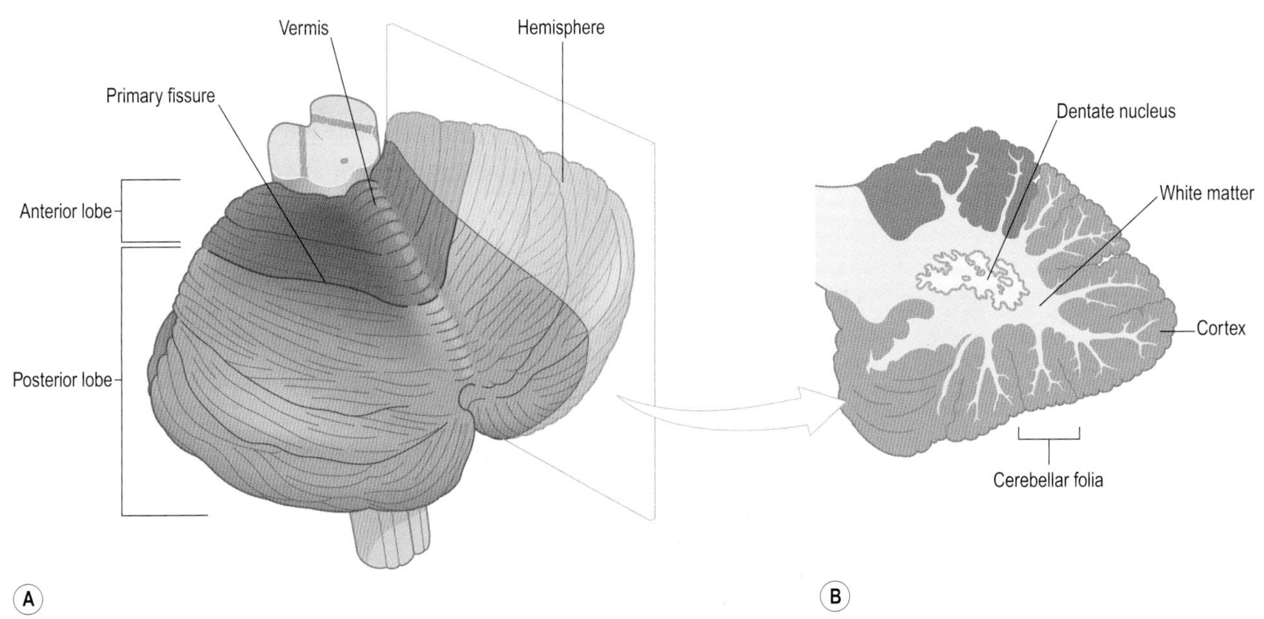

Fig. 1.20 **Gross anatomy of the cerebellum. (A)** Oblique view of the cerebellum from the posterolateral aspect, showing its intimate relationship to the brain stem. The division of the cerebellar hemispheres and vermis into anterior and posterior lobes is illustrated. The small flocculonodular lobe is not visible in this view (it can only be seen from the anterior aspect); **(B)** An oblique slice through the cerebellar hemisphere showing the cortex, white matter and dentate nucleus.

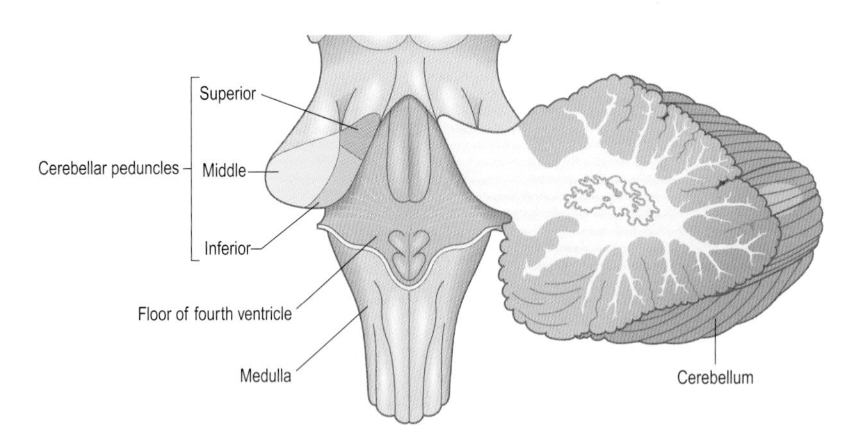

Fig. 1.21 **Posterior view of the brain stem with the left half of the cerebellum removed, exposing the diamond-shaped floor of the fourth ventricle.** The three cerebellar peduncles have been cut (on the left-hand side) and are therefore seen in transverse section. [NB: The inferior cerebellar peduncle ascends vertically through the medulla and then passes directly backwards into the cerebellum, making a 90-degree bend.]

The motor and premotor areas of the frontal lobe project to the basal pons (on the same side) via the **frontopontine pathway**. The pontine nuclei then give rise to **transverse pontine fibres** which project to the contralateral cerebellar hemisphere (via the middle cerebellar peduncle). Each frontal lobe thus projects to the contralateral cerebellar hemisphere. The cerebellum is therefore 'uncrossed' (with respect to the cerebrum) so that unilateral cerebellar damage affects coordination on the same (**ipsilateral**) side of the body.

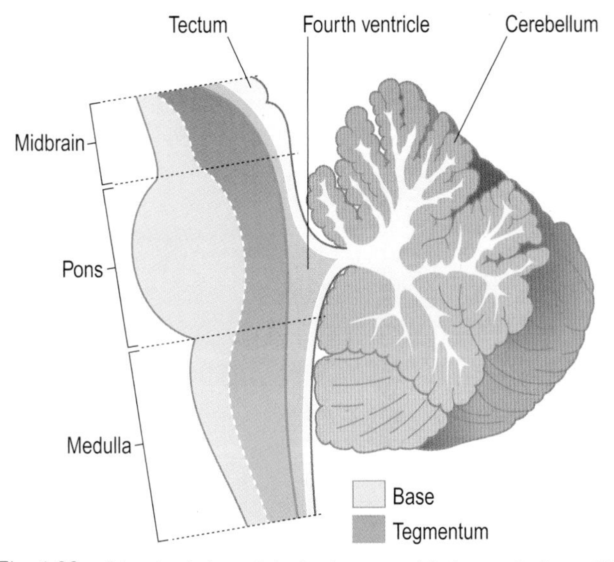

Fig. 1.22 **Midsagittal view of the brain stem with the cerebellum still attached, illustrating the basal and tegmental regions.** Note that the midbrain also has a 'roof plate' (the tectum) that lies dorsal to the cerebral aqueduct, but there is no corresponding region in the pons or medulla.

Key Points

- The cerebellum is composed of the cerebellar hemispheres and vermis. It is divided into a small anterior lobe and a large posterior lobe by the primary fissure.
- Like the cerebrum, the cerebellum has an outer cortical layer (thrown into parallel ridges called folia) and a central core of white matter. The main efferent structure is the dentate nucleus.
- The cerebellum is connected to the brain stem by three pairs of white matter bundles: the superior, middle and inferior cerebellar peduncles. These fibre systems connect to the midbrain, pons and medulla respectively.
- The main functions of the cerebellum include the maintenance of balance, posture, muscle tone and coordination. Lesions cause ipsilateral incoordination.

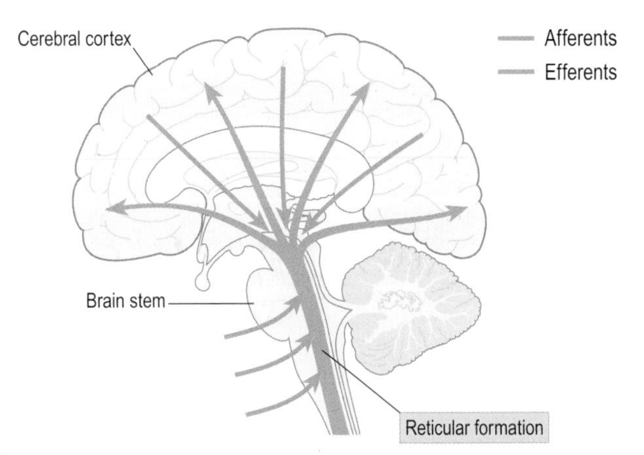

Fig 1.23 **The afferent and efferent projections of the ascending reticular activating system (ARAS).** These connections contribute to wakefulness and coma.

Brain stem

The cerebrum and cerebellum are both attached to the brain stem, which is composed of the **midbrain**, **pons** and **medulla oblongata** (discussed separately in Ch. 3).

Taken as a whole, the brain stem can be divided into two longitudinal regions called the **base** and **tegmentum** (Fig. 1.22). In other animals, such as rodents, the base of the brain stem lies inferiorly and the tegmentum is above it (Latin: tegmentum, a covering). Since humans are bipedal (and stand upright) the 'base' is anterior to the tegmentum.

The **basilar** region is composed mainly of descending axons, such as the **pyramids** of the medulla which contain the primary motor pathway or **pyramidal tract**. The **tegmentum** is the central core of the brain stem. It contains the nuclei of the lower ten cranial nerves (III–XII) and a diffuse network of neurons referred to as the **reticular formation** (described below). The brain stem transmits several **long tracts**, including ascending (sensory) and descending (motor) pathways.

Reticular formation

The **reticular formation** forms a polysynaptic network in the tegmentum of the brain stem. It contains the so-called **vital centres** (respiratory and cardiovascular) and mediates the airway-protective **brain stem reflexes** (e.g. cough, sneeze, gag). It also coordinates several stereotyped actions concerned with feeding, via connections with the cranial nerve nuclei. These include salivating, chewing, swallowing and vomiting. Other activities include control of: (i) bladder emptying (the **micturition reflex**); (ii) conjugate gaze (via the **vertical** and **horizontal gaze centres** of the midbrain and pons); and (iii) posture, muscle tone and gait.

The **ascending reticular activating system** (**ARAS**) is a diffuse projection that arises from the rostral brain stem. It receives afferents from each of the sensory systems and influences cortical excitability by release of excitatory neurotransmitters including **acetylcholine** and **noradrenaline** (Fig. 1.23). Activity in this system is influenced by general and special sensory afferents and is vital for maintaining wakefulness. For this reason, brain stem damage may result in **coma** (Clinical Box 1.1).

Diffuse neurochemical systems

A number of small brain stem nuclei give rise to extremely diffuse neurochemical projections that influence the entire CNS (Fig. 1.24). These diffuse modulatory systems release the neurotransmitters **serotonin**, **noradrenaline**, **dopamine** and **acetylcholine** via synaptic terminals distributed

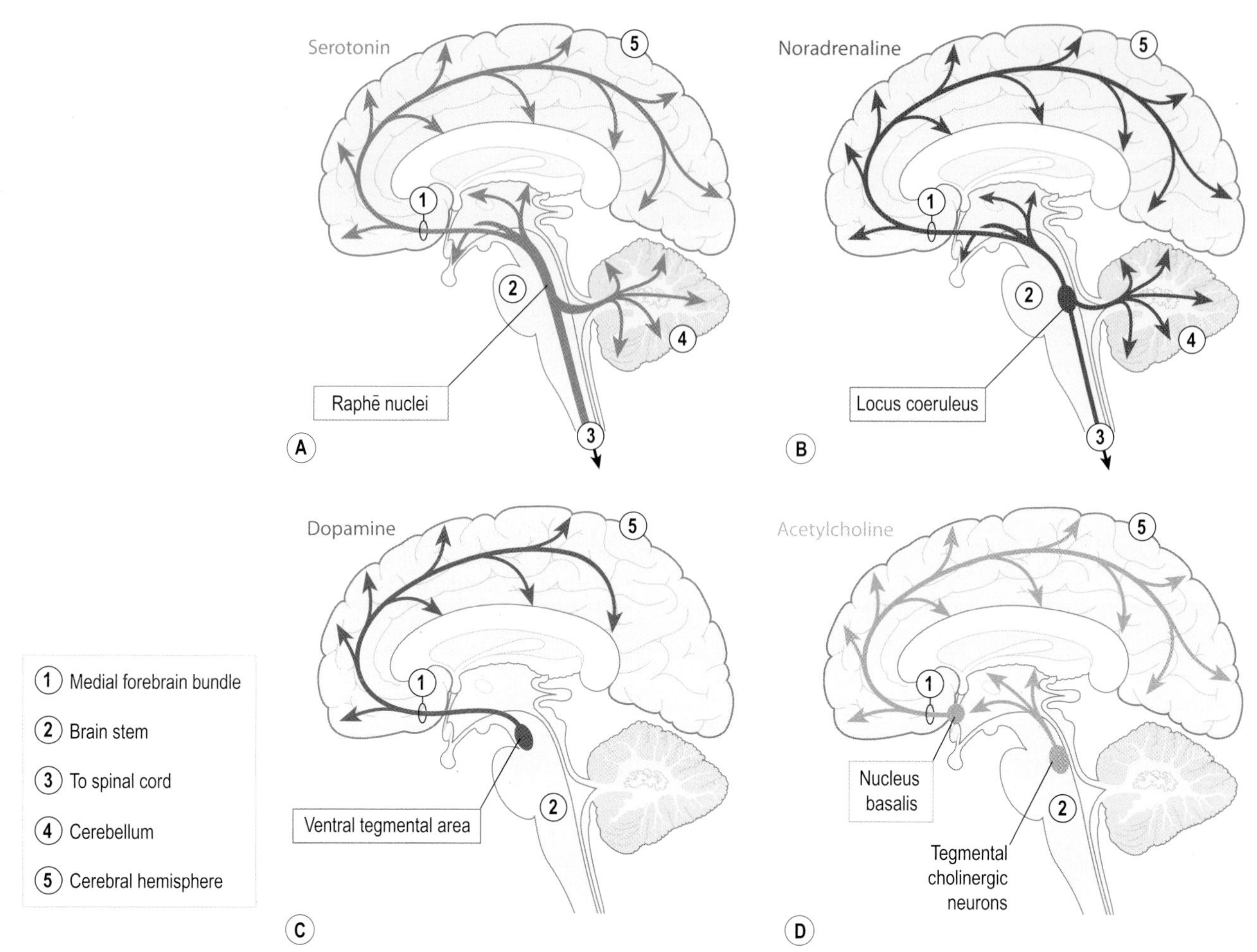

Fig. 1.24 **The diffuse neurochemical systems. (A)** Serotonergic fibres originate in the midline raphē nuclei (pronounced 'RAFF-ay'); **(B)** The paired loci coerulei (singular: locus coeruleus) of the rostral pons give rise to noradrenergic fibres; **(C)** Dopamine is released throughout the cerebral cortex, limbic lobe and amygdala by fibres originating in the ventral tegmental area of the midbrain; the substantia nigra (another midbrain dopaminergic nucleus that is part of the basal ganglia) projects only to the corpus striatum and is not a diffuse projection system; **(D)** There are several cholinergic nuclei that give rise to diffuse projections, including those within the nucleus basalis (of the basal forebrain) and the tegmentum of the rostral brain stem.

throughout the brain and spinal cord. The main pathways travel together between the brain stem and the cerebral hemisphere within the **medial forebrain bundle**.

The suffix '**-ergic**' is used to refer to fibres releasing a common neurotransmitter such that those releasing serotonin are said to be 'serotonergic' and those releasing noradrenaline are referred to as 'noradrenergic'. Coordinated activity in these diffuse projections influences neural functions on a global scale, including **arousal**, **vigilance**, **sleep–wake cycles** and **mood** (Clinical Box 1.2).

Clinical Box 1.1: Coma and brain stem death

Interference with the ascending reticular activating system (e.g. following brain stem injury) may cause **coma**. This is defined as a profound state of unconsciousness characterized by lack of responsiveness to external stimuli and absence of sleep–wake cycles. More severe damage can result in loss of spontaneous respiration and cardiovascular drive which is not compatible with survival. This is termed **brain stem death**. Artificial ventilation can prolong life, but if the brain stem is irreversibly damaged, recovery will not be possible.

Clinical Box 1.2: Amines and depression

During the 1960s a theory emerged which aimed to explain depression as a disorder of neurotransmitter chemistry. It had been noted that some patients receiving the drug **reserpine** for the treatment of high blood pressure became depressed or even suicidal. It was also known that the mechanism of action of reserpine was to deplete neurons of **amine neurotransmitters.** Later, attempts to produce new agents for the treatment of tuberculosis lead to the development of the drug **iproniazid** which turned out to have mood-elevating properties. The mechanism appeared to be potentiation of endogenous amines via inhibition of a key enzyme responsible for their degradation (**monoamine oxidase, MAO**). Thus it was postulated that depression might represent a deficiency of CNS amines such as serotonin and noradrenaline, which came to be known as the **biogenic amine hypothesis**. Indeed, all modern anti-depressant agents appear to potentiate these neurotransmitter systems. However, despite rapid changes at central synapses, there is a delay of around 2–4 weeks before symptoms start to improve. This suggests that 'knock-on' effects in neuronal biochemistry may be responsible for the symptomatic benefit. Nevertheless, it is important to exercise caution when attempting to extrapolate a theory of disease causation from the mechanism of a drug used to treat it: analogous to repairing a pair of spectacles with a dab of glue and then concluding that they must have been 'glue-deficient'.

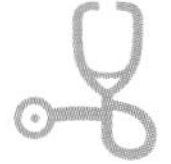

Key Points

- The brain stem is composed of the midbrain, pons and medulla.
- The tegmentum of the brain stem contains the nuclei of cranial nerves III–XII, the reticular formation and several ascending (sensory) tracts. The base contains descending (motor) tracts.
- The reticular formation maintains normal cardiorespiratory function, mediates airway-protective brain stem reflexes and is involved in wakefulness and coma.
- The diffuse neurochemical systems arise from small nuclei in the brain stem and base of the cerebral hemisphere. They release the transmitters serotonin, noradrenaline, dopamine and acetylcholine throughout the CNS and contribute to mood, arousal and sleep–wake cycles.
- Other brain stem centres mediate conjugate gaze, regulation of bladder emptying and the maintenance of normal muscle tone, posture and gait.

The spinal cord

The spinal cord is a slender continuation of the brain stem which is contained within the bony **spinal canal**. It is 40–50 cm in length, up to 1.5 cm in width and contains around a billion neurons. A lateral view of the spinal cord shows the **cervical** and **lumbar enlargements** which are required for the considerable sensory and motor supply to the upper and lower limbs (Fig. 1.25).

The spinal cord is significantly shorter than the vertebral column and terminates at the lower border of the first lumbar vertebra (L1/2) as the tapering **conus medullaris**. A consequence of this length-discrepancy is that the upper roots leave the cord horizontally, but the lower roots follow a progressively more oblique course. Below the conus medullaris, the roots form an almost-vertical leash called the **cauda equina** (Latin: horse's tail).

The 31 pairs of spinal nerves are attached to the cord via the **dorsal (sensory)** and **ventral (motor) roots** which arise from a series of rootlets. Each dorsal root bears a **dorsal root ganglion** which contains the cell bodies of sensory neurons.

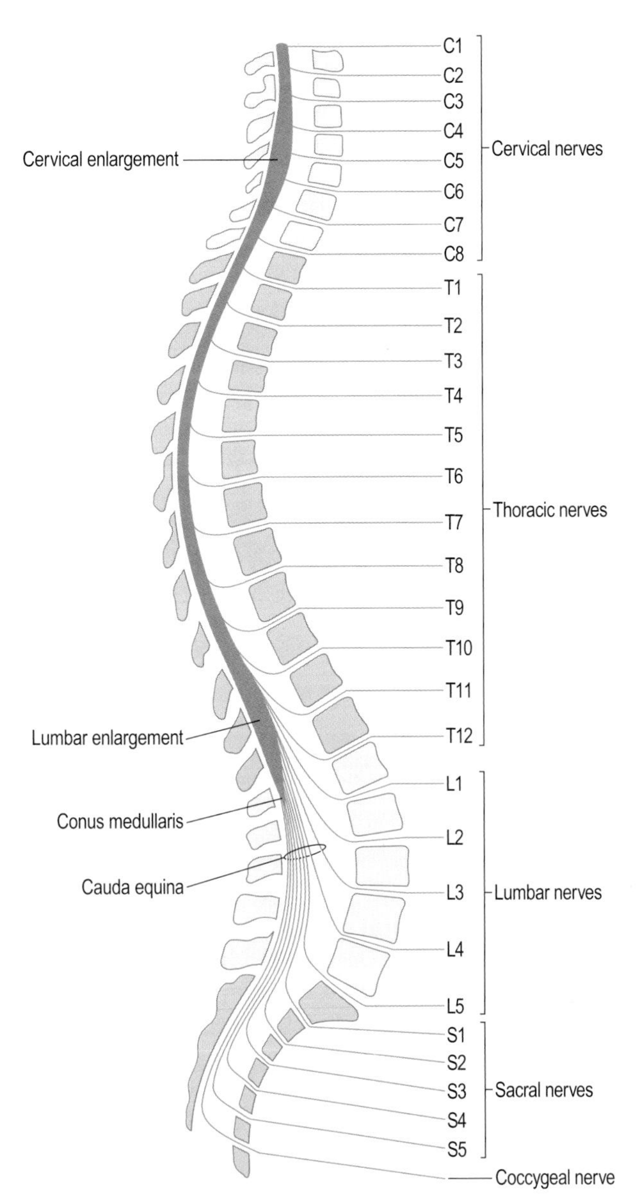

Fig. 1.25 **The relationships between the vertebral column, spinal cord and spinal nerves.** The cervical nerves emerge above their corresponding vertebrae, apart from the C8 nerve which emerges below the seventh cervical vertebra. This is because there are eight cervical nerves but only seven vertebrae. All other spinal nerves (thoracic, lumbar and sacral) exit below their corresponding vertebrae. The spinal cord ends at the conus medullaris (at the level of the L1/L2 disc).

Internal anatomy

The spinal cord contains a central, H-shaped core of grey matter (with **dorsal** and **ventral horns**) that is surrounded by a thick layer of white matter. The spinal cord white matter is arranged in three longitudinal **columns** that contain ascending and descending pathways (Fig. 1.26).

The posterior columns are located between the dorsal roots and are separated by the **dorsal median sulcus**. The anterior columns lie between the ventral roots and are separated by the more substantial **ventral median fissure**. The lateral columns are situated between the attachments of the dorsal and ventral nerve roots on each side of the cord.

Spinal **reflexes** contribute to normal muscle tone and mediate a number of simple motor responses (e.g. withdrawal from a painful stimulus). The spinal cord also contains more complex neuronal networks called **central pattern**

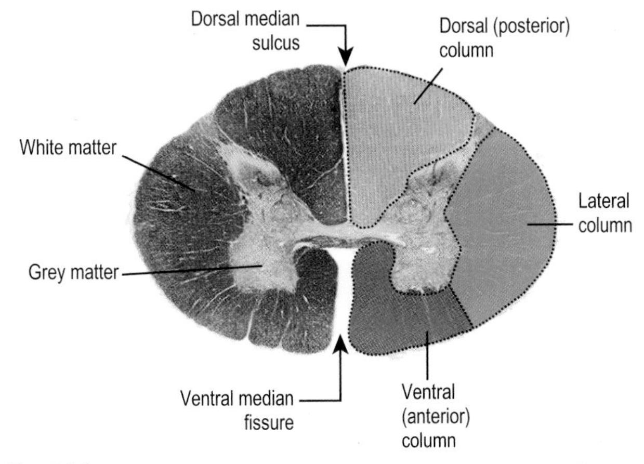

Fig. 1.26 **A transverse section through the lumbar spinal cord.** Modified from Nolte: The Human Brain in Photographs and Diagrams 3e (Mosby 2007) with permission.

generators (**CPGs**). These coordinate semi-automatic actions such as walking and are recruited and modulated by descending projections from the brain.

> *Key Points*
>
> - The spinal cord is a continuation of the brain stem which occupies the bony spinal canal. It terminates at the lower border of the first lumbar vertebra as the conus medullaris.
> - The cervical and lumbar enlargements of the spinal cord reflect the considerable sensory and motor supply to the upper and lower limbs.
> - The spinal cord gives rise to the ventral (motor) roots and dorsal (sensory) roots which unite to form the mixed spinal nerves. The dorsal roots bear the dorsal root (sensory) ganglia.
> - The spinal cord transmits nerve impulses to and from the brain and mediates several important reflexes. It also coordinates more complex motor sequences (e.g. those required for walking).

Protective coverings of the CNS

The central nervous system is protected by the bones of the skull and spinal column and by three layers of investing membranes. In addition, a fluid-filled space around the brain and spinal cord provides a cushioning or 'shock-absorbing' effect.

The skull and vertebral column

The skull is composed of the **cranium** (which encases the brain), together with the **facial skeleton** and **mandible** (lower jaw). The brain lies within the cranial cavity, resting on the **skull base**. It is covered by the dome-like **cranial vault**. The bones that make up the skull vault are the **calvaria** (singular: calvarium) (Fig. 1.27). They include the frontal, parietal, occipital and temporal bones, after which the underlying lobes of the cerebral hemispheres are named. The calvarial bones unite at the **cranial sutures**, but this process is not complete until about 18 months of age.

The **skull base** accommodates the ventral part of the brain and can be divided into three broad recesses or **fossae** (singular: fossa). The frontal and temporal lobes lie in the anterior and middle fossae respectively, whereas the brain stem and cerebellum occupy the posterior fossa. The brain stem becomes continuous with the spinal cord via a large opening in the skull base, the **foramen magnum**. The cranial fossae contain numerous openings by which the cranial nerves reach their target structures in the head and neck.

The spinal cord is protected by the **vertebral column**, which is composed of multiple separate **vertebrae** that align to form the hollow **vertebral canal**. The joints, ligaments and muscles attached to the vertebral column provide the necessary stability and protection for the spinal cord, whilst at the same time permitting a good deal of mobility (Fig. 1.28).

Cranial and spinal meninges

In addition to its bony coverings, the central nervous system is invested by three layers of protective membranes, the **meninges** (singular: meninx) (Fig. 1.29).

The outermost layer is the **dura mater** (Latin: dura, tough). This is a tough fibrous membrane that is tightly adherent to the inside of the skull and is fused with the periosteum. The dura extends through the foramen magnum to surround the spinal cord as the **dural sac** which terminates at the level of the second sacral vertebra (S2). The dural sac is separated from the bones of the vertebral column by an **extradural venous plexus**, which is embedded in fatty connective tissue.

Closely apposed and loosely attached to the dura is the **arachnoid mater** (Greek: arachnoid, resembling a cobweb).

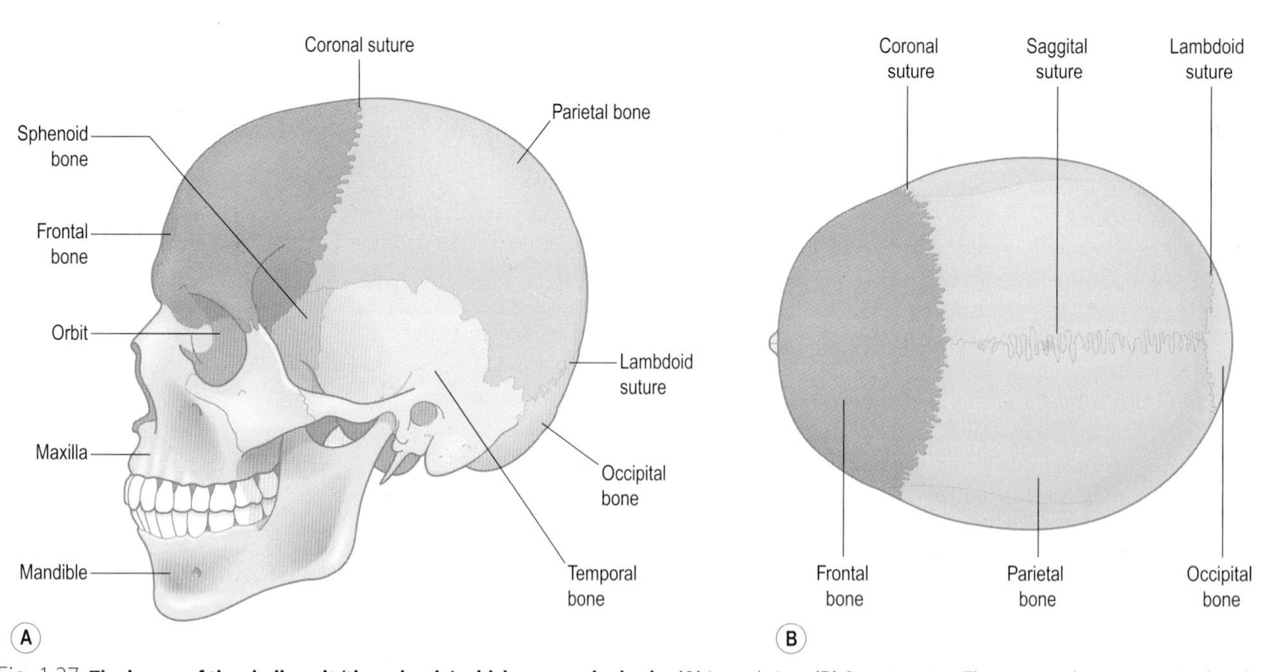

Fig. 1.27 **The bones of the skull vault (the calvaria) which encase the brain. (A)** Lateral view; **(B)** Superior view. The separate bones are united at the cranial sutures.

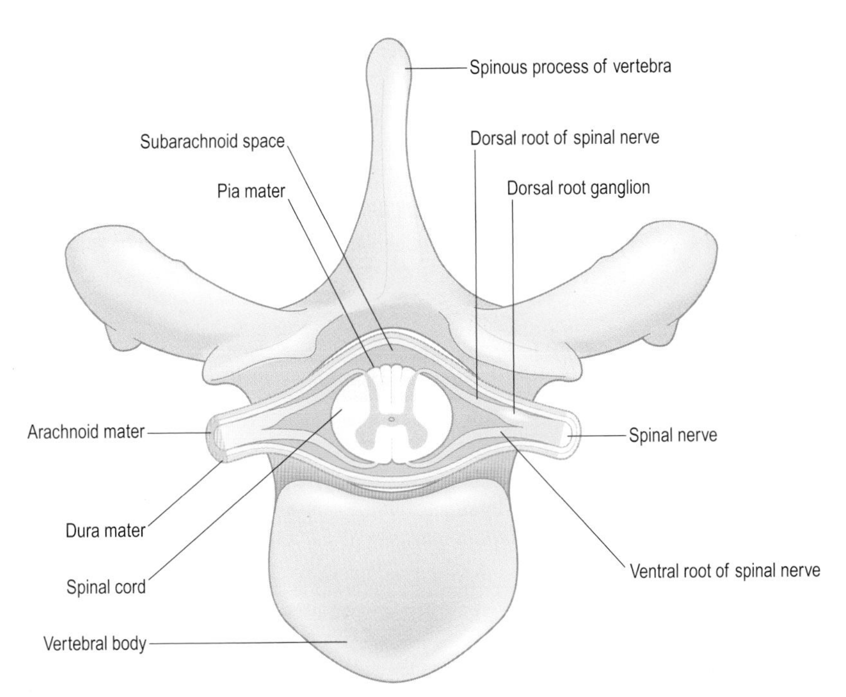

Fig. 1.28 **Transverse section through the thoracic spine illustrating the relationships between the spinal cord, meninges and vertebral column.**

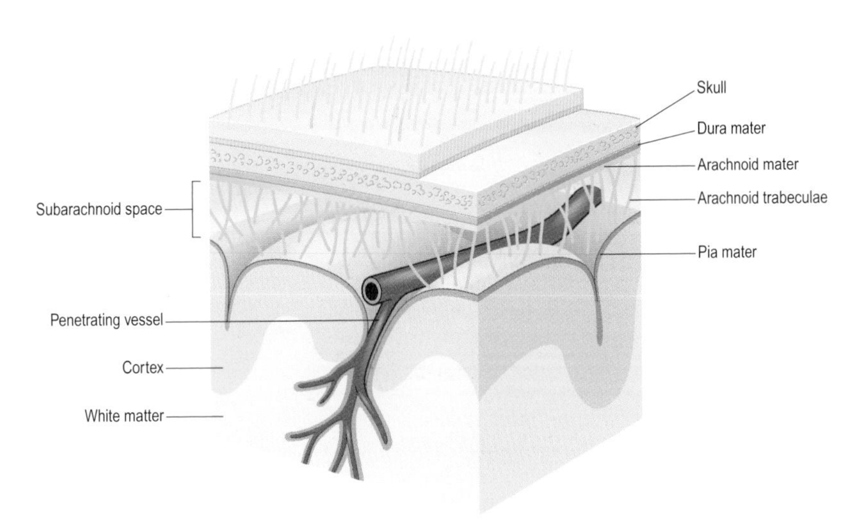

Fig. 1.29 **The relationship of the meninges to the surface of the brain.** Note that the cerebral arteries occupy the fluid-filled subarachnoid space and that penetrating blood vessels are invested by a sheath of pia mater as they plunge into the CNS tissue.

The dura-arachnoid represents a double layer that lines the skull and forms the dural sac.

The innermost membrane is the **pia mater** (Latin: pia, delicate). This is a thin layer of vascular connective tissue that is intimately associated with the surface of the brain and spinal cord, diving down into every sulcus and fissure. A sheath of pia mater also invests the arteries as they penetrate the substance of the brain and spinal cord.

Subarachnoid space

The arrangement of the three meningeal layers creates the **subarachnoid space** between the arachnoid and pia. The subarachnoid space is filled with **cerebrospinal fluid (CSF)** and is in continuity with the cerebral ventricles via three openings at the base of the brain (see Ch. 2). Thus the surface of the CNS is bathed in cerebrospinal fluid, which contains dissolved oxygen and glucose that helps to nourish neural tissues.

The subarachnoid space also has a protective role since it offers buoyancy and cushions against sudden head movements. Further support is provided by fine fibrous connections between the arachnoid and pia (the **arachnoid trabeculae**) which effectively suspend the brain like puppet strings. Since the CSF is intimately related to the brain and spinal cord it is sometimes sampled clinically to look for evidence of infection, metabolic derangements or tumours (Clinical Box 1.3).

Dural compartments

Double-layered folds of dura form two incomplete partitions inside the skull, dividing it up like the inside of an egg box (Fig. 1.31).

The **falx cerebri** is a sickle-shaped fold of dura (Latin: falx, sickle) that lies between the cerebral hemispheres, in the longitudinal fissure. The **tentorium cerebelli** is between the cerebrum and cerebellum, occupying the transverse fissure; it thus arches over the cerebellar hemispheres and posterior fossa in a tent-like fashion, rising to a peak in the midline. A gap in the tentorium (the **tentorial hiatus**) allows the brain stem to pass through. The region above the tentorium, containing the cerebral

Clinical Box 1.3: Lumbar puncture

A sample of cerebrospinal fluid can be helpful in the assessment of patients with infectious, inflammatory, metabolic or toxic CNS disorders. Tumours can also be diagnosed (very rarely) if the specimen contains malignant cells. The sample is obtained from the spinal subarachnoid space via a **lumbar puncture** (Fig. 1.30). A needle is inserted between the third and fourth lumbar vertebrae under local anaesthetic (well below L1/L2, where the spinal cord ends) and advanced through the dural sac into the subarachnoid space, pushing aside the nerve roots of the cauda equina. The CSF pressure is measured and approximately 10–20 mL of clear, colourless fluid is collected for analysis. Damage to the spinal cord or nerve roots is extremely rare and most patients complain only of a mild headache following the procedure (attributed to low CSF pressure).

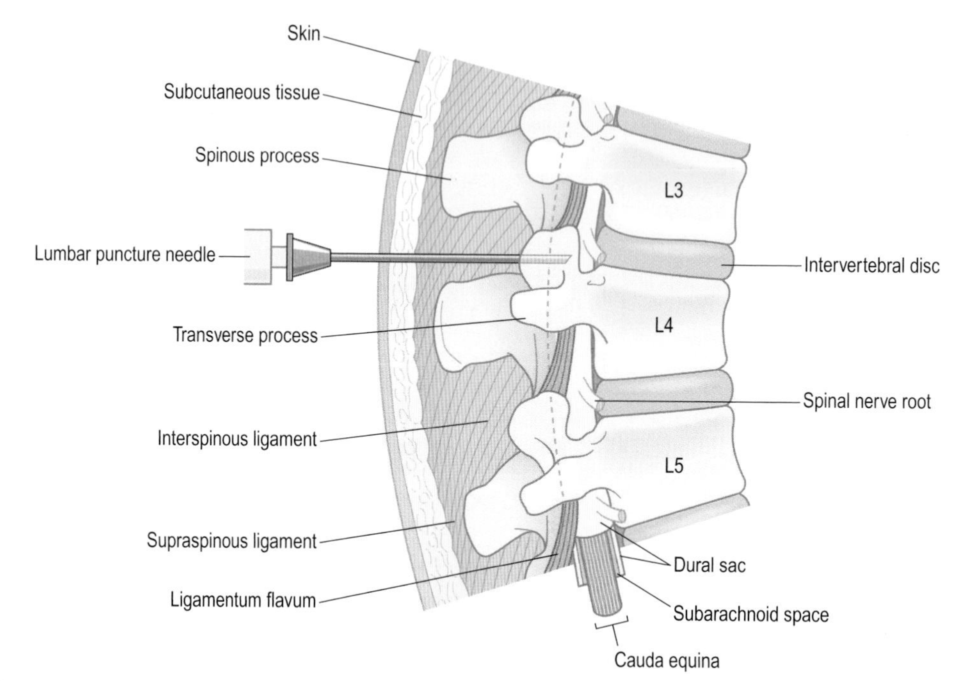

Fig. 1.30 **Lumbar puncture.** The patient is positioned with the spinal column in flexion to separate the lumbar vertebrae. The needle passes in turn through the skin, subcutaneous tissue, supraspinous and interspinous ligaments and the ligamentum flavum before entering the CSF-filled dural sac.

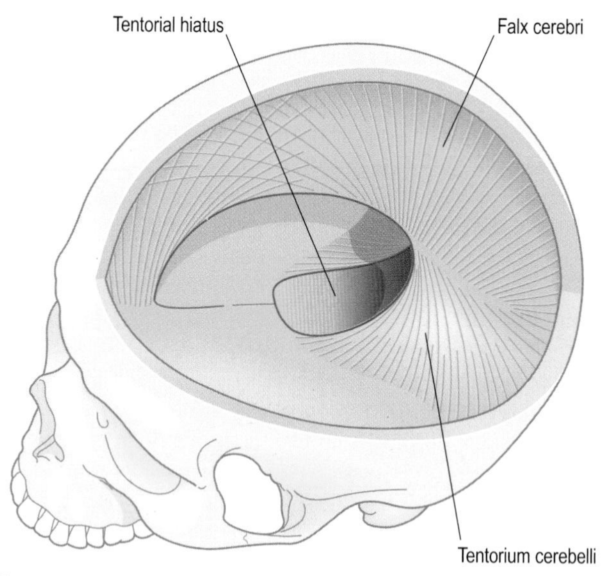

Fig. 1.31 **The interior of the skull, illustrating the position of the two major dural partitions: the falx cerebri and tentorium cerebelli.**

hemispheres, is the **supratentorial compartment**; the area below, occupied by the brain stem and cerebellum, is the **posterior fossa**.

The cranial dura contains a number of blood-filled channels that run along the free and attached margins of the falx cerebri and tentorium cerebelli (Fig. 1.32). These are the **dural venous sinuses**, into which the cerebral veins empty. The cerebral arteries are discussed in Chapter 10, in the context of stroke.

Subarachnoid cisterns

The depth of the subarachnoid space varies from place to place within the CNS and in some areas is significantly expanded to create a CSF-filled **cistern** (Fig. 1.33). The largest example is the **cisterna magna** which is located between the cerebellum and medulla. It is occasionally tapped for a CSF sample when a lumbar puncture proves technically difficult.

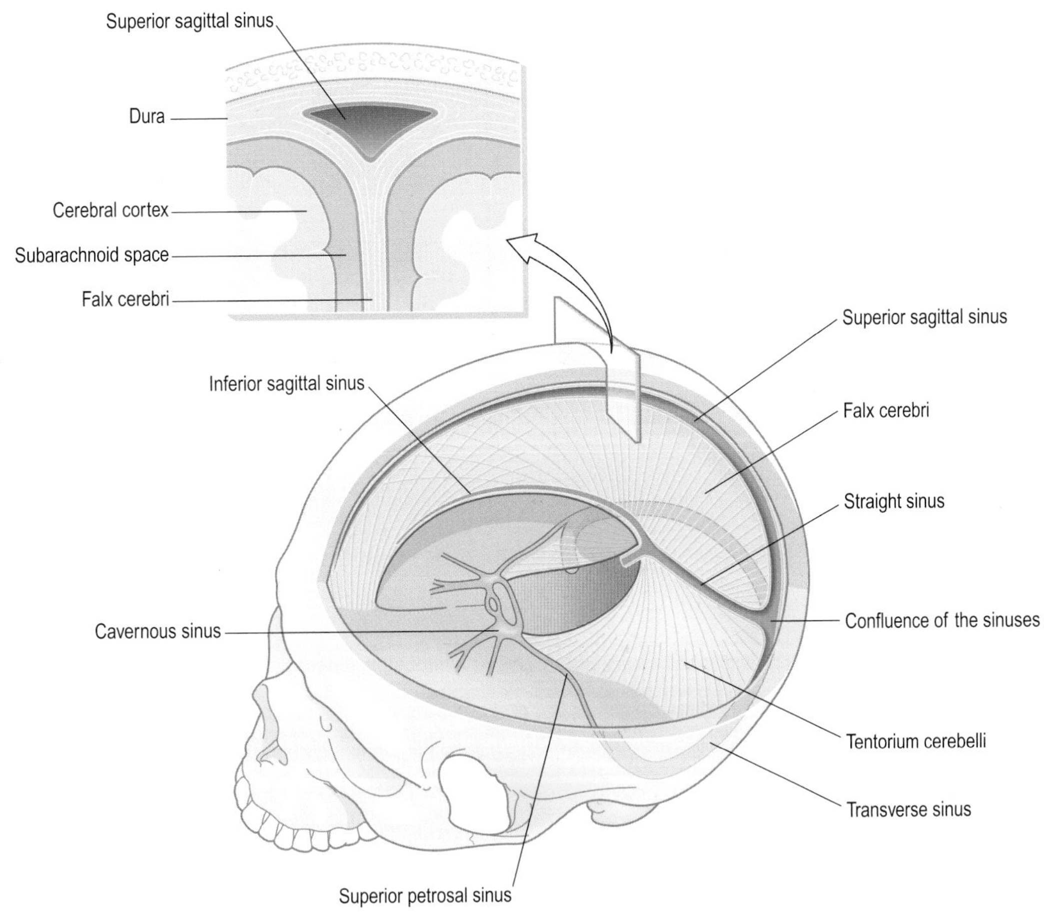

Fig. 1.32 **The dural venous sinuses.** Blood from the superficial and deep cerebral veins drains into the dural venous sinuses. It flows from anterior to posterior, towards the confluence of the sinuses, before entering the transverse and sigmoid sinuses, which empty into the jugular veins in the neck.

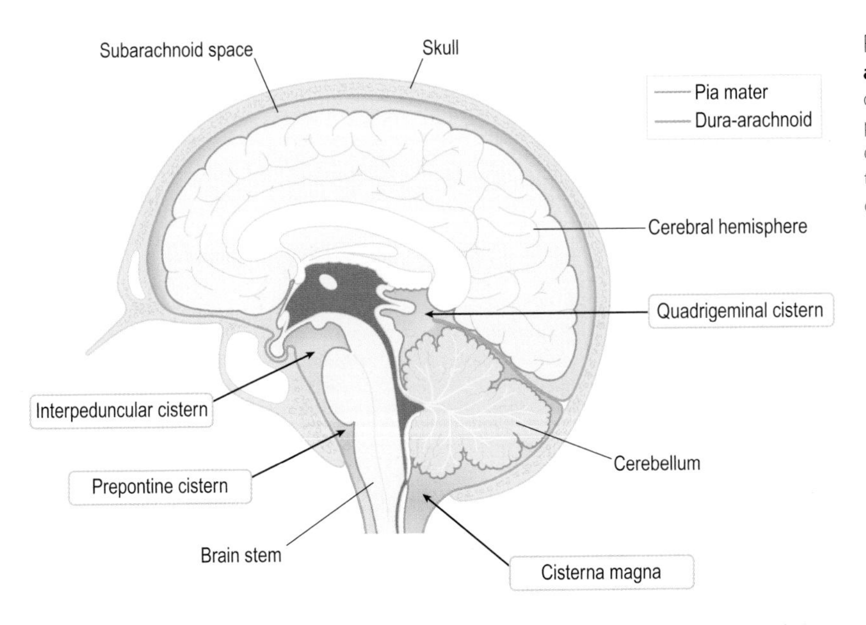

Fig. 1.33 **The basal cisterns represent expanded areas of the subarachnoid space.** CSF-filled cisterns occur wherever the surface of the brain (covered by pia) is some distance from the overlying skull (lined by dura-arachnoid). The cisterna magna is the largest of the basal cisterns and is also known as the cerebellomedullary cistern.

Key Points

- The central nervous system is protected by the bones of the skull and vertebral column.
- The brain is contained within and protected by the cranium. It is divided into the base (with anterior, middle and posterior cranial fossae) and the calvaria (which make up the vault or skull-cap).
- The brain and spinal cord are also protected by three layers of investing membranes (meninges): the dura, arachnoid and pia mater.
- The cranial meninges give rise to two dural partitions: the falx cerebri (within the longitudinal fissure) and the tentorium cerebelli (within the transverse fissure).
- The CSF-filled subarachnoid space surrounds the brain and spinal cord. This provides buoyancy and helps to cushion the brain from sudden head movements.
- A sample of CSF can be obtained via a lumbar puncture. A needle is passed between the L3 and L4 vertebrae, well below the level at which the spinal cord terminates, to enter the dural sac.

Chapter 2
Development of the brain

CHAPTER CONTENTS

Neural tube formation

The central nervous system is derived from the **neural tube**, which appears during the fourth week after fertilization. At this early stage the embryo takes the form of a **trilaminar germ disc**, lying in the floor of the amniotic sac (Fig. 2.1). The germ disc is composed of three layers of tissue from which all the structures of the body originate:

- The **ectoderm** (Greek: ektos, outside) contributes mainly to the skin, but also gives rise to the central and peripheral nervous systems.
- The **mesoderm** (Greek: misos, middle) is the origin of the cardiovascular, musculoskeletal, urinary and reproductive systems.
- The **endoderm** (Greek: endon, within) contributes chiefly to the respiratory and gastrointestinal tracts, including the liver, gallbladder and pancreas.

The process by which the embryonic ectoderm gives rise to the neural tube is called **primary neurulation** (Fig. 2.2). It is initiated by the **notochord**, a rod-like mesodermal structure that helps to define the longitudinal axis of the embryo. The notochord releases soluble mediators including cell adhesion molecules and trophic factors, which influence the overlying ectoderm. This process is termed **neural induction**.

Ultrasound studies show that in humans the neural tube begins to form at around 21-23 days after fertilization, when the embryo is just 2–3 mm in length. The first change (which occurs at about day 18) is the appearance of the **neural plate**, a broad area of thickening in the dorsal ectoderm. A shallow longitudinal depression termed the **neural groove** separates the neural plate into paired **neural folds** which gradually roll up to form a cylinder. The neural folds ultimately meet in the midline and unite to create the neural tube and **neural canal**. Fusion begins in the presumptive cervical region and proceeds both rostrally and caudally in a 'zipper-like' fashion. The open ends of the neural tube are called the cranial and caudal **neuropores**, which have normally closed by the beginning of week five. Disorders resulting from faulty neural tube closure are discussed in Clinical Box 2.1.

The sacral and coccygeal segments derive from the **caudal eminence**, a solid mass of cells that arises just below the developing neural tube and ultimately fuses with it. A central cavity forms within the caudal eminence and becomes continuous with the central canal of the spinal cord. This process is termed **secondary neurulation**.

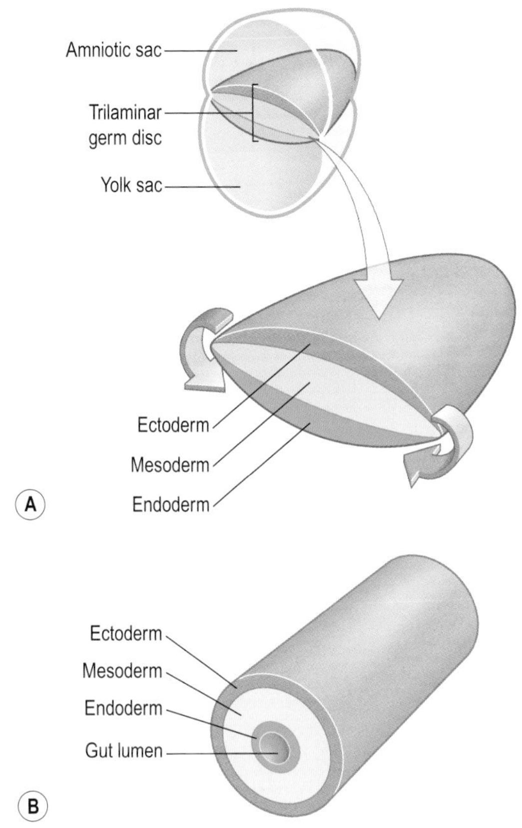

Fig. 2.1 **The trilaminar germ disc in the floor of the amniotic sac, bisected in the coronal plane. (A)** The germ disc is composed of three primitive germ layers from which all body tissues are derived. A complex process of folding (not illustrated) transforms the germ disc so that the ectoderm comes to lie on the outside and the endoderm lines the gut lumen; **(B)** The body can be represented in cartoon form as a hollow cylinder with the mouth at one end and the anus at the other.

Origin of neurons and glial cells

The wall of the neural tube can be divided into three concentric zones (Fig. 2.3). The **ventricular zone** is closest to the fluid-filled neural canal (which will become the cerebral ventricles) and is composed of proliferating neural progenitor cells. These include **neuroblasts** (neuronal precursors) and **glioblasts** (glial precursors) that give rise to most of the specialized cells of the central nervous system. **Microglia** are the resident **phagocytes** of the brain, but originate from the bone marrow and are of mesodermal rather than ectodermal lineage.

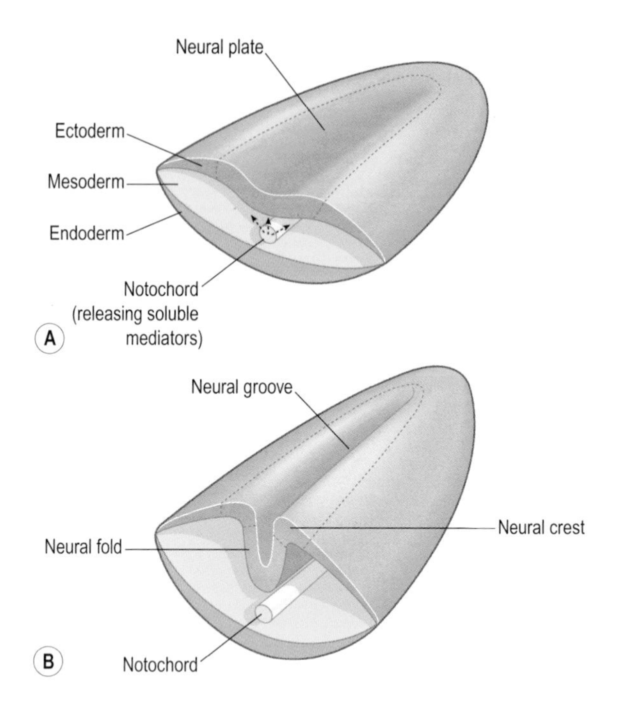

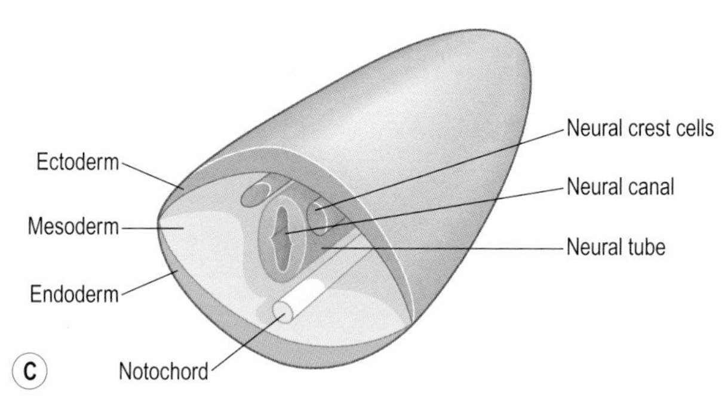

Fig. 2.2 **The origin of the neural tube and neural crest. (A)** The mesodermal notochord releases soluble mediators that induce neural tube formation in the overlying ectoderm (neural induction); **(B)** The neural tube forms from the paired neural folds which flank the neural groove; **(C)** The neural crest cells detach from the dorsolateral margins of the neural tube and will give rise to much of the peripheral nervous system, including the spinal and autonomic ganglia.

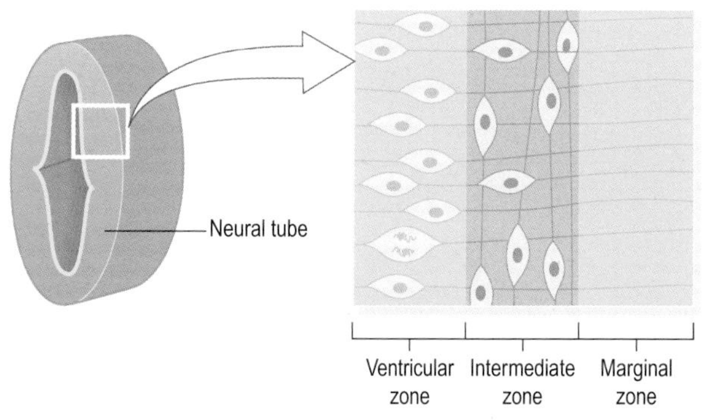

Fig. 2.3 **Transverse section through the neural tube, illustrating the ventricular, intermediate and marginal zones.** Cell division (mitosis) occurs in the ventricular zone, giving rise to neurons and glia.

Cells that have arisen in the ventricular zone migrate outwards through the wall of the neural tube. This is facilitated by **radial glia** which provide a 'scaffold' along which cells are able to crawl, guided by signalling molecules. Neurons and glial cells accumulate in the **intermediate zone** of the neural tube where they extend processes and begin to make connections with other cells. The outermost layer is the **marginal zone**. It is relatively cell-poor and is mainly composed of neuronal and glial processes.

Clinical Box 2.1: Neural tube defects

Incomplete closure of the neural tube is responsible for a group of developmental disorders called **neural tube defects**. The incidence is approximately 1 in 500 live births. The most common form is **spina bifida** which results in malformation of the lower spinal cord due to abnormal caudal neuropore closure. The severity is variable, ranging from little or no neurological impairment to paralysis of the lower limbs with lack of bladder and bowel control. An asymptomatic partial form that only affects the vertebral arches (**spina bifida occulta**) is present in up to 10% of the population. Defective closure of the cranial neuropore can lead to **anencephaly** in which the forebrain fails to develop (Greek: a-, without; enkephalos, brain). Anencephalic fetuses are often stillborn, but may survive for a few hours after birth. It has been shown that **folic acid** supplements in women of child-bearing age reduce the incidence of neural tube defects by around 70%.

Formation of the cerebral cortex

The three-layered arrangement of the neural tube is modified extensively to form the brain. In the developing cerebral hemispheres there is a second (superficial) neuronal layer called the **cortical plate** which is the precursor of the cerebral cortex. Beneath it is a transient structure called the **subplate**.

Cortical neurons arise in the ventricular zone (referred to as the **germinal matrix** in the brain) and migrate along radial glia to enter the cortical plate – or form transient connections within the subplate. Those neurons that will ultimately occupy the deepest of the six cortical laminae arrive first, with more superficial layers being added in sequential waves of **neurogenesis** and **migration**. This means that the cerebral cortex is constructed 'inside-out'.

Proper neuronal migration depends on a layer of **Cajal–Retzius** cells (pronounced: ka-HARL) located in the most superficial part of the cerebral cortex. The outward migration of newly formed neurons is regulated by the protein **reelin**, a molecular 'stop-signal' that is secreted by Cajal–Retzius cells. This ensures that neurons reach the appropriate layer of the cerebral cortex.

In the cerebral hemispheres the majority of neurons ultimately vacate the intermediate zone or undergo **programmed cell death** (see Ch. 8) and this region eventually becomes the subcortical white matter. Up to 50% of neurons produced in the developing brain fail to (i) reach their intended targets or (ii) make appropriate functional connections and are consequently deleted by programmed cell death.

Sensory and motor areas

The neural tube has two functional divisions, separated by the **sulcus limitans** (Fig. 2.4A). The **basal plate** occupies the ventral portion of the neural tube (anterior to the sulcus limitans) and is predominantly a motor structure; the **alar plate** is located dorsally and is sensory. This dorsal–ventral division between sensory and motor areas is reflected in the adult spinal cord, with sensory fibres entering via the dorsal roots and motor fibres emerging in the ventral roots (Fig. 2.4B). It is echoed throughout the central nervous system

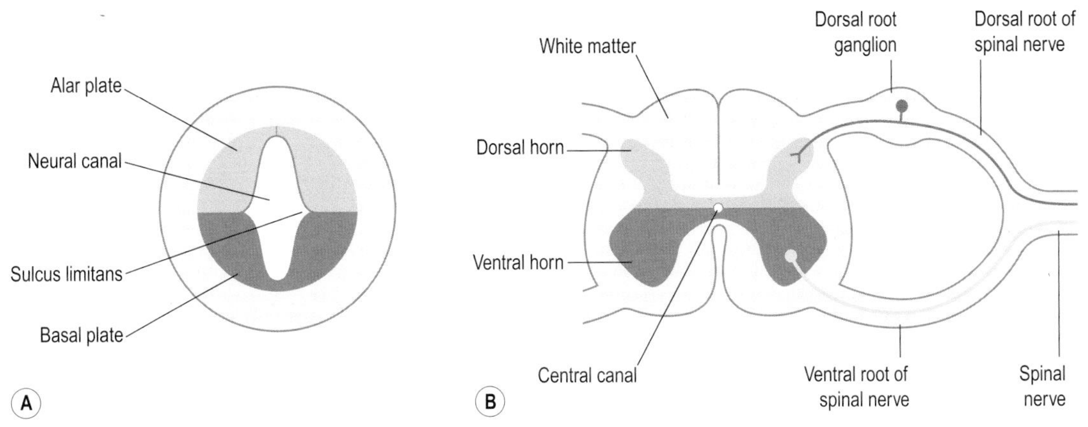

Fig. 2.4 **Transverse sections through (A) the developing neural tube and (B) the adult spinal cord.** The basal (motor) plate is separated from the alar (sensory) plate by the sulcus limitans.

so that motor structures (e.g. cortical areas, tracts, nuclei) tend to be anterior to sensory structures.

The neural crest

The peripheral nervous system is mainly derived from the **neural crest**. This is a population of cells that detaches from the lateral margins of the neural plate during neurulation (see Fig. 2.2). Neural crest cells that come to lie dorsolateral to the neural tube ultimately become the primary sensory neurons of the **dorsal root ganglia**. These neurons are initially **bipolar** but their central and peripheral processes fuse at a common T-shaped extension of the cell body to form a single continuous axon. For this reason they are described as **pseudounipolar** (Greek: pseudo-, false). The central processes of the dorsal root ganglion cells innervate the alar (sensory) plate of the neural tube, whereas the peripheral processes enter the **spinal nerves** at each segmental level (see Fig. 2.4B).

The ventral roots of the spinal nerves represent the axons of basal plate motor neurons. The primary sensory neurons of **cranial nerve ganglia** are also crest-derived, although not all cranial nerves carry sensory fibres. Other neural crest derivatives include the ganglia of the **autonomic nervous system**, peripheral **Schwann cells** and the inner two **meningeal layers** (pia and arachnoid). In contrast, the dura is a mesodermal derivative. The neural crest also gives rise to non-neural structures including skin melanocytes and components of the laryngeal cartilages and teeth.

Key Points

- The brain and spinal cord develop from the neural tube, which is derived from the ectoderm. The neural folds rise up on either side of the neural groove and fuse to form a cylinder.
- The wall of the neural tube is divided into three concentric zones spanned by radial glia. The ventricular zone contains proliferating progenitor cells that give rise to neurons and glia.
- The neural tube is divided by the sulcus limitans into a basal (motor) plate anteriorly and an alar (sensory) plate posteriorly.
- The neural crest arises from the dorsolateral margins of the neural tube and gives rise to most of the peripheral nervous system including neurons of the cranial, spinal and autonomic ganglia.
- Folic acid supplementation in women of child-bearing age reduces the incidence of neural tube defects such as spina bifida and anencephaly by 70%.

Divisions of the brain

The three fundamental divisions of the brain can be identified in the neural plate as early as week three, before the neural tube has closed. They are illustrated schematically (at a later stage of development) in Fig. 2.5:

- The **prosencephalon** (Greek: pro, before) is the precursor of the **forebrain** and will give rise to the cerebral hemispheres, basal ganglia and thalamic region (diencephalon).
- The **mesencephalon** corresponds to the adult **midbrain**.
- The **rhombencephalon** (Greek: rhomboeides, shaped like a rhombus) gives rise to the **hindbrain**, which includes the pons, medulla and cerebellum.

During weeks four and five the neural tube closes and the cranial portion undergoes an impressive transformation, differentiating into five regions that will become the major anatomical divisions of the adult brain (Fig. 2.6). Each of these components contains a fluid-filled cavity or channel that corresponds to the lumen of the neural tube (Fig. 2.7).

The forebrain (or **cerebrum**) gives rise to two large vesicles which are the forerunners of the cerebral hemispheres. These balloon out on either side of the forebrain in the most cranial

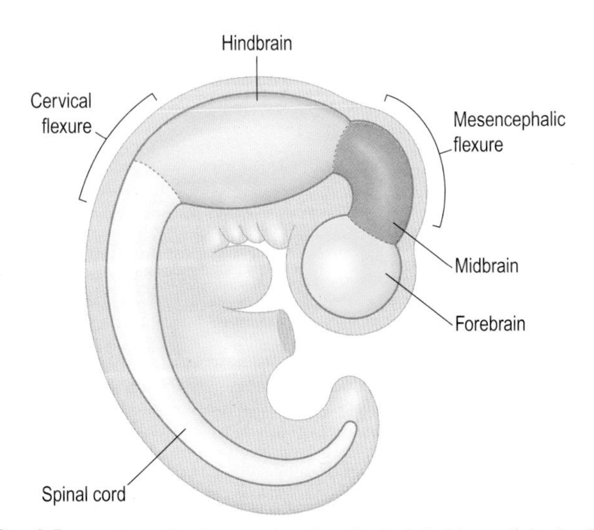

Fig. 2.5 **The three fundamental embryological divisions of the brain:** forebrain (prosencephalon), midbrain (mesencephalon) and hindbrain (rhombencephalon). Note the two forward-flexures that contribute to the change in the longitudinal axis of the nervous system.

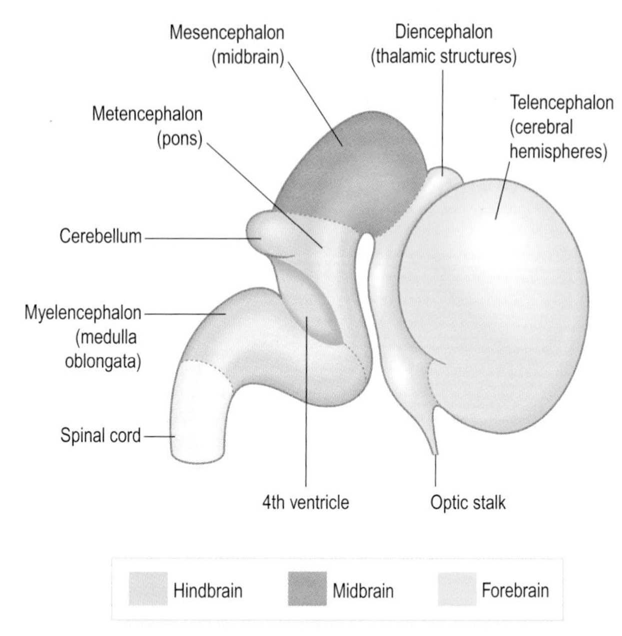

Fig. 2.6 **The five major anatomical divisions of the brain can be identified by the end of the fifth week post-fertilization.** At this stage the embryo is around 10 mm in length.

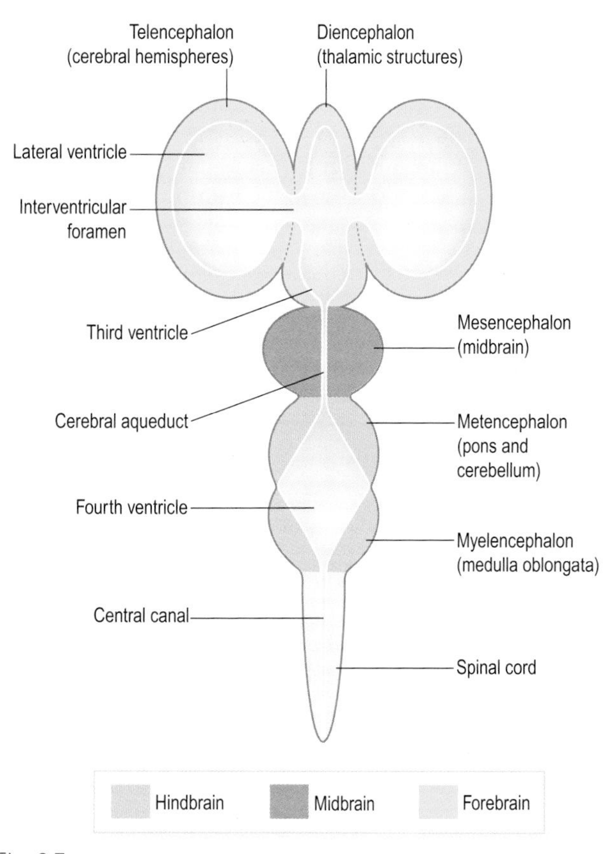

Fig. 2.7 **The brain and ventricular system.** Each part of the brain contains a fluid-filled cavity or channel corresponding to the lumen of the neural tube.

part of the neural tube and collectively make up the **telencephalon** (Greek: telos, end). In humans, the telencephalon undergoes massive expansion and comes to dominate the entire brain. The remaining midline portion of the forebrain, situated between the cerebral hemispheres, is the **diencephalon** (Greek: dia, between). This part of the cerebrum will become the thalamus, hypothalamus and a number of related structures surrounding the cavity of the third ventricle (including the pineal gland).

The hindbrain also differentiates into two parts. The upper portion becomes the **metencephalon**, which is the precursor of the pons and cerebellum and makes up the bulk of the hindbrain (Greek: meta, behind). The lower part gives rise to the **myelencephalon**, which corresponds to the medulla.

In contrast, the **mesencephalon** does not subdivide further. Instead, it retains a somewhat tubular structure as the adult midbrain, traversed by a narrow cerebral aqueduct.

Key Points

- The three fundamental divisions of the brain are the prosencephalon (forebrain), mesencephalon (midbrain) and rhombencephalon (hindbrain).
- These give rise to five divisions that correspond to the principal anatomical components of the brain: telencephalon, diencephalon, mesencephalon, metencephalon, myelencephalon.
- The forebrain (cerebrum) includes the telencephalon (cerebral hemispheres) and diencephalon (thalamic region). The hindbrain includes the metencephalon (pons, cerebellum) and myelencephalon (medulla). The mesencephalon (midbrain) is not further subdivided.

Flexures and the neuraxis

The neural tube develops three **flexures** (bends). Two forward-flexures (**cervical** and **mesencephalic**; Figs 2.5 & 2.6) contribute to the change in the longitudinal axis of the nervous system (the **neuraxis**). This is vertical in the spinal cord but horizontal in the cerebral hemispheres. The 90-degree bend in the human neuraxis contrasts with that of other animals (partly because of our upright, bipedal stance) and alters the meaning of certain anatomical terms (Fig. 2.8).

The **pontine flexure** bends in the opposite direction to the other two and marks the boundary between the pons and medulla. It also causes the neural tube to split along its relatively weak line of fusion and 'gape open' posteriorly (Fig. 2.9; see also Fig. 2.6). The pontine flexure thus contributes to the rhomboid shape of the fourth ventricle, which is the origin of the term **rhombencephalon**.

Expansion of the telencephalon

The cerebral hemispheres and lateral ventricles become C-shaped as a result of the non-uniform expansion of the telencephalon (Fig. 2.10). As the frontal, parietal, temporal and occipital lobes grow the telencephalon expands like an inflating balloon. A small island of tissue overlying the basal ganglia expands comparatively little and is progressively 'swallowed up' by the surrounding frontal, parietal and temporal lobes. This region corresponds to the **insula**, which is hidden within the depths of the lateral sulcus in the mature brain (Latin: insula, island).

As the telencephalon continues to expand it eventually envelops and fuses with the diencephalon. Once this has happened, axons can pass directly between the cerebral hemispheres and brain stem, traversing the basal ganglia and partially dividing them (see Ch. 3). Many internal hemispheric structures are distorted by the expansion of the cerebral

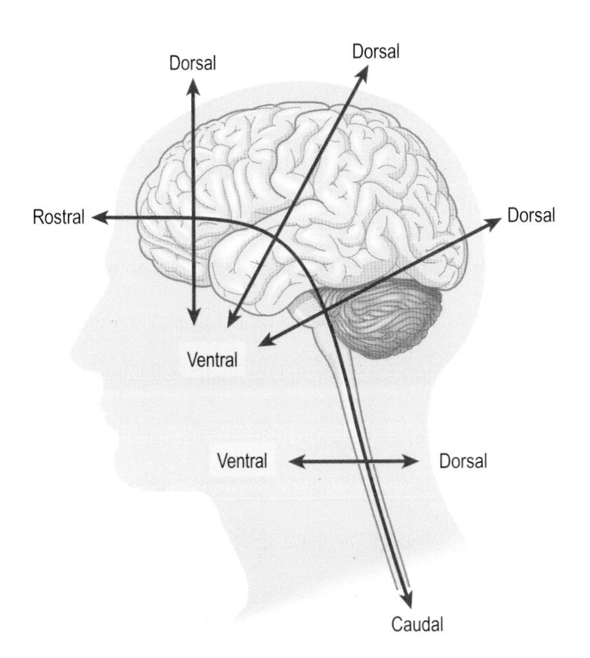

Fig. 2.8 **The human neuraxis is approximately vertical in the spinal cord and almost horizontal in the brain.** This is partly due to our upright, bipedal posture and alters the meaning of certain directional terms in the dorsoventral and rostrocaudal axes (i.e. in the spinal cord, dorsal = posterior and ventral = anterior; whereas in the brain, dorsal = superior and ventral = inferior).

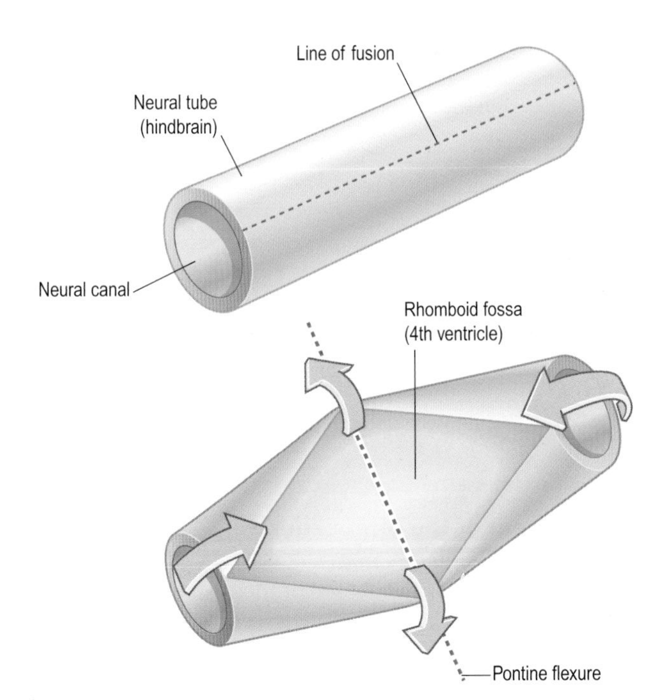

Fig. 2.9 **How the pontine flexure causes the neural tube to 'splay open' posteriorly, creating the rhomboid fossa (the floor of the fourth ventricle).** The neural tube is seen from the posterior aspect. This view would normally be obscured by the cerebellum which covers the rhomboid fossa and contributes to the roof of the fourth ventricle. [This can be reproduced by bending a piece of rolled-up A4 paper.]

hemispheres and take on the same C-shaped profile as the lateral ventricles. These include the **hippocampus** and its outflow pathway, the **fornix** (Fig. 2.11) which are involved in memory formation (see Ch. 3).

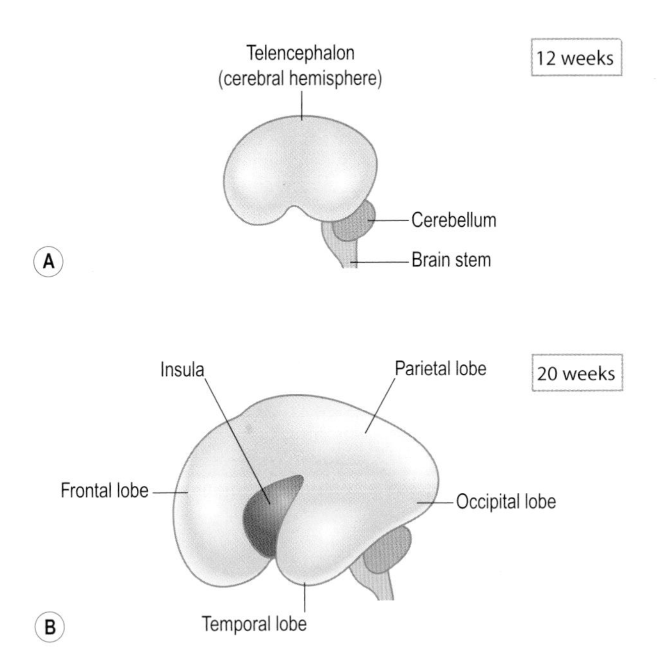

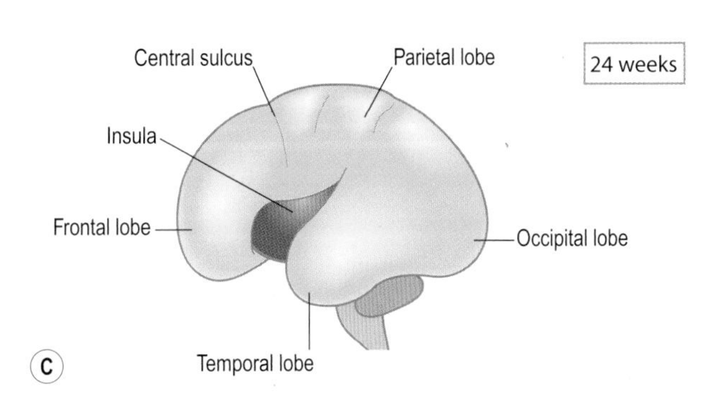

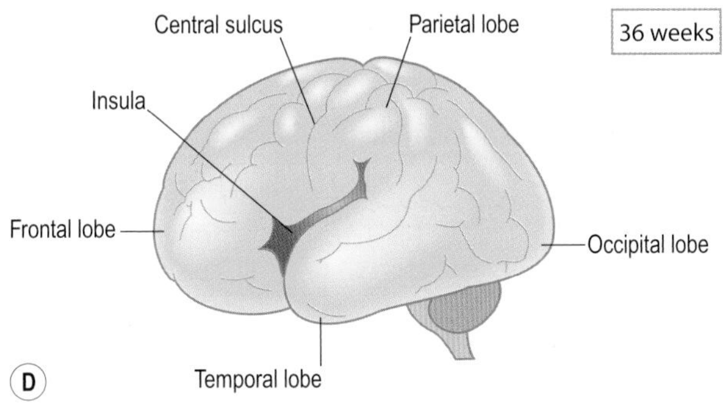

Fig. 2.10 **The dramatic expansion of the telencephalon and the origin of the insula. (A)** At 12 weeks the surface of the brain is still smooth; **(B)** By 20 weeks the four lobes are just discernible and the insula can be seen within the lateral sulcus; **(C)** The central sulcus is evident at 24 weeks, marking the boundary between the frontal and parietal lobes; **(D)** By 36 weeks the surface convolutions are well-developed and the insula is mostly hidden within the lateral sulcus.

Formation of gyri and sulci

Gyral development is maximal in the third trimester. At 24 weeks after fertilization the surface of the fetal brain is almost smooth, apart from the **lateral** and **central sulci**. The normal arrangement of gyri and sulci gradually emerges over the following weeks and the pattern of surface convolutions

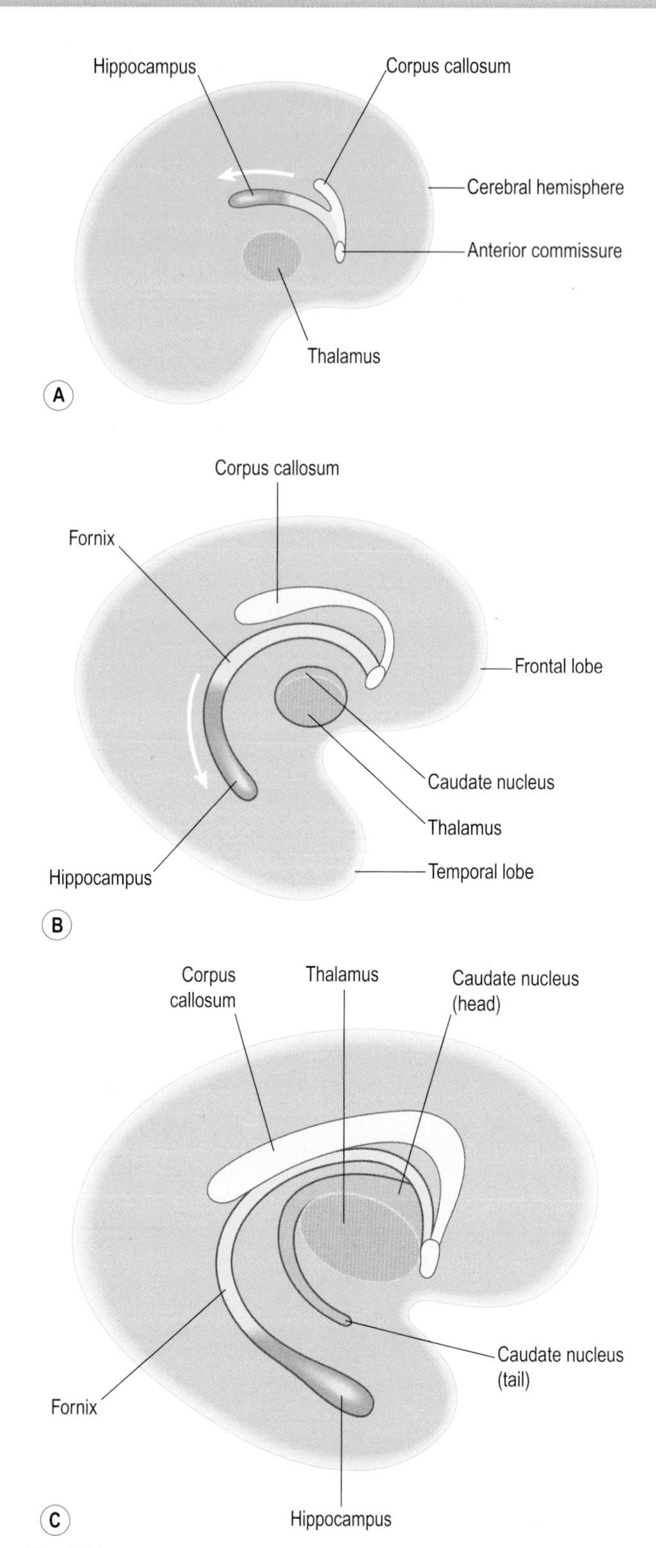

Fig. 2.11 **The descent of the hippocampus during expansion of the telencephalon. (A)** The hippocampus originates as a dorsal midline structure, superior to the thalamus and in other species remains in this position; **(B)** As the human telencephalon expands, the hippocampus is carried downwards and forwards, coming to lie in the floor of the temporal lobe; **(C)** The hippocampus leaves behind an arching trail of white matter, the fornix, which echoes the C-shaped curvature of the cerebral hemisphere and lateral ventricle. Modified from Fitzgerald: Clinical Neuroanatomy and Neuroscience 5e (2006) with permission.

in the term fetus is similar to that of the adult. However, neural development at birth is far from complete and the mass of the brain is only around 350 g (in comparison to the adult mass of 1350 g). In particular, the cerebral hemispheres are poorly myelinated in the neonate.

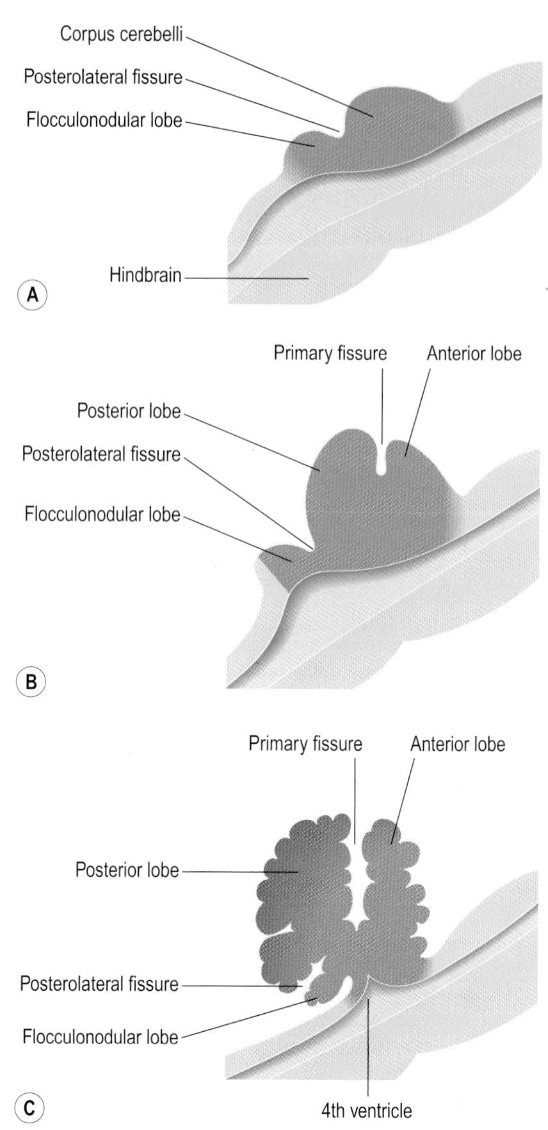

Fig. 2.12 **Development of the cerebellum. (A)** The cerebellum arises from the alar plate of the metencephalon and is initially divided into the corpus cerebelli and flocculonodular lobe by the posterolateral fissure; **(B, C)** The primary fissure further subdivides the corpus cerebelli into anterior and posterior lobes. In the mature human brain, the flocculonodular lobe is very small.

Development of the cerebellum

The cerebellum originates from a dorsal outgrowth of the metencephalon (in the hindbrain). It thus overlies the pons and fourth ventricle (Fig. 2.12). The alar (sensory) plates of the metencephalon (including the **rhombic lips**, which overhang the upper part of the fourth ventricle) fuse to form the **cerebellar plate**. Expansion of the cerebellar plate gives rise to the cerebellar hemispheres and vermis which eventually cover the rhomboid fossa, forming the roof of the fourth ventricle. In keeping with its origin as an alar (sensory) plate derivative, the cerebellum has many more afferent than efferent connections and has no direct role in movement initiation.

The cerebellum is initially divided into the **corpus cerebelli** and the **flocculonodular lobe** by the **posterolateral fissure**. The main body of the cerebellum (Latin: corpus, body) is then subdivided into a small anterior lobe and much larger posterior lobe by the **primary fissure**. The narrow midline portion of the adult cerebellum is called the **vermis** which is said to resemble a segmented worm (Latin: vermis, worm). This is flanked on either side by the **cerebellar hemispheres**.

> ### *Key Points*
> - The cervical and mesencephalic flexures contribute to the shift in the axis of the nervous system from vertical (in the spinal cord) to horizontal (in the brain).
> - The pontine flexure causes the neural tube to 'gape open' along its weak line of fusion, contributing to the shape of the rhomboid fossa (floor of the fourth ventricle).
> - The cerebellum arises from the alar (sensory) plate of the metencephalon. It is divided into anterior, posterior and flocculonodular lobes by the primary and posterolateral fissures.

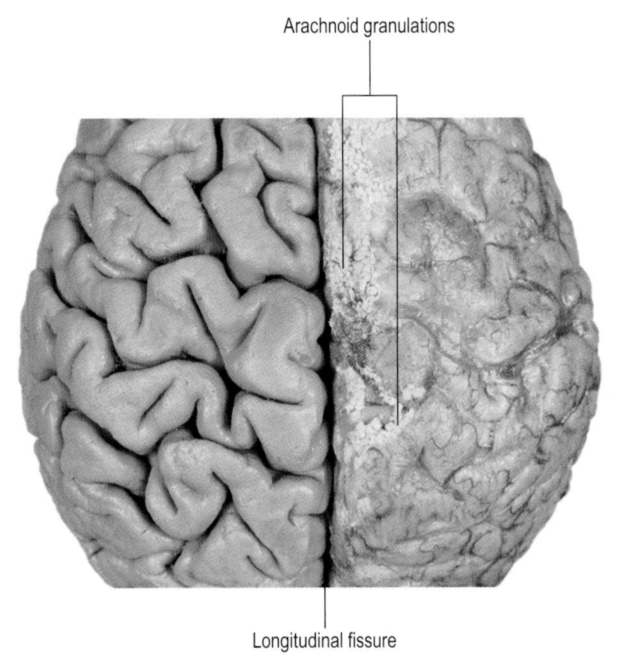

Fig. 2.14 **The dorsal surface of the cerebral hemispheres.** The tough, leathery dura is not seen in this image (it is tightly adherent to the periosteum and is usually left inside the skull when the brain is removed) but the pia and arachnoid membranes are present on the right-hand side, including the arachnoid granulations. On the left side, the membranes have been stripped to reveal the underlying gyri and sulci. From Crossman: Neuroanatomy ICT 4e (Churchill Livingstone 2010) with permission.

Ventricular system

The fluid-filled cavity of the neural tube is represented in the adult brain by the **ventricular system**. This consists of four interconnected cavities or **ventricles** which contain around 30 mL of colourless **cerebrospinal fluid (CSF)** (Fig. 2.13).

The **lateral ventricles** are C-shaped cavities within the cerebral hemispheres. Each lateral ventricle has a central **body** and three **horns** (frontal, occipital and temporal). The point at which the body joins with both the occipital and temporal horns is called the **trigone** (or **atrium**).

The slot-like **third ventricle** occupies the diencephalon (thalamic region). The two thalami form the upper part of the lateral wall, whereas the hypothalamus forms the floor and lower part of the lateral wall. The third ventricle is so narrow that in 80% of people the two thalami 'kiss' across the water, forming the **thalamic interconnexus**, but no axons are exchanged. This gives the third ventricle its distinctive shape which resembles a distorted ring-doughnut (the central 'hole' is where the two thalami touch). The lateral ventricles communicate with the third ventricle via the paired **interventricular foramina** (singular: foramen) which creates a Y-shaped profile on coronal views.

The **fourth ventricle** is situated between the brain stem and cerebellum. Its diamond-shaped floor corresponds to the posterior surfaces of the pons and medulla. The third and fourth ventricles communicate via the **cerebral aqueduct**, a narrow channel that passes through the midbrain.

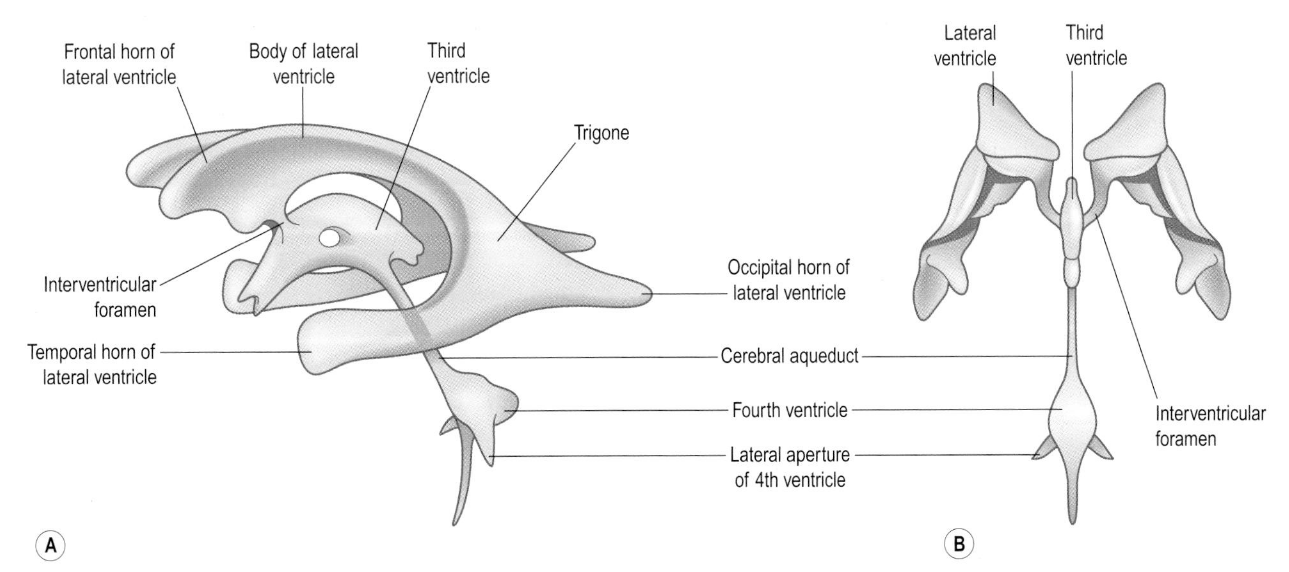

Fig. 2.13 **The ventricular system. (A)** Lateral aspect; **(B)** Anterior aspect.

Circulation of CSF

The **choroid plexuses** are highly vascular structures that project into each of the ventricles and continuously produce cerebrospinal fluid by active secretion from the blood.

CSF escapes from the fourth ventricle (to the subarachnoid space) via three openings: the single median aperture and the two lateral apertures. It is ultimately reabsorbed into the venous system via the **arachnoid granulations** which run along the superior aspect of the cerebral hemispheres (Fig. 2.14). These correspond to the **arachnoid villi**, finger-like projections into a large venous channel called the **superior sagittal sinus**. These structures allow the reabsorption of CSF into the venous circulation.

The total volume of intracranial CSF is around 140 mL, most of which is in the subarachnoid space; the spinal CSF volume is more variable and difficult to estimate. Due to a constant cycle of production and reabsorption, the CSF is replaced up to four times each day.

Interference with CSF production or drainage can lead to **ventricular dilation** and **raised intracranial pressure** (Clinical Box 2.2).

Key Points

- Each division of the adult brain contains a fluid-filled cavity or channel corresponding to the lumen of the embryonic neural tube. This constitutes the ventricular system.
- The lateral and third ventricles are connected via the (left and right) interventricular foramina, whereas the third and fourth ventricles are linked by the (single) cerebral aqueduct.
- CSF is produced within each ventricle by the choroid plexuses. It escapes from the fourth ventricle via the median and lateral apertures to reach the subarachnoid space.
- CSF is reabsorbed into the venous system (at the superior sagittal sinus) via the arachnoid villi. Enlargement of the ventricular system is called hydrocephalus, which can be treated by shunting.

Clinical Box 2.2: Hydrocephalus

Enlargement of the ventricles due to accumulation of CSF is termed **hydrocephalus** (Greek: hydro, water; kephalē, head) (Fig. 2.15). This is usually associated with **raised intracranial pressure** which can lead to progressive brain damage. In infants with congenital hydrocephalus the cranium may become grossly enlarged since fusion of the skull bones is not complete until 18 months of age. **Obstructive hydrocephalus** is caused by occlusion of one of the CSF drainage channels and leads to dilation of that portion of the ventricular system above the level of the blockage. **Communicating hydrocephalus** results in dilation of the entire ventricular system; it is due either to inadequate reabsorption of CSF or (very rarely) excessive production by a choroid plexus tumour. Hydrocephalus can be treated surgically by the insertion of a **shunt** which diverts excess CSF, usually to the abdominal peritoneum (Fig. 2.16). A pressure-operated valve and sometimes also an anti-siphon device are incorporated into the system to ensure appropriate one-way flow. Unfortunately shunts are prone to infection, blockage, disconnection and valve malfunction and frequently need to be replaced (the failure rate is around 80% at 12 years).

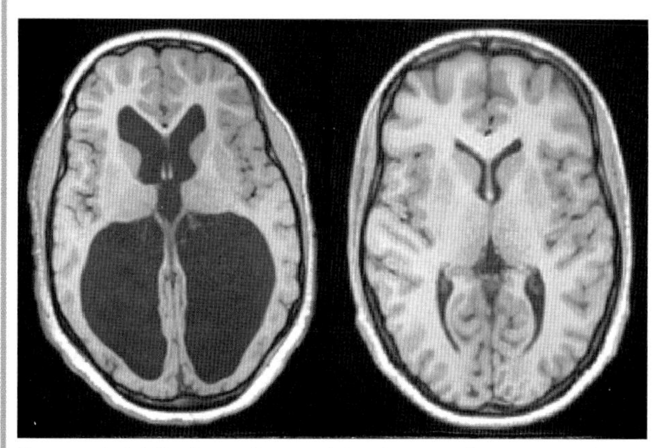

Fig. 2.15 **Axial (horizontal) T1-weighted magnetic resonance image (MRI) of the brain in a patient with hydrocephalus (left) and a normal control (right).** The images are taken at approximately the same level and show gross dilatation of the lateral ventricles in the patient with hydrocephalus. This is usually associated with raised intracranial pressure which may lead to progressive brain damage, if left untreated. Courtesy of Dr Gemma Northam.

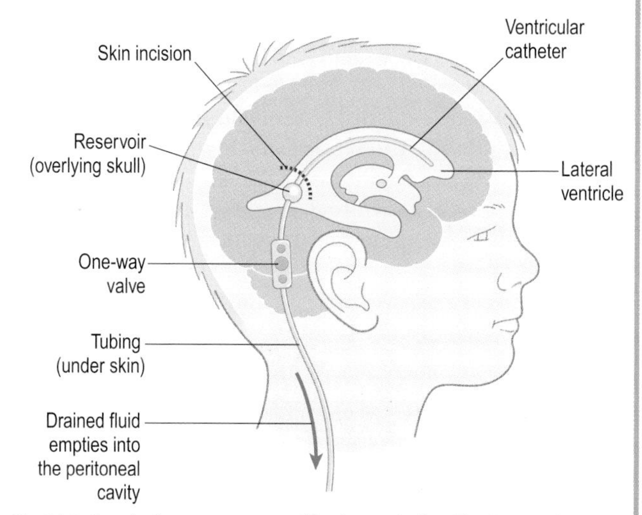

Fig. 2.16 **Surgical management of hydrocephalus.** This Figure shows a child with an implanted ventriculoperitoneal (VP) shunt. The distal end of the shunt tubing is tunnelled under the skin and implanted into the abdomen to allow excess CSF to drain into the peritoneal cavity.

Chapter 3
Functional neuroanatomy

This chapter examines the functional anatomy of the brain, focusing on the cerebral cortex, basal ganglia, hippocampus and amygdala. The main functional divisions of the thalamic region, brain stem and cerebellum are also discussed. Sensory and motor pathways of the CNS are described in Chapter 4. The blood supply to the brain is discussed in Chapter 10, in the context of stroke.

Cerebral cortex

This section describes the gyri and sulci of the cerebral hemispheres (Figs 3.1–3.3) and the main functional areas of the cerebral cortex (Fig. 3.4). **Brodmann areas (BA)** are indicated in brackets if they have important functional or clinical associations (these are numbered cortical regions, defined by microscopic differences in the structure of the cerebral cortex; see Chapter 5).

Frontal lobe

The frontal lobe is anterior to the **central sulcus** and above the **lateral sulcus**. It accounts for around 40% of the cortical surface area and contributes to movement, behaviour, personality and language. It has lateral, medial and inferior surfaces.

Lateral aspect (Figs 3.1 and 3.4A)

The **precentral gyrus** ribbons forward over the cerebral convexity, immediately anterior to the central sulcus. It corresponds to the **primary motor cortex (BA 4)** which contains an inverted, point-to-point or **somatotopic map** of the opposite half of the body (Greek: soma, body; topos, place). The representation of each body part in the **motor strip** is proportional to the precision of movement control. This means that the areas for the hands, face and tongue are disproportionately large (Fig. 3.5). A useful landmark for identifying the motor cortex is the **motor hand area** which resembles an inverted capital omega (Fig. 3.6).

The remainder of the lateral frontal lobe consists of the **superior, middle** and **inferior frontal gyri** which run from anterior to posterior. The region in front of the motor strip is the **lateral premotor area (BA 6)** but it does not correspond to any particular gyral or sulcal boundaries. The premotor cortex also contains an inverted body map and is concerned with preparation and execution of movement sequences, particularly those that occur in response to an external trigger (e.g. catching a ball, rather than throwing one). More anteriorly, the **frontal eye field (BA 8)** is a cortical centre for attention and gaze which directs both eyes towards the contralateral visual field. The frontal eye field and the remainder of the lateral frontal lobe belong to the **prefrontal cortex**, which is discussed separately below.

> *Key Points*
>
> - The frontal lobe is anterior to the central sulcus and above the lateral sulcus. It is the largest of the four main lobes, accounting for 40% of the cortical surface area.
> - The precentral gyrus corresponds to the primary motor cortex. It contains an inverted somatotopic (point-to-point) representation of the opposite half of the body.
> - A useful landmark for identifying the primary motor cortex is the hand area, which resembles an inverted capital omega.
> - The lateral premotor area lies in front of the motor strip and is concerned with the preparation and execution of motor sequences, particularly those that are externally triggered.

Medial aspect (Figs 3.2 and 3.4B)

The superior frontal gyrus and precentral gyrus both continue onto the medial surface of the hemisphere. The boundary between the superior frontal gyrus and the underlying limbic lobe is the **cingulate sulcus**. This runs parallel to the corpus callosum before turning upwards to the superior margin of the hemisphere as the **pars marginalis** (marginal part). The central sulcus lies immediately anterior to the pars marginalis and slopes downwards and backwards towards it at an angle of approximately 90 degrees. The **paracentral lobule** is a U-shaped convolution on the medial surface of the hemisphere that loops underneath the central sulcus. It therefore straddles the boundary between the frontal and parietal lobes. The paracentral lobule includes the primary motor and sensory areas for the lower limbs and genitalia.

The **supplementary motor area (SMA)** is just in front of the paracentral lobule. It contains a map of both sides of the body and tends to be recruited with its counterpart in the opposite hemisphere (e.g. when the hands are working together to manipulate an object). In contrast to the lateral premotor area, the SMA (or 'medial premotor area') is particularly concerned with **internally generated** (self-initiated) actions, rather than those that occur in response to an external event. The SMA is underactive in **Parkinson's disease**, in which voluntary movements are initiated with effort and performed slowly (Ch. 13). Just anterior to the SMA, there is a small medial extension of the frontal eye field.

Inferior (orbitofrontal) aspect (Fig. 3.3)

The inferior part of the frontal lobe is the **orbital cortex**, which overlies the orbital cavity. The **olfactory sulcus** divides

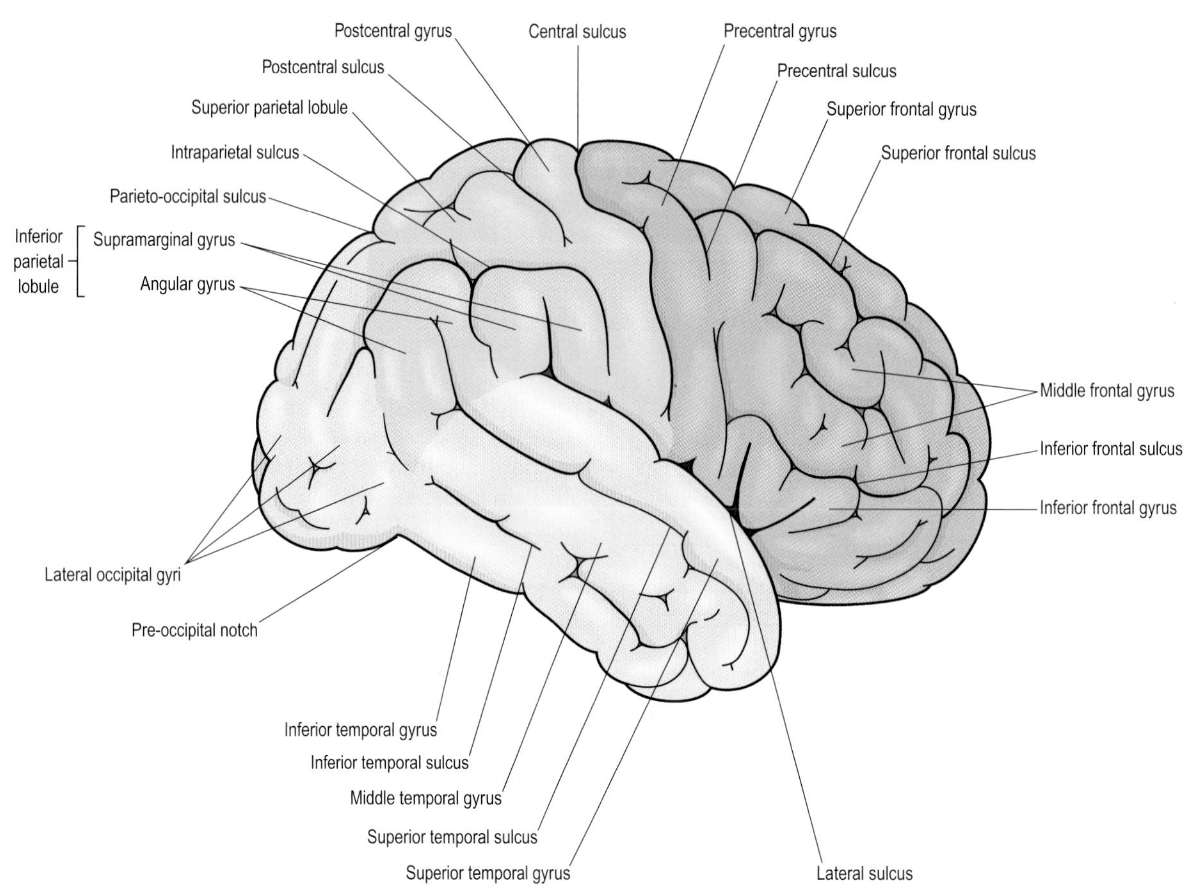

Fig. 3.1 **Lateral view of the cerebral hemisphere, showing the main named gyri and sulci.**

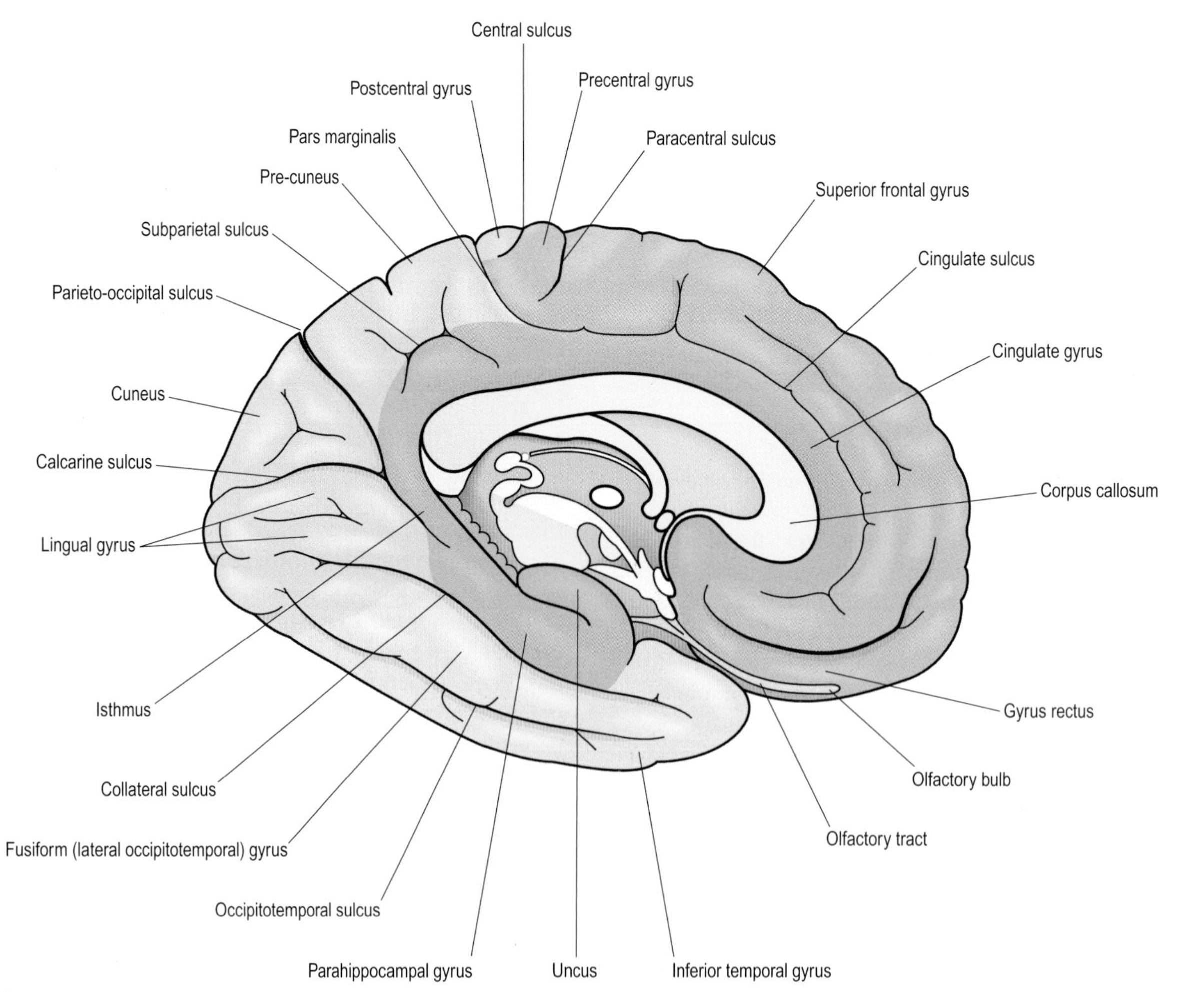

Fig. 3.2 **Medial view of the cerebral hemisphere, showing the main named gyri and sulci.**

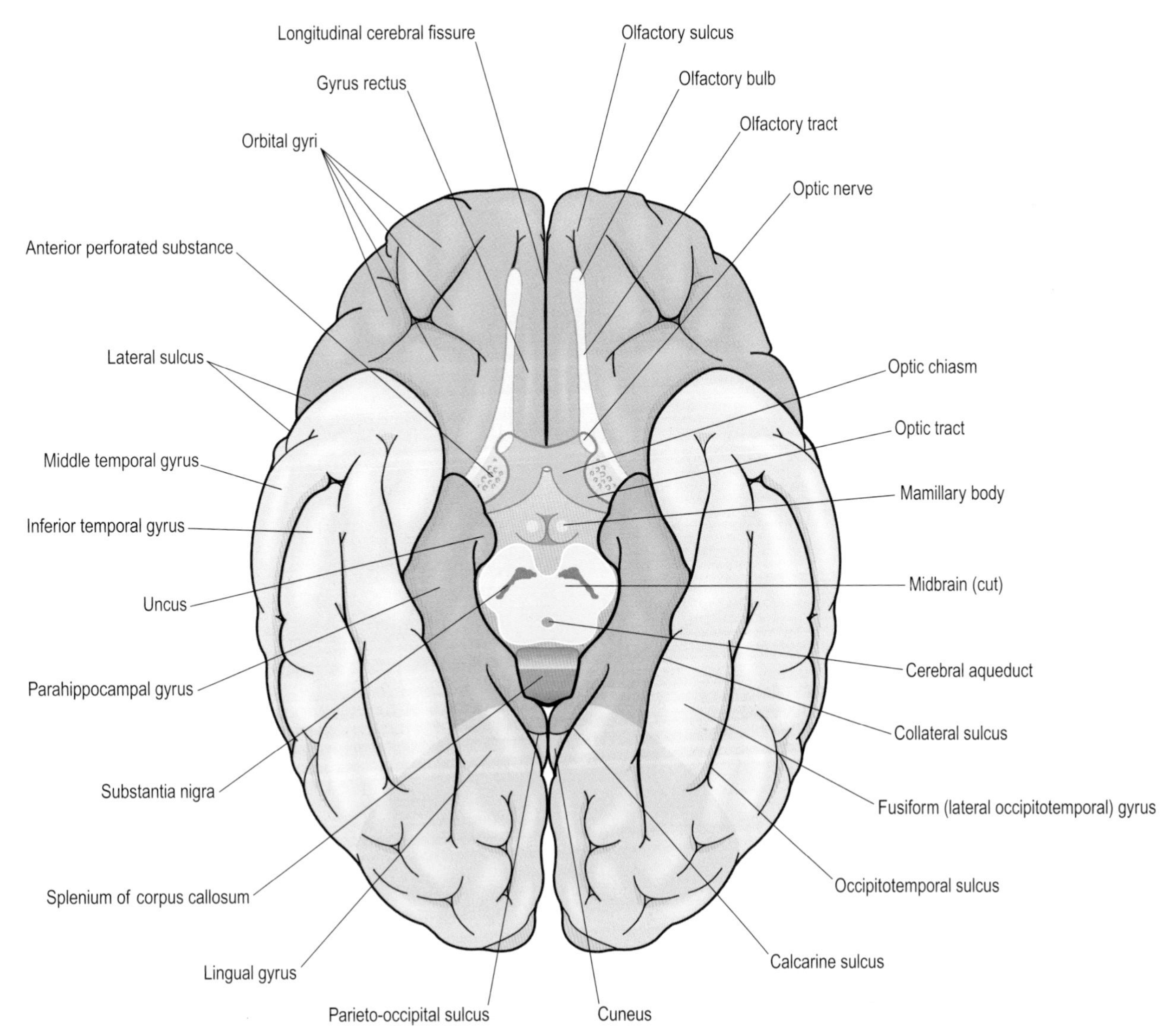

Fig. 3.3 **Inferior view of the cerebral hemispheres, showing the main named gyri and sulci.**

the orbital region into two parts. There is a small medial portion that is narrow and rectangular, called the **gyrus rectus** (Latin: rectus, straight) and a much larger lateral orbital region that contains an H-shaped sulcus. The orbital region belongs to the **prefrontal cortex**.

Prefrontal cortex (Figs 3.3 and 3.4)

The large portion of the frontal lobe anterior to the motor and premotor areas is the **prefrontal cortex** and is involved in personality, behaviour, language and intellect. It is divided into lateral, orbital and medial parts:

- The **dorsolateral prefrontal cortex** (**DLPFC**) is concerned with organizing and planning behaviour in pursuit of short-, medium- and long-term goals.
- The **orbitofrontal cortex** (**OFC**) has a predominantly inhibitory role, preventing inappropriate behaviour (e.g. during social interactions) and facilitating moderation, restraint and tact.
- The **medial prefrontal cortex** (**mPFC**) is concerned with mood, motivation and emotion. It is part of the so-called 'default network' of the brain (areas that are active during quiet contemplation).

The prefrontal cortex includes **Broca's area** (discussed below, in the context of language) and the frontal eye fields (see above). The effects of prefrontal cortex lesions are discussed in Clinical Box 3.1.

> ### *Key Points*
>
> - On the medial surface of the hemisphere the pars marginalis of the cingulate sulcus is a good landmark for finding the central sulcus, which lies immediately anterior to it.
> - The paracentral lobule is a U-shaped convolution that loops below the medial part of the central sulcus and includes the motor (anterior) and sensory (posterior) areas for the lower limbs.
> - The supplementary motor area (SMA) is just anterior to the paracentral lobule. It is involved in self-initiated (voluntary) actions and is underactive in Parkinson's disease.
> - The prefrontal cortex is the large portion of the the frontal lobe that is anterior to the motor and premotor areas. It is involved in personality, behaviour, language and intellect.

Parietal lobe

The parietal lobe is posterior to the central sulcus and above the lateral sulcus. Its posterior boundary is the **parieto-occipital sulcus**, which is only visible from the medial aspect of the cerebral hemisphere. The parietal lobe is concerned with somatosensory and visuospatial perception. It has lateral and medial surfaces.

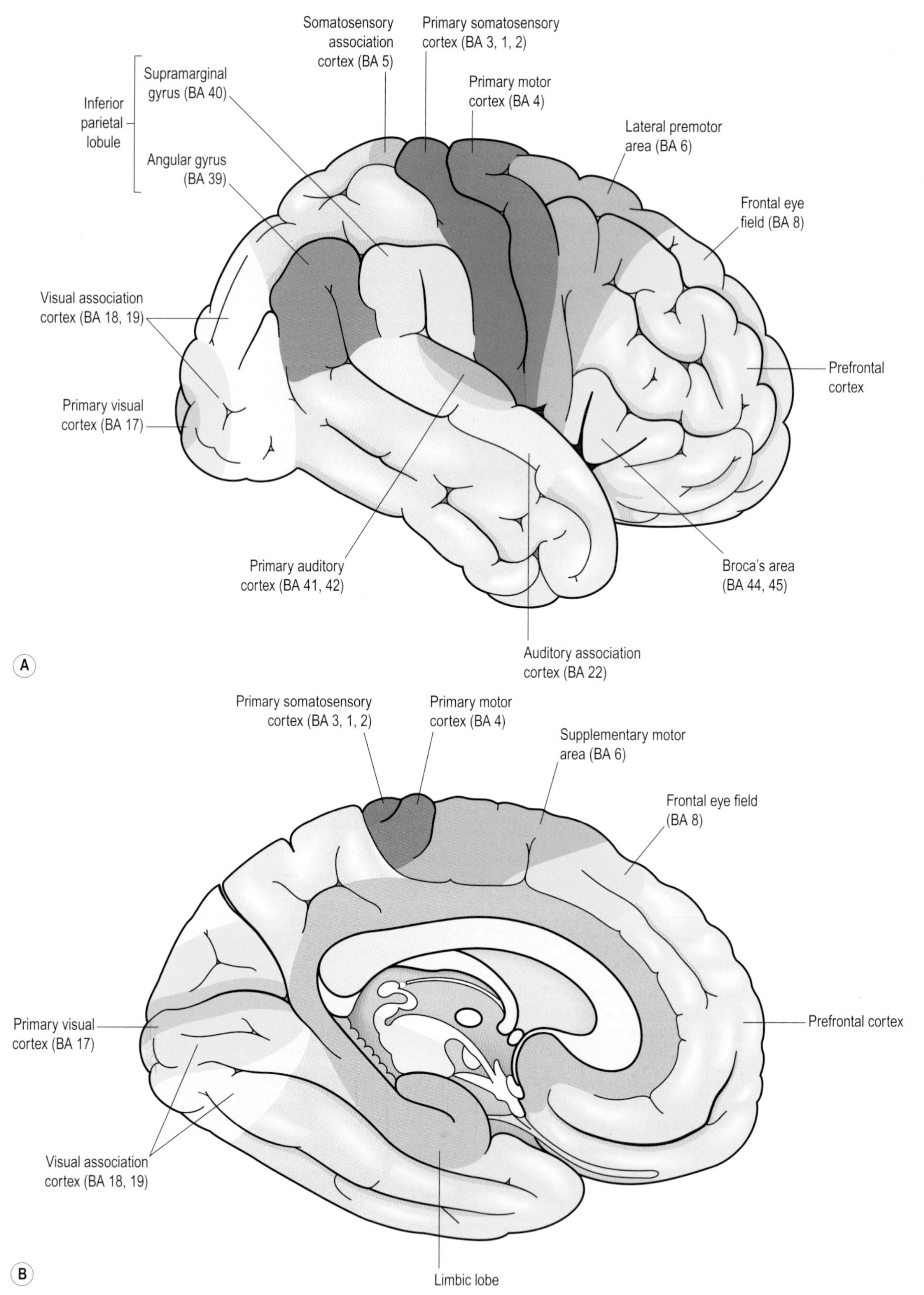

Fig. 3.4 **The main functional areas of the cerebral hemispheres shown from (A) lateral and (B) medial aspects.** Brodmann areas are indicated in brackets (apart from the prefrontal cortex and limbic lobe, which are large regions that incorporate numerous cortical functional zones).

Lateral aspect (Figs 3.1 and 3.4A)

The **postcentral gyrus** is immediately posterior to the central sulcus, behind and parallel to the motor strip. It corresponds to the **primary somatosensory cortex** (**BA 3, 1** and **2**). The **sensory strip** contains an inverted map of the opposite side of the body that mirrors that of the motor strip, but the relative proportions of the body parts reflect the degree of tactile sensitivity.

The remainder of the lateral parietal lobe is divided into **superior** and **inferior parietal lobules** by the

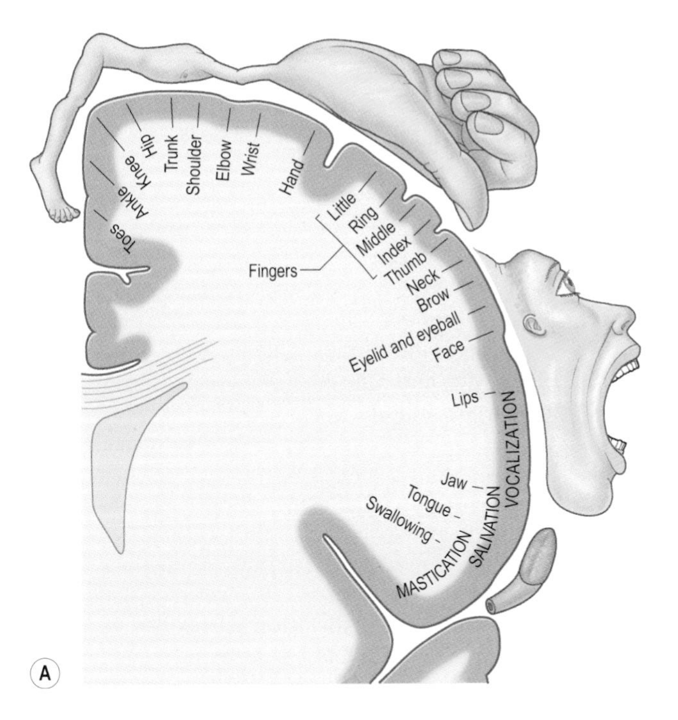

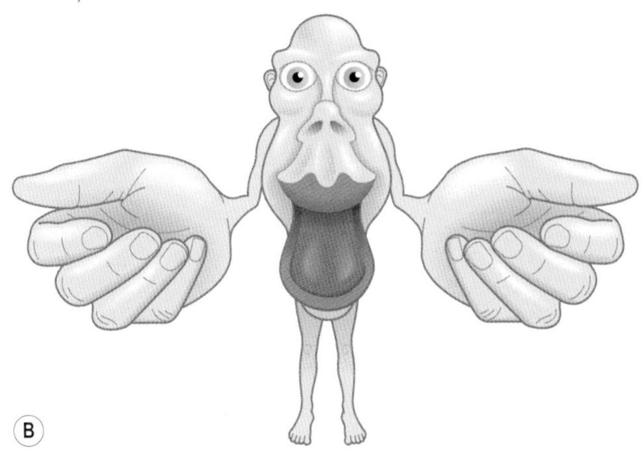

Fig. 3.5 **The primary motor cortex. (A)** The motor strip contains an orderly somatotopic (point-to-point) representation of the contralateral half of the body, from the toes (medially) to the face and tongue (laterally). The size of the cortical representation for each body part reflects the precision of motor control, so that the areas for the hands, face and tongue are disproportionately large; **(B)** This can be represented graphically as a 'homunculus'. Adapted from Matthew Levy, Bruce Koeppen, Bruce Stanton: Berne & Levy Principles of Physiology 4e (Mosby 2006) with permission.

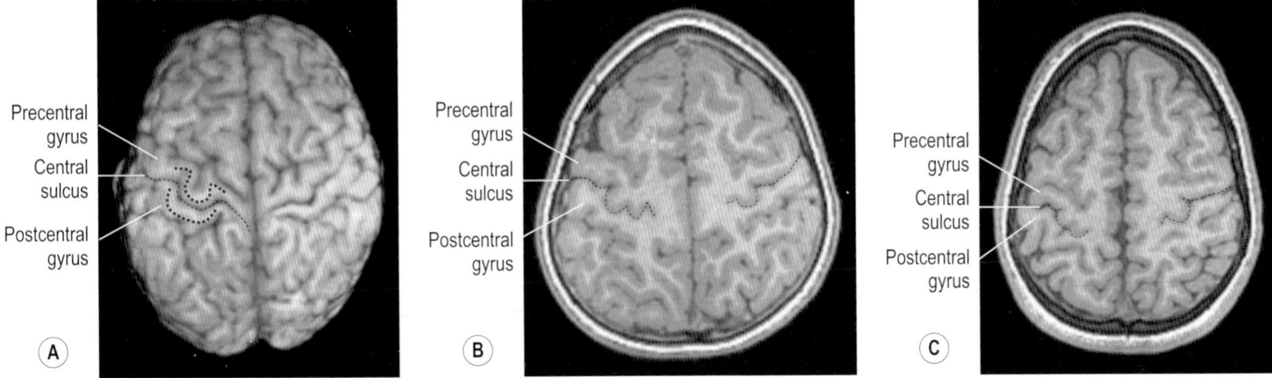

Fig. 3.6 **The motor hand area of the precentral gyrus. (A)** On the superior surface of the brain, the convolution corresponding to the 'hand area' of the primary motor cortex often resembles an inverted capital omega (Ω) as shown here in a surface rendering of the brain (obtained from a volumetric MRI scan). The motor hand area (in the precentral gyrus) is indicated by the red dashed line. The sensory hand area (of the postcentral gyrus) is shown in blue; **(B)** In axial sections (in this case, a T1-weighted MRI scan in the same individual) the 'hand area' of the primary motor cortex can be seen projecting backwards (red dashed line). Its shape often resembles a door-knob, as seen on the right-hand side in this individual; **(C)** Another example (in a different person). [Note: it is more common for the 'hand-knob' to be single (Ω-shaped) rather than double (ω-shaped).] Courtesy of Dr Gemma Northam.

Clinical Box 3.1: Prefrontal cortex lesions

Damage (or disease) affecting the prefontal region leads to changes in personality, behaviour and intellect. Orbitofrontal lesions tend to cause **disinhibited behaviour,** so that patients may become rude, inappropriate or tactless. There may be **impaired judgement** and decision-making, with **lack of restraint,** leading to rash or imprudent behaviour (accompanied by unconcern or **lack of insight**). Dorsolateral prefrontal lesions are more likely to cause impairment of **executive functions** (planning, organizing, decision-making) and there may be compulsive repetition of thoughts or actions, termed **perseveration.** Medial prefrontal lesions are associated with emotional changes such as **apathy, loss of empathy** or **abulia** (the opposite of ebullience) with reduced initiative, motivation and drive.

intraparietal sulcus. This is a deep cleft at right angles to the central sulcus. The **somatosensory association cortex** (**BA 5**) is a small area in the superior parietal lobule, just behind the sensory strip. Lesions here may lead to **astereognosia**: the inability to recognize objects by touch (Greek: a-, without; stereos, solid; gnosis, knowledge). The **posterior parietal cortex** (**BA 7**) has close links with the occipital lobe and is concerned with visuospatial perception and attention (Clinical Box 3.2). This includes the representation and manipulation of objects (e.g. using a knife and fork) and the perception of movement (e.g. judging the approach of a moving vehicle). Certain semi-automatic movements are initiated by projections from the parietal cortex to the lateral premotor area (Clinical Box 3.3).

The inferior parietal lobule is a multimodal **association area** which lies at the junction of the visual, auditory and somatosensory cortices. It consists of the **supramarginal gyrus** (**BA 40**) anteriorly and the **angular gyrus** (**BA 39**)

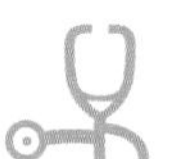

Clinical Box 3.2: Neglect syndromes

Lesions of the non-dominant (usually the right) parietal lobe may cause **hemispatial neglect,** in which the opposite (usually the left) side of the world is ignored, despite normal vision (e.g. eating food from one side of a plate, applying makeup to one half of the face). A related phenomenon is **sensory inattention,** in which a stimulus on the affected side may not be noticed if there is a competing stimulus on the other side (e.g. fingers moving in the left and right visual fields). This phenomenon is called **extinction.** Some neglect patients have associated neurological impairments such as limb paralysis but are unaware of their deficits and may deny that they exist. This is termed **anosognosia** (Greek: a-, without; nosos, disease; gnosis, knowledge).

Clinical Box 3.3: Apraxia

The word 'praxis' is used in neurology to describe certain types of effortless, **semi-automatic movement** (such as using a pair of scissors or tying shoelaces). Patients with apraxia may be able to do these things in context, but struggle when asked to mime them (Greek: a-, without; praxis, deed or action). This phenomenon is referred to as **voluntary-automatic dissociation.** In a simplistic sense, apraxia represents damage to or 'disconnection' between the **posterior parietal cortex** (which is involved in movement initiation) and the **lateral premotor area** (which has a more direct role in movement preparation/execution).

posteriorly. The inferior parietal lobule contributes to aspects of receptive **language** such as phonology, reading and spelling, particularly in the language-dominant hemisphere. It is also involved in spatial and symbolic representation of abstract concepts including quantity and number.

Medial aspect (Figs 3.2 and 3.4B)

The superior parietal lobule continues onto the medial surface of the hemisphere as the **precuneus.** This rectangular-shaped area is involved in mental imagery and recall of personal experiences. Like the medial prefrontal cortex, it is part of the 'default network' of the brain and is engaged during activities such as daydreaming and introspection. The **postcentral gyrus** ('sensory strip') also continues onto the medial surface of the hemisphere, making up the posterior part of the paracentral lobule (representing the lower half of the body).

Occipital lobe

The occipital lobe is posterior to the **preoccipital notch** and the **parieto-occipital sulcus.** It is concerned entirely with vision and has medial, lateral and inferior surfaces.

Medial aspect (Figs 3.2 and 3.4B)

The **calcarine sulcus** follows an undulating course from the parieto-occipital sulcus anteriorly to the occipital pole posteriorly. It is a deep cleft which extends to the occipital horn of the lateral ventricle. The wedge-shaped region above the calcarine sulcus is the **cuneus** (Latin: cuneus, wedge) which represents the lower quadrant of the opposite visual field. The tongue-like **lingual gyrus** is below the calcarine sulcus (Latin: lingua, tongue) and represents the upper quadrant of the opposite visual field.

Much of the **primary visual cortex** (**BA 17**) is hidden from view within the banks of the calcarine sulcus. Central vision is represented towards the occipital pole, peripheral vision more anteriorly. The primary visual cortex is flanked above and below by **visual association cortex** (**BA 18** and **19**) located within the cuneus and lingual gyrus.

Lateral and inferior aspects (Figs 3.1–3.4)

The gyral pattern is variable in the lateral occipital region but it is possible to identify **superior**, **middle** and **inferior occipital gyri** which converge on the occipital pole. These consist mainly of visual association cortex. The inferior occipital surface is described together with the inferior aspect of the temporal lobe, with which it is continuous.

Central visual pathways (Figs 3.7 and 3.8)

The retina contains a point-to-point (**retinotopic**) representation of the visual fields which is maintained throughout the central visual pathways. Its **retinal ganglion cells** give rise to over a million axons that leave the posterior pole of the eye as the **optic nerve**. The two optic nerves then unite to form the **optic chiasm**. Posterior to the chiasm, the **optic tracts** continue on each side to the **lateral geniculate nucleus** (**LGN**) of the thalamus where they synapse. Thalamocortical neurons then project to the primary visual cortex, via the **optic radiations**.

The optic chiasm (Fig. 3.7)

The central visual pathways are **crossed**. This means that the right visual field is represented in the left occipital lobe and vice versa. Since light travels in straight lines and enters the eye via the small aperture of the pupil, objects in the *right* visual field project to the *left* half of each retina (coloured red

Key Points

- The parietal lobe is posterior to the central sulcus and above the lateral sulcus. Its posterior boundary (with the occipital lobe) is the parieto-occipital sulcus.
- The postcentral gyrus corresponds to the primary somatosensory cortex and contains an inverted map of the contralateral body, mirroring that of the motor strip.
- The superior parietal lobule has close links with the occipital lobe and is involved in aspects of attention and visuospatial perception, including the representation and manipulation of objects.
- The inferior parietal lobule consists of the angular and supramarginal gyri. These contribute to reading, writing and arithmetic in the language-dominant hemisphere.
- Posterior parietal lobe lesions may cause a neglect syndrome or sensory inattention, with impaired attention to stimuli in the contralateral half of the visual field.
- Apraxia may be caused by lesions in the (i) dominant posterior parietal cortex, (ii) lateral premotor area or (iii) in white matter pathways connecting the two regions.

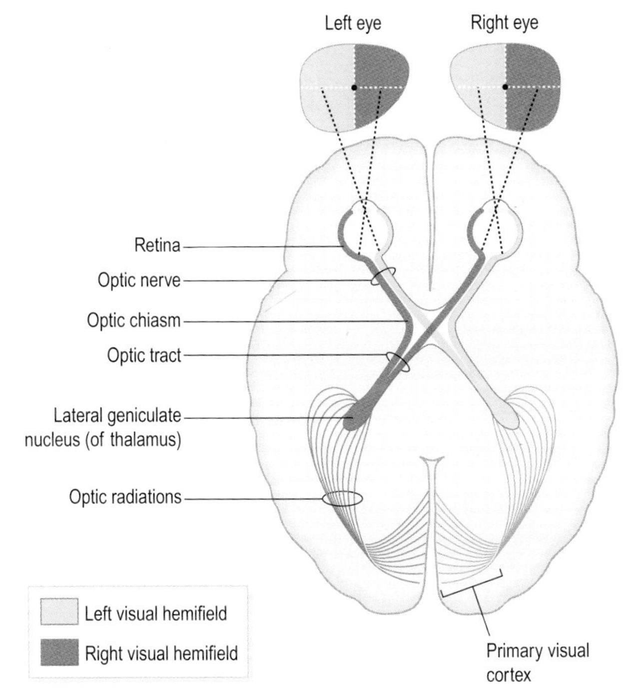

Fig. 3.7 **The central visual pathways.** The visual fields of each eye are illustrated separately in this figure, but in reality they overlap extensively to allow for binocular vision (and contributing to depth perception).

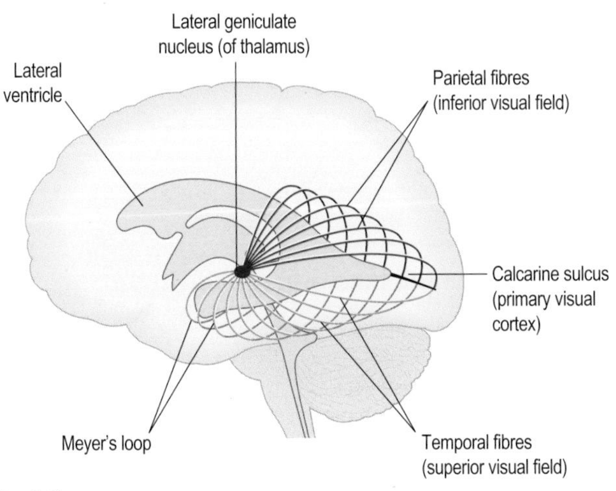

Fig. 3.8 **The optic radiations.**

in Fig. 3.7). Axons originating from the left half of each retina must therefore project to the left cerebral hemisphere. For this to happen, nerve fibres from the inner half of the retina must cross the midline to enter the opposite optic tract. This takes place at the **optic chiasm**, named for its resemblance to the Greek letter chi.

The primary visual cortex

Visual information is segregated into three separate 'channels' (concerned with form, motion and colour) by the **primary visual cortex (V1)** and **visual association cortices (V2, V3… and higher)**. Two parallel visual 'streams' dealing with different aspects of visual perception arise from the occipital lobe. The dorsal or **parietal lobe stream** is concerned with the location and movement of objects and their positions relative to the body (the 'where' pathway). The ventral or **temporal lobe stream** synthesizes information about form and colour, allowing objects to be recognized (the 'what' pathway). Central visual pathway lesions are discussed in Clinical Box 3.4.

Clinical Box 3.4: Visual pathway lesions

A discrete lesion in the central visual pathway may cause a small blind spot or **scotoma** (Greek: scotos, darkness) or a larger **visual field defect.** The effects of lesions at different locations in the central visual pathway are illustrated in Fig. 3.9:

- **Monocular blindness** or unilateral visual loss is caused by disease of the eye or optic nerve on one side, anterior to the optic chiasm.
- **Bitemporal hemianopia** means loss of the outer (temporal) half of the visual field in *both* eyes. It is usually due to a lesion of the optic chiasm (e.g. compression due to a pituitary gland tumour).
- **Hemianopia** is loss of vision in a hemifield (the left or right half of the visual field in *both* eyes), due to a lesion posterior to the optic chiasm.
- **Quadrantanopia** is blindness in the superior or inferior quadrant of one hemifield. The lesion may be in the optic radiations or visual cortex.

Field defects that are the same in both eyes are referred to as **homonymous**, those that are not identical in each eye are described as **heteronymous**. There is often **sparing of central (macular) vision**, since the macula (i) is represented in both hemispheres and (ii) this part of the cortex is supplied by two cerebral arteries (see Ch. 10).

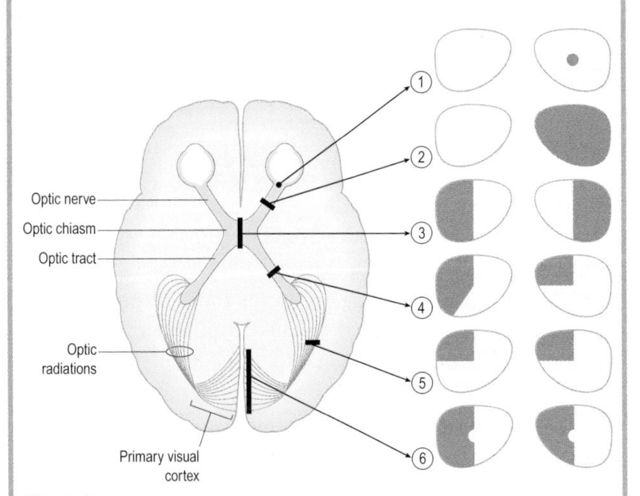

Fig. 3.9 **Visual pathway lesions.** The effects of lesions in various parts of the central visual pathway are illustrated. The visual fields of the left and right eyes are shown in pale yellow and the areas of reduced or absent vision are shown as purple shading. [The defects depicted are as follows: (1) = small scotoma (blind spot) in the right eye; (2) = monocular blindness, right eye; (3) = bitemporal hemianopia or 'tunnel vision'; (4) = heteronymous left-sided field defect; (5) = left superior quadrantanopia, homonymous field defect; (6) = left hemianopia with macular (central) sparing.]

Temporal lobe

The temporal lobe lies below the lateral sulcus and is angled downwards and forwards to resemble the thumb of a boxing glove. Its posterior boundary (with the occipital lobe) is the **pre-occipital notch**. The temporal lobe is involved in hearing, speech comprehension and visual recognition. It has superior, lateral and inferior surfaces.

Key Points

- The occipital lobe lies posterior to the preoccipital notch and the parieto-occipital sulcus. It is concerned entirely with vision and contains the primary visual cortex within the calcarine sulcus.
- The upper and lower halves of the contralateral visual field are represented in the lingual gyrus and cuneus, respectively.
- The first part of the central visual pathway consists of the optic nerve, chiasm and tract. It originates in the retina and terminates in the lateral geniculate nucleus (LGN) of the thalamus.
- At the optic chiasm, fibres originating from the inner (nasal) half of each retina cross the midline to ensure that information from each visual hemifield reaches the contralateral hemisphere.
- The LGN projects to the primary visual cortex (V1) via the optic radiations. Higher-order visual association areas (V2, V3, etc.) are progressively further away from the primary visual cortex.
- The dorsal visual stream ('where' pathway) projects to the parietal lobe. The ventral visual stream ('what' pathway) projects to the temporal lobe.

Superior aspect (Fig 3.10)

The superior surface of the temporal lobe is hidden within the lateral sulcus and includes the **transverse temporal gyri**. These finger-like convolutions run obliquely (posteriorly and medially) and include the **primary auditory cortex** (**BA 41** and **42**). The auditory cortex contains a **tonotopic** map that represents the audible frequency spectrum (low frequencies laterally, high frequencies medially).

Projections reach the auditory cortex from the **medial geniculate nucleus** (**MGN**) of the thalamus via the **auditory radiations**. The primary auditory cortex receives projections from both ears. This means that a temporal lobe lesion would not be expected to cause contralateral deafness in the same way that an occipital lobe lesion might cause contralateral loss of sight.

The surrounding cortex, which continues onto the lateral surface of the temporal lobe is the **auditory association area** (**BA 22**). In the language-dominant hemisphere this is specialized for the comprehension of speech sounds.

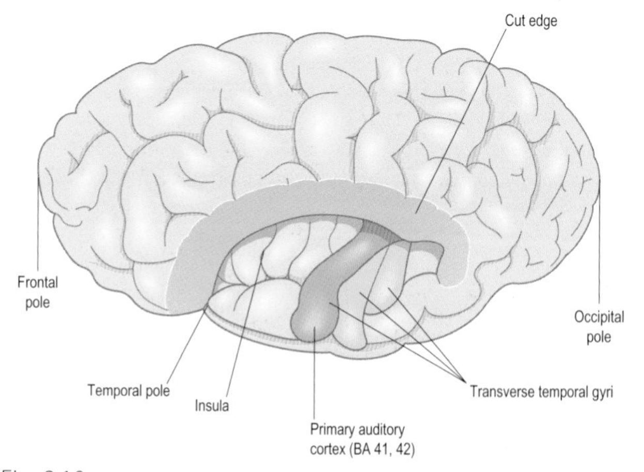

Fig. 3.10 **A dissection showing the superior surface of the temporal lobe and primary auditory cortex.** This view shows the superolateral aspect of the left cerebral hemisphere with the frontal and parietal opercula dissected away to reveal the superior surface of the temporal lobe (including the transverse temporal gyri and primary auditory cortex). Part of the insula can also be seen.

Lateral aspect (Figs 3.1 and 3.4A)

The lateral temporal lobe has **superior**, **middle** and **inferior temporal gyri**, separated by the superior and inferior temporal sulci. The superior temporal sulcus is parallel to the lateral sulcus and is generally uninterrupted, whilst the inferior temporal sulcus is usually broken up into segments. The lateral temporal lobe consists of visual and auditory association cortex.

Inferior aspect (Fig. 3.3)

On the inferior aspect of the hemisphere, the occipital and temporal lobes form a continuous, uninterrupted surface that is composed of the medial and lateral occipitotemporal gyri. The **medial occipitotemporal gyrus** is medial to the collateral sulcus. The portion lying within the occipital lobe is also known as the lingual gyrus, whereas the part contained in the temporal lobe is the parahippocampal gyrus. The **lateral occipitotemporal gyrus** runs alongside, between the collateral sulcus medially and occipitotemporal sulcus laterally. The anterior and posterior ends of the lateral occipitotemporal gyrus are usually tapered to give it a 'spindle' shape. It is therefore also known as the **fusiform gyrus** (Latin: fusiform, shaped like a spindle). It receives projections from the occipital lobe (part of the 'what pathway') and appears to be involved in the recognition of complex visual patterns. It contributes to **reading** (in the language-dominant hemisphere) and **face recognition** (in the non-dominant hemisphere) (Clinical Box 3.5).

Clinical Box 3.5: Visual agnosia

Lateral and inferior temporal lobe lesions may interfere with object recognition, despite otherwise normal vision, which is called **visual agnosia** (Greek: a-, without; gnosis, knowledge). The two main types are illustrated in Fig. 3.11. **Apperceptive agnosia** is a problem with the early stages of recognition, interfering with the ability to perceive objects. **Associative agnosia** involves the later stages of recognition. Objects are seen normally and can be described in detail, but do not look familiar and can only be recognized and named using other senses (e.g. touch, smell). Sometimes agnosia affects specific categories of object (e.g. foodstuffs, living things, tools). Damage to the non-dominant fusiform gyrus, in the inferior temporal region, may cause selective visual agnosia for faces, termed **prosopagnosia** (Greek: prosop, face; a-, without; gnosis, knowledge).

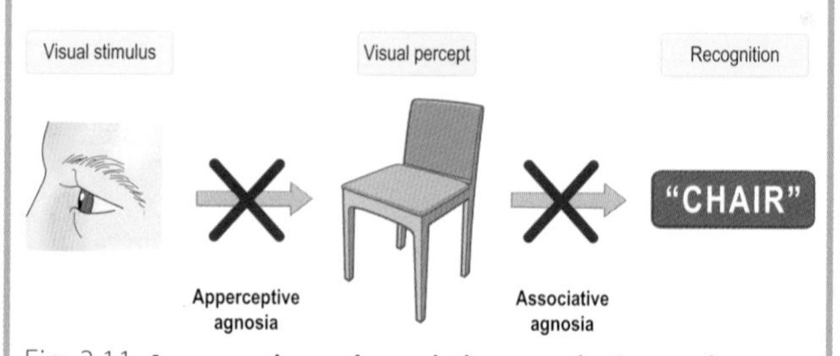

Fig. 3.11 **Apperceptive and associative agnosia.** See text for explanation.

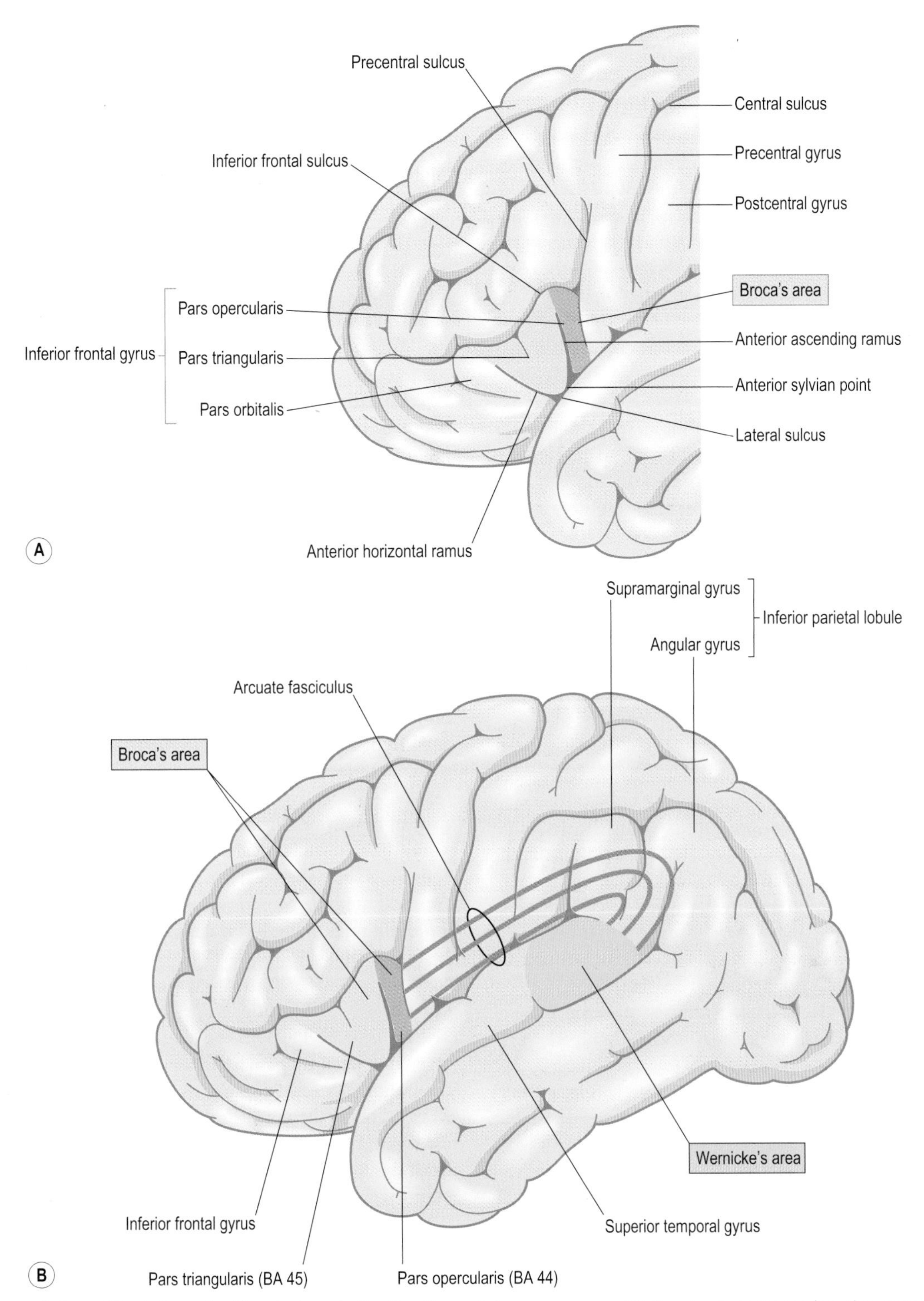

Fig. 3.12 **Lateral view of the left cerebral hemisphere indicating the main language areas. (A)** Broca's area corresponds to the opercular and triangular parts of the inferior frontal gyrus (i.e. the pars opercularis and pars triangularis, coloured orange and yellow in the figure). These are defined by the ascending and horizontal branches (rami) of the lateral sulcus, which arise from an enlargement of the lateral sulcus called the anterior sylvian point; **(B)** The anterior and posterior language areas are linked by the arcuate fasciculus, which is the main language-associated white matter bundle.

Key Points

- The temporal lobe lies below the lateral sulcus and its posterior border (with the occipital lobe) is the preoccipital notch.
- The superior surface of the temporal lobe (normally hidden within the lateral sulcus) includes the transverse temporal gyri, which contain the primary auditory cortex.
- The lateral temporal region includes the auditory association cortex. It also has close links with the occipital lobe and contributes to visual recognition.

Language areas (Fig. 3.12)

Language is represented in the left cerebral hemisphere in 95% of right-handed people and in 70% of those who are left-handed. Pure right-hemisphere language is uncommon, probably occurring in less than 2% of the population. This means that most people who are not strongly left-lateralized for language tend to have a bilateral cortical representation.

Broca's area

Broca's area is involved in the expressive aspects of spoken and written language (production of sentences constrained by the rules of grammar and syntax). It corresponds to the opercular and triangular parts of the **inferior frontal gyrus** (**BA 44** and **45**) (Fig. 3.12A). As illustrated in the figure, these are defined by two rami (branches) of the lateral sulcus (one ascending, one horizontal) which 'slice into' the inferior frontal gyrus. In keeping with its role in speech and language, Broca's area is immediately anterior to the motor and premotor representations of the face, tongue and larynx. A homologous area in the opposite hemisphere is involved in **non-verbal communication** such as facial expression, gesticulation and modulation of the rate, rhythm and intonation of speech.

Wernicke's area

Wernicke's area (pronounced: VER-nikker) corresponds to the posterior third of the superior temporal gyrus and is part of the auditory association cortex (Fig. 3.12B). It lies at the junction of the visual and auditory cortices and is involved in transforming the visual impression of letters (**graphemes**) into mental representations of speech sounds (**phonemes**). It is therefore important for speech comprehension and reading. The non-dominant homologue of Wernicke's area is involved in understanding intonation and emphasis (the 'music' of speech) which can alter the meaning of words considerably. Some patients with non-dominant temporal lobe lesions may therefore have monotone, 'robotic' speech or fail to grasp nuances of intonation (termed **aprosodia**).

Language pathways

The two main language areas are connected by the **arcuate fasciculus**, a large white matter bundle that arches around the lateral sulcus (Latin: arcus, bow) (Fig. 3.12B).

One component, the long segment, passes directly between Broca's and Wernicke's areas. There is also an indirect pathway (composed of two short segments) which connects the anterior and posterior language areas via the inferior parietal lobule. Collectively, these pathways make up the **dorsal language stream** which is concerned with the **phonological** aspects of language.

A second language-associated pathway interconnects the anterior and lateral temporal lobe with the inferior frontal lobe via the hook-shaped **uncinate fasciculus** (Latin: uncus, hook) (see Ch. 1, Fig. 1.18). This has been referred to as the **ventral language stream** and is more concerned with **semantic** aspects of language (the meaning of words and concepts). Language disorders are discussed in Clinical Box 3.6.

Key Points

- Wernicke's area lies at the temporoparietal junction and is involved in language comprehension. Lesions cause a fluent aphasia with impaired understanding of spoken and written language.
- Broca's area includes the opercular and triangular parts of the inferior frontal gyrus and is involved in the expressive aspects of language. Lesions cause a non-fluent (motor) aphasia.
- The dorsal language stream connects Broca's and Wernicke's areas (via the direct and indirect components of the arcuate fasciculus) and is concerned with phonology.
- The ventral language stream connects the anterior and lateral temporal lobe with the inferior frontal lobe (via the uncinate fasciculus) and is concerned with semantics.

Clinical Box 3.6: Dysphasia

Dysphasia is an acquired disorder of spoken and written language (Greek: dys-, disordered; phasis, utterance). Lesions involving Broca's area cause **expressive dysphasia**, which is non-fluent. Speech is hesitant, fragmented and 'telegraphic', with word-finding difficulty and a paucity of grammatical elements such as verbs and prepositions. Since comprehension is relatively spared, patients tend to become frustrated as they struggle to express themselves. **Receptive dysphasia** results from lesions in Wernicke's area. Speech is fluent but makes little sense, consisting of word fragments, substitutions and **neologisms** (nonsense words). Since comprehension is affected, patients may be unaware of their own errors. A combination of receptive and expressive features is called **global dysphasia** (or **aphasia**). Specific problems repeating sentences (e.g. 'no ifs, ands or buts') despite normal fluency and comprehension is termed **conduction aphasia**. It is usually attributed to a lesion in the arcuate fasciculus which is said to 'disconnect' the two primary language areas.

Limbic lobe and insula

The limbic lobe is a ring-shaped convolution surrounding the medial border of the cerebral hemisphere (Latin: limbus, border) (Fig. 3.13). It is primarily concerned with **emotion** and **memory**. The anterior insula, posterior orbitofrontal cortex and temporal pole have similar functional roles and are referred to as **paralimbic areas**. The **hippocampus** (a cortical region that belongs to the limbic lobe) and the **amygdala** (a subcortical structure involved in emotional responses) are discussed separately below. The outdated term 'limbic system' is sometimes used as vague shorthand for 'emotional brain' but it has no proper definition and is best avoided.

Parts of the limbic lobe

The limbic lobe includes the cingulate and parahippocampal gyri, connected by an underlying core of white matter called the **cingulum** (or cingulum bundle). The **cingulate gyrus** wraps around the corpus callosum on the medial surface of the cerebral hemisphere (Latin: cingulum, belt). It is separated from the overlying frontal lobe by the cingulate sulcus. The boundary with the parietal lobe is the **subparietal sulcus**. Posteriorly, the cingulate gyrus tapers to a narrow **isthmus** (pronounced: IZ-muss) behind the splenium of the corpus callosum. The limbic lobe continues into the medial temporal region as the **parahippocampal gyrus** (medial to the collateral sulcus). This ends in a hook-shaped fold of cortex called the **uncus** (Latin: hook).

The insula

The **insula** is an 'island' of cortex hidden in the depths of the lateral sulcus (Latin: insula, island) which can be exposed by retracting the overhanging **opercula** of the frontal, parietal and temporal lobes (Latin: operculum, lid) (Fig. 3.14; see also Ch. 2, Fig. 2.10). It is divided into anterior (visceral) and posterior (somatic) parts by the **central sulcus** of the insula. The anterior insula receives projections from the olfactory bulb and is part of the **primary olfactory cortex**. It is also involved in nausea, vomiting, disgust and pain perception, including the accompanying visceral and autonomic phenomena. Studies using **functional magnetic resonance**

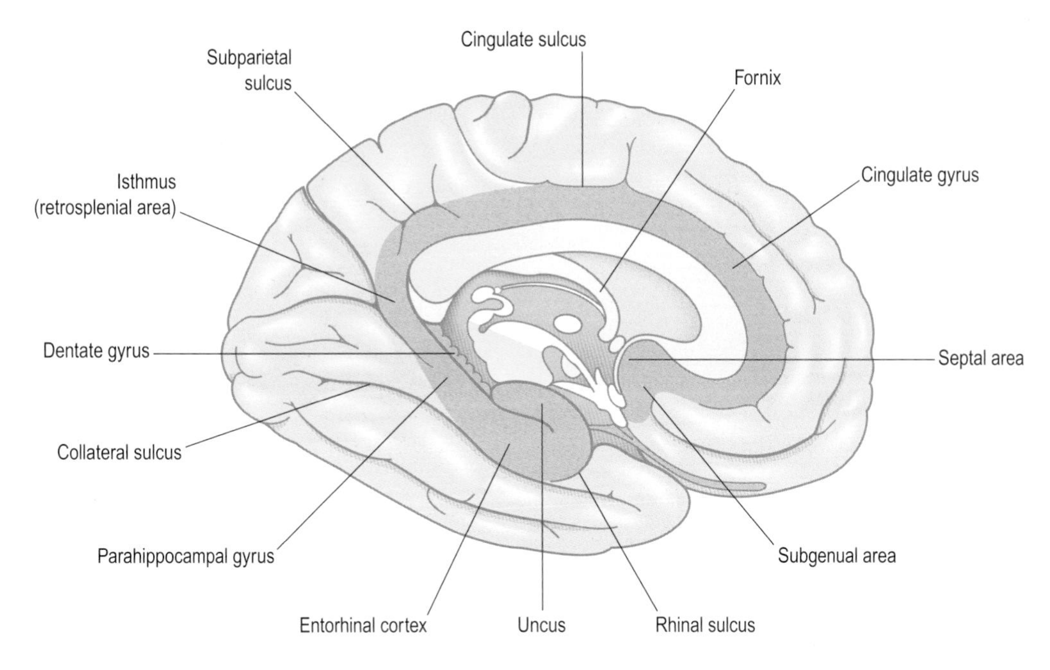

Fig. 3.13 **Medial aspect of the cerebral hemisphere, illustrating the limbic lobe.**. The brain stem has been removed and the 'teeth' of the dentate gyrus can be seen (Latin: dentālis, bearing teeth). The septal area is also indicated. This is connected to numerous brain regions that are involved in mood, emotion and reward-based learning.

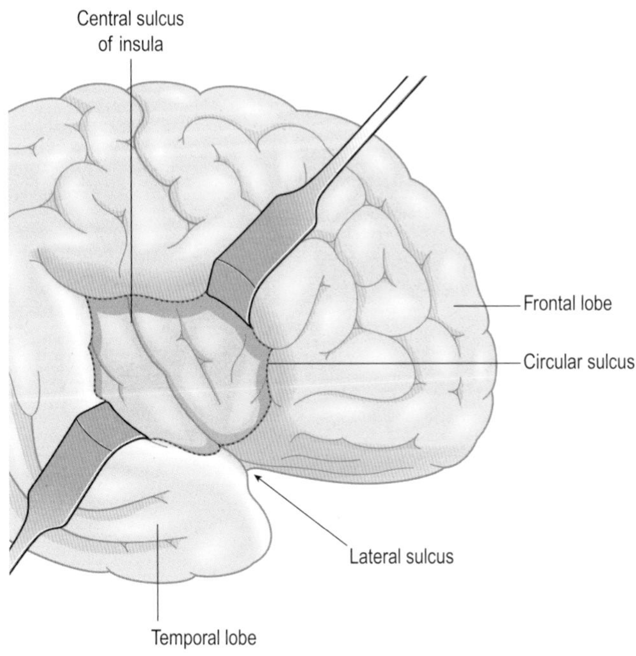

Fig. 3.14 **The insula.** The frontal, parietal and temporal opercula have been retracted to reveal the insula, which is normally hidden within the depths of the lateral sulcus, overlying the basal ganglia.

imaging (fMRI) suggest that the anterior insula, which is immediately adjacent to Broca's area, may also be involved in language. The posterior insula integrates non-visceral (somatic) information related to touch, vision and hearing.

Key Points

- The limbic lobe is a ring-shaped convolution at the medial border (limbus) of the cerebral hemisphere. It includes the cingulate gyrus, parahippocampal gyrus and hippocampus.
- The insula is an 'island' of cortex buried within the lateral sulcus, divided into anterior (visceral) and posterior (somatic) parts by the central sulcus of the insula.
- The limbic lobe and anterior insula are involved in mood, memory and olfaction.

Hippocampus and amygdala

The hippocampus is a cortical region (belonging to the limbic lobe) that is involved in memory formation and spatial navigation. The amygdala is a subcortical structure (a group of nuclei) that is concerned with emotional responses and learning.

Hippocampus

The hippocampus occupies the temporal horn of the lateral ventricle. It is therefore 'submerged' in cerebrospinal fluid and forms a longitudinal bulge in the ventricular floor (Fig. 3.15A). The hippocampus is covered by a thin sheet of white matter called the **alveus**, which derives from the Latin for 'river bed'. The name hippocampus continues the aquatic theme, reflecting its resemblance to a sea horse (Fig. 3.15B). The term derives ultimately from a creature in Greek mythology that is part horse, part fish (Greek: hippos, horse; kampos, sea monster).

Parts of the hippocampus

The hippocampus is formed by an S-shaped fold of relatively simple three-layered cortex that is continuous with the neighbouring **parahippocampal gyrus** (Greek: para-, beside). It is composed of **allocortex** (see Ch. 5) which is thinner and less complex than the six-layered neocortex that is found in 90% of the cerebral hemisphere. Its relationship to the lateral ventricle and parahippocampal gyrus are illustrated in Figure 3.16A. The hippocampus consists of the **dentate gyrus** and **Ammon's horn** (within the ventricle) together with the **subiculum** below (Latin: subicere, to support) (Fig. 3.16B). Ammon's horn (also referred to as the **hippocampus proper**) contains large pyramidal neurons arranged in three zones called CA1, CA2 and CA3. The terminology derives from the Latin form of Ammon's horn, **cornu ammonis (CA)** and refers to an Egyptian deity with ram's horns.

Afferent and efferent connections

The major afferent projection into the hippocampus is the **perforant path**. This originates in the **entorhinal cortex (BA 28)** in the anterior part of the parahippocampal gyrus. It terminates on granule cells in the dentate gyrus of the hippocampus. The axons of dentate granule cells (called

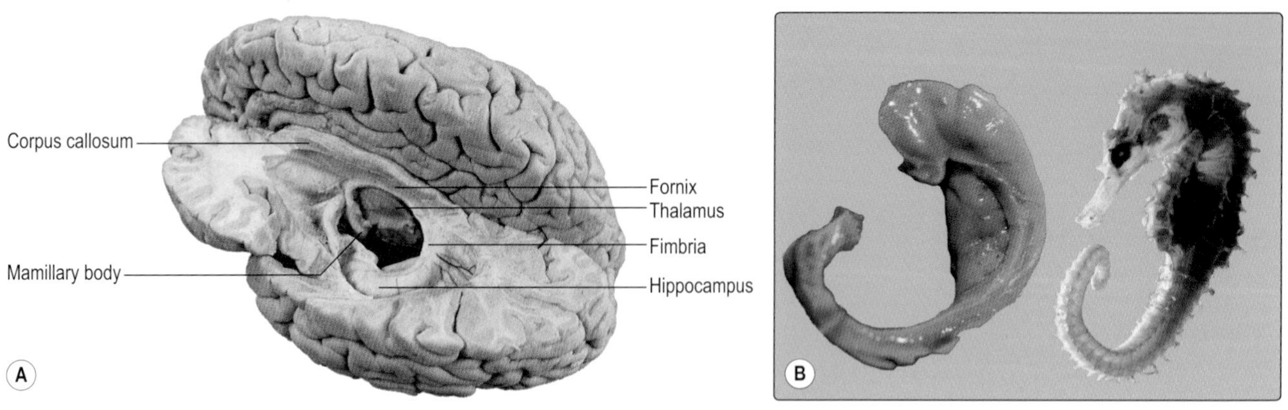

Fig. 3.15 **Gross anatomy of the hippocampus. (A)** Dissection of the left cerebral hemisphere showing the hippocampus in the floor of the temporal horn of the lateral ventricle. The fornix, a major outflow pathway of the hippocampus, can be seen arching up towards the midline (below the corpus callosum) before terminating in the mamillary body in the floor of the third ventricle. From Standring: Gray's Anatomy 40e (2008: Churchill Livingstone) with permission; **(B)** When the hippocampus and fornix are dissected free from the brain they resemble a seahorse (*Hippocampus* spp). Courtesy of Professor László Seress.

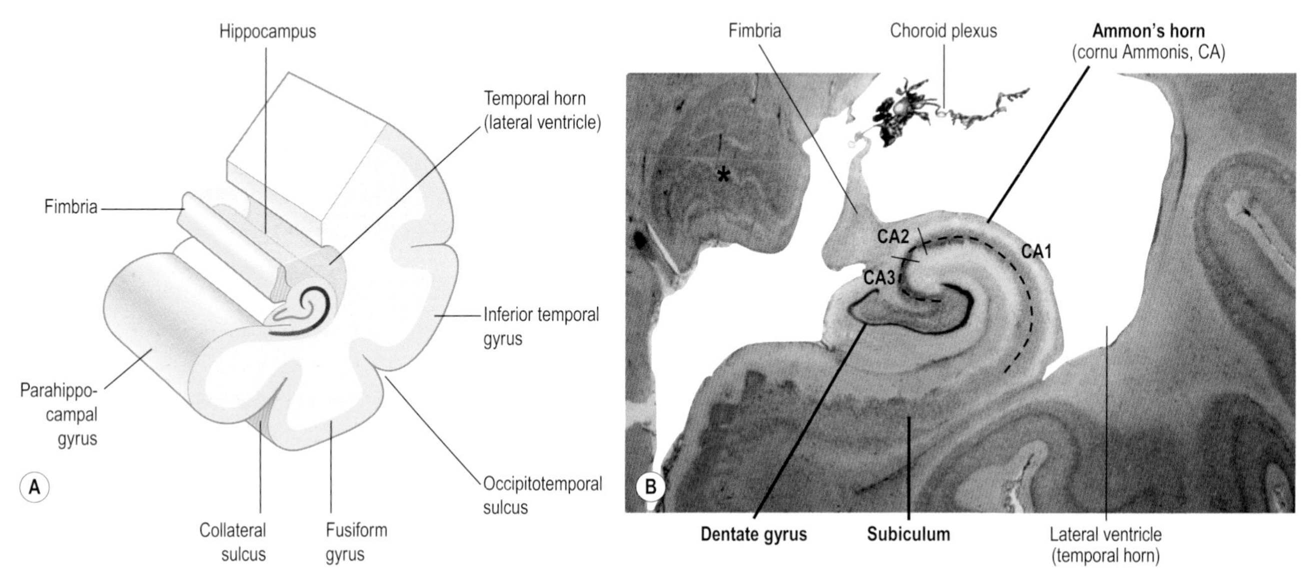

Fig. 3.16 **Parts of the hippocampus. (A)** Illustration of the hippocampus (viewed from the medial aspect) and its relationship to the parahippocampal gyrus and temporal horn of the lateral ventricle [blue = dentate gyrus, red = Ammon's horn, purple = subiculum]; **(B)** Microscopic structure of the hippocampus showing the main parts, including the subsectors of Ammon's horn, CA1-CA3 [Nissl stain]. From Weller, R: Advances in Clinical Neuroscience and Rehabilitation, Vol 7 (Whitehouse Publishing 2008) with permission. *Indicates the lateral geniculate nucleus (LGN) of the thalamus.

mossy fibres) project in turn to CA3 pyramidal cells. These give rise to long axons that project out of the hippocampus (to the hypothalamus and brain stem). The intrinsic connections of the hippocampus also project back to the entorhinal cortex to form a closed loop that is important in memory formation. The term **hippocampal formation** is used to describe the entorhinal cortex together with the hippocampus.

Fimbria and fornix

Hippocampal efferent fibres gather in the **fimbria**, which runs along the medial border of the hippocampus (Latin: fimbria, fringe) (see Fig. 3.16). The fimbria emerges from the posterior aspect of the hippocampus to be renamed the **fornix**. This is a white, cord-like structure that sweeps up to the midline and forms an arch below the corpus callosum (Latin: fornix, arch) (see Fig. 3.15A). The fornix terminates in the **mamillary bodies** (of the hypothalamus) in the floor of the third ventricle (Latin: mamilla, nipple). The mamillary bodies project in turn to the cingulate gyrus (via a 'relay station' in the **anterior thalamus**) and a complete loop can be traced back to the entorhinal cortex via the cingulum bundle (Fig. 3.17).

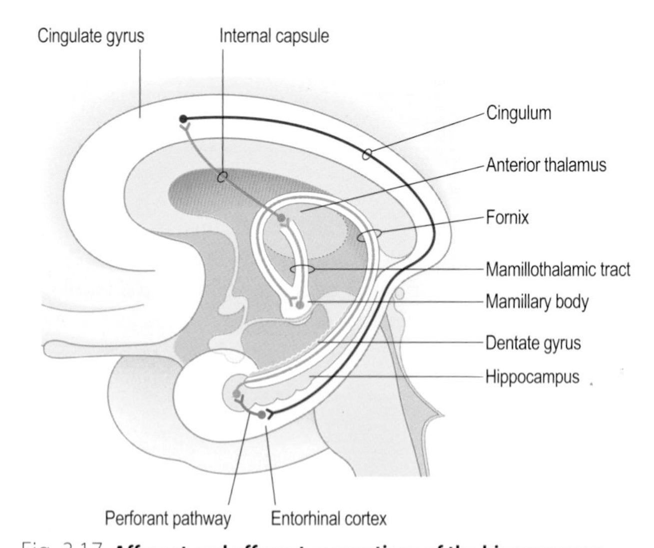

Fig. 3.17 **Afferent and efferent connections of the hippocampus.** The main afferent projection into the hippocampus is the perforant path (blue) which arises from the entorhinal cortex in the anterior part of the parahippocampal gyrus; the main outflow projection is the fornix (pink) which arches up towards the midline before terminating in the mamillary body of the hypothalamus.

Functions of the hippocampus

The hippocampus is involved in the formation of new memories and is particularly important for the recollection of personal experiences, termed **episodic memory**; this is in contrast to **semantic memory** which has to do with abstract knowledge and facts (Clinical Box 3.7). The hippocampus also stores **spatial maps** of the environment (e.g. familiar towns, streets and buildings) that we use to navigate. In keeping with this role, it has been found to be significantly larger in licensed **London taxi drivers**. The effects of hippocampal lesions are discussed in Clinical Boxes 3.8 and 3.9.

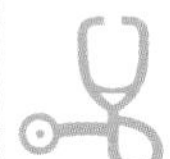

Clinical Box 3.7: Classification of memory

Memory can be categorized as **short-term** (minutes, hours) or **long-term** (weeks, months, years). Long-term memories are further classified as **declarative** and **non-declarative**. Declarative (or **explicit**) memories are those which can be put into words. They are further sub-divided into semantic and episodic types. **Semantic memory** includes abstract facts and information, whereas **episodic memory** is a personal record of day-to-day experiences. Non-declarative (**implicit**) memory includes various forms of semi-automatic learning that are only partially accessible to consciousness. An example is **procedural memory** which is important for learning motor skills. The term **working memory** refers to the ability to 'hold in mind', pay attention to and manipulate several pieces of information at once.

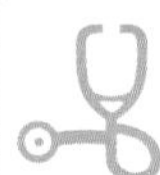

Clinical Box 3.8: Hippocampal lesions and memory

Patients with extensive bilateral hippocampal lesions lose the ability to form new memories (**anterograde amnesia**), with a particularly marked deficit in **episodic memory**. In contrast, their **procedural memory** is usually normal, which means that it is still possible to learn new skills. For instance, it would be possible to train a person with medial temporal lobe amnesia to play the piano, but they would not be aware that they had received any lessons. Some pre-existing memories may also be lost following hippocampal damage (**retrograde amnesia**), occasionally extending over several years. The hippocampus may therefore store memories temporarily prior to **consolidation** in the neocortex. In Alzheimer's disease (the most common form of dementia; see Ch. 12) there is severe degeneration of the hippocampus and entorhinal cortex, which is associated with profound disturbance of episodic memory and spatial navigation (e.g. forgetting recent conversations or getting lost in familiar places).

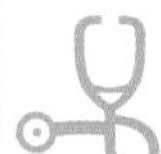

Clinical Box 3.9: The Wernicke–Korsakoff syndrome

Wernicke's encephalopathy is an acute neurological syndrome characterized by confusion, incoordination and gaze paralysis (ophthalmoplegia). It is usually seen in alcoholics in association with **vitamin B1** (**thiamine**) deficiency. Pathological changes include small haemorrhages in the mamillary bodies, interrupting connections with both hippocampi. Repeated episodes may cause **Korsakoff's psychosis**, a syndrome of profound **anterograde amnesia** with **confabulation** (creation of fictitious memories which the patient thinks are real).

Amygdala

The amygdala is an almond-shaped mass of grey matter in the anterior part of the medial temporal region that is concerned with **emotional responses** (Greek: amygdalum, almond). It lies just in front of the hippocampus, close to the temporal pole, and blends with the medial temporal cortex (see Fig. 3.21). Although the amygdala is involved in all types of emotional response (both 'positive' and 'negative'), it is particularly important in situations that elicit anxiety, fear or rage. The amygdala has three main nuclear groups (Fig. 3.18):

- The **basolateral group** is the largest division in the human brain. It receives particularly strong projections from the visual and auditory association areas of the temporal lobe.
- The **corticomedial group** mainly receives sensory afferents from the olfactory bulb. It is therefore more important in macrosmatic animals (those with a keen sense of smell).
- The **central nucleus** elicits emotional responses by projecting to the hypothalamus and autonomic nuclei of the brain stem via the **stria terminalis** (Fig. 3.19).

The amygdala integrates diverse sensory, cognitive and other information to help determine the **emotional significance** of a particular situation. An important role is the identification of potentially harmful circumstances and triggering appropriate autonomic responses (e.g. a 'fight or flight' reaction) via projections to the hypothalamus and brain stem. It has therefore been described as a **danger detector**. The orbital region of the **prefrontal cortex** exerts a moderating influence on the amygdala which can alter or inhibit emotional responses based on context or previous experience (e.g. fleeing from a snake encountered on a forest floor, but not in a zoo or pet shop).

The amygdala is also involved in **implicit learning**, particularly during emotionally charged situations (**fear conditioning**). This may be of relevance in **anxiety**

Key Points

- The hippocampus (dentate gyrus, Ammon's horn and subiculum) is part of the cerebral cortex and belongs to the limbic lobe. It is composed of an S-shaped fold of three-layered allocortex in the temporal horn of the lateral ventricle.
- The dentate gyrus is the afferent (or 'input') portion of the hippocampus and receives a major projection from the entorhinal cortex, called the perforant path.
- The term 'hippocampal formation' is used to refer to the hippocampus together with the entorhinal cortex. These structures are involved in episodic memory formation and spatial navigation.
- The fornix is a major outflow pathway of the hippocampus, which arches under the corpus callosum and terminates (on each side) in the mamillary body of the hypothalamus.
- Lesions of the hippocampus, fornix or mamillary bodies may be associated with anterograde amnesia, sometimes with confabulation (creation of fictitious memories).

disorders including **phobias** and **post-traumatic stress disorder** (**PTSD**). Other roles include the recognition of emotional facial expressions which help us to understand what other people are thinking and feeling (referred to as **theory of mind** or **ToM**). This is vital for normal social interactions and is disturbed in **autism**.

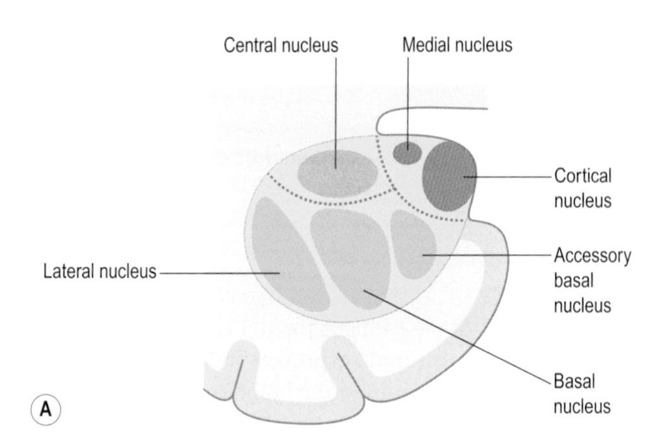

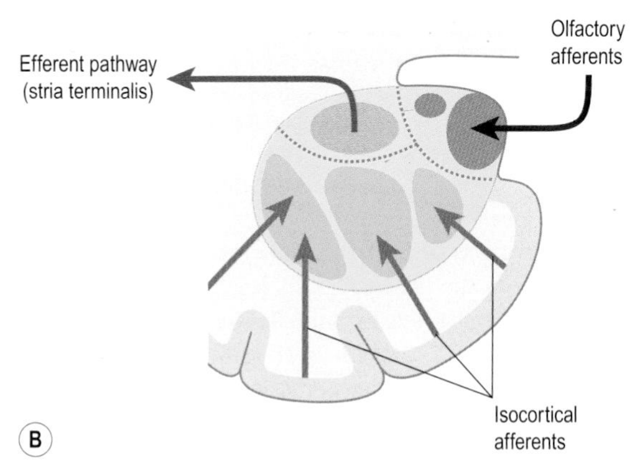

Fig. 3.18 **The amygdala. (A)** The three major nuclear groups of the amygdala are illustrated (corticomedial, basolateral and central) with their main subnuclei labelled; **(B)** The corticomedial and basolateral nuclei receive olfactory and non-olfactory afferents, respectively. The central nucleus gives rise to a major efferent projection, the stria terminalis.

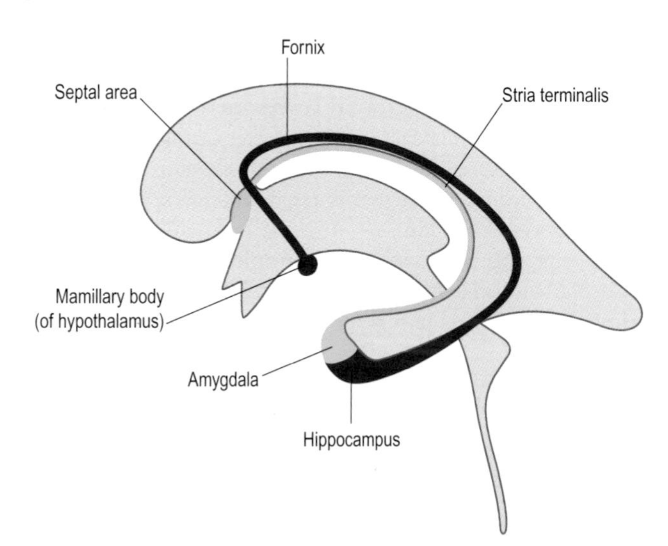

Fig. 3.19 **The positions of the amygdala and hippocampus relative to the lateral ventricle, together with their main outflow pathways: the stria terminalis and fornix.** The targets of the stria terminalis and fornix are similar, including the hypothalamus, brain stem and limbic ('emotion-related') part of the basal ganglia. Both pathways also project to the septal area (illustrated here; see also Fig. 3.13) which is involved in mood, emotion and reward-based learning.

Key Points

- The amygdala is an almond-shaped mass of grey matter in the medial temporal region (just anterior to the hippocampus) that is primarily concerned with emotional responses. It is made up of several sub-nuclei.
- The corticomedial and basolateral groups receive olfactory and non-olfactory afferents respectively, providing information about events and social interactions. The central group projects to the hypothalamus via the stria terminalis, which enables it to influence the activities of the autonomic nervous system and endocrine system.
- The amygdala is involved in determining the emotional significance of events and generating an appropriate emotional response, moderated by projections from the orbitofrontal cortex.
- It is involved in all types of emotional response, but is particularly important in situations that provoke anxiety, fear or rage and has been described as a 'danger detector'.

Basal ganglia

The basal ganglia are a collection of deep hemispheric nuclei (strictly speaking, the term 'ganglia' is a misnomer) that contribute to voluntary movement, cognition and behaviour. Their involvement in movement control is illustrated by **Parkinson's disease**, the most common basal ganglia disorder (Ch. 13). The largest component of the basal ganglia is the corpus striatum.

Corpus striatum (Fig. 3.20)

This is a large mass of grey matter in the base of the cerebral hemisphere that is intimately related to the lateral ventricle and internal capsule. The name derives from its striated appearance in cross section, due to the presence of myelinated fibres arranged in small bundles. The corpus striatum is composed of the caudate and lentiform nuclei.

Caudate nucleus

The **caudate nucleus** is a large C-shaped structure with a head, body and tail, that nestles into the inner curvature of the lateral ventricle (Latin: cauda, tail). On coronal sections the head and body of the caudate nucleus can be seen bulging into the side wall of the lateral ventricle, whilst its slender tail sweeps down into the temporal lobe to occupy the roof of the temporal horn.

Lentiform nucleus

The **lentiform nucleus** lies beneath the insula. It is said to resemble a lens (Latin: lentiform, lens-shaped) but is best regarded as a cone with the base underlying the insula and a blunt apex pointing towards the midline (Fig. 3.21). The outer portion of the lentiform nucleus, immediately beneath the insula, is the **putamen** (Latin: putamen, husk or shell). The inner part is the **globus pallidus** which has internal and external segments. The globus pallidus is so named because of its pallid (pale) appearance in comparison to the dark grey colour of the caudate nucleus and putamen. This is due to the presence of myelinated fibres forming the internal connections of the basal ganglia.

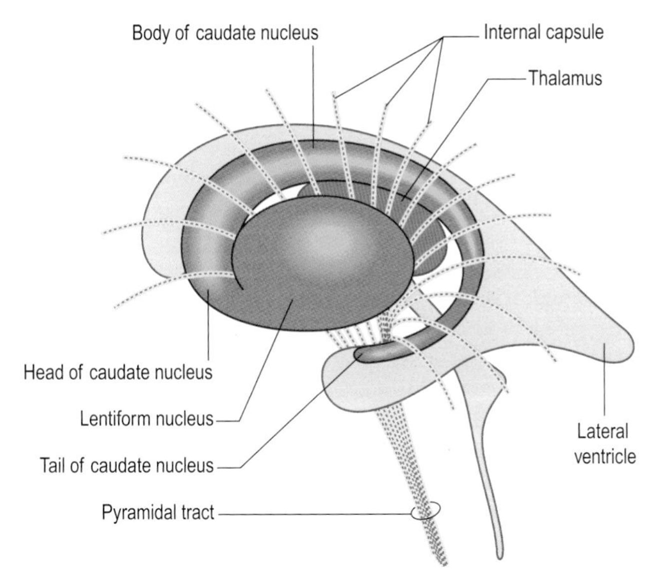

Fig. 3.20 **The corpus striatum is composed of the C-shaped caudate nucleus and the cone-shaped lentiform nucleus.** These two nuclei are largely divided by the white matter of the internal capsule, but are fused anteriorly (as shown in the figure). Note that in this view only the base of the cone-shaped lentiform nucleus can be seen; its blunt apex is pointing towards the midline (compare with coronal view in Fig. 3.21).

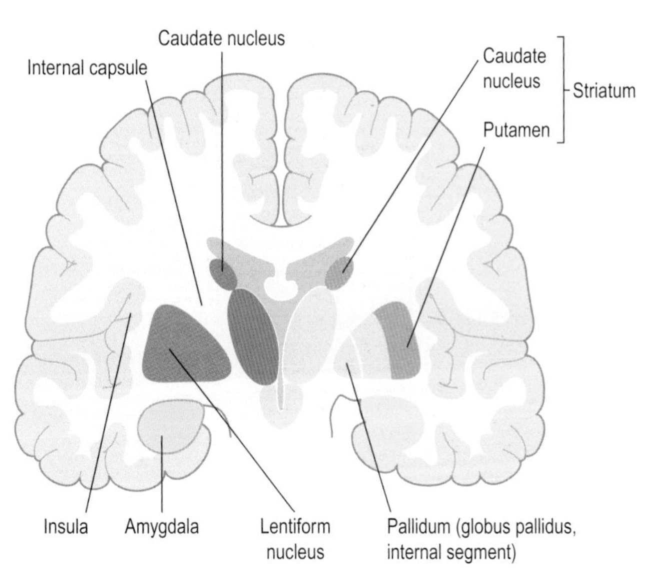

Fig. 3.21 **Coronal section through the corpus striatum.** The left side of the figure shows the caudate and lentiform nuclei, separated by the white matter of the internal capsule; the amygdala can be seen below the cone-shaped lentiform nucleus, in the medial temporal region. The right side of the figure shows the functional sub-divisions of the corpus striatum. The 'input' region (striatum) consists of the caudate nucleus and putamen, which is shown in dark grey. The 'output' region (pallidum) consists of the internal segment of the globus pallidus, shown in light grey.

Internal capsule

The internal capsule is a thick sheet of white matter consisting of **projection fibres** (see Ch. 1, Fig. 1.17) passing to and from the cerebral cortex. It makes a sharp 'knee-bend' or **genu** around the apex of the lentiform nucleus (Latin: genu, knee). This gives it a V-shape when viewed in axial (horizontal) section (Fig. 3.22). There is therefore an **anterior limb** (between the lentiform nucleus and the head of the caudate nucleus) and a **posterior limb** (between the lentiform nucleus and the thalamus).

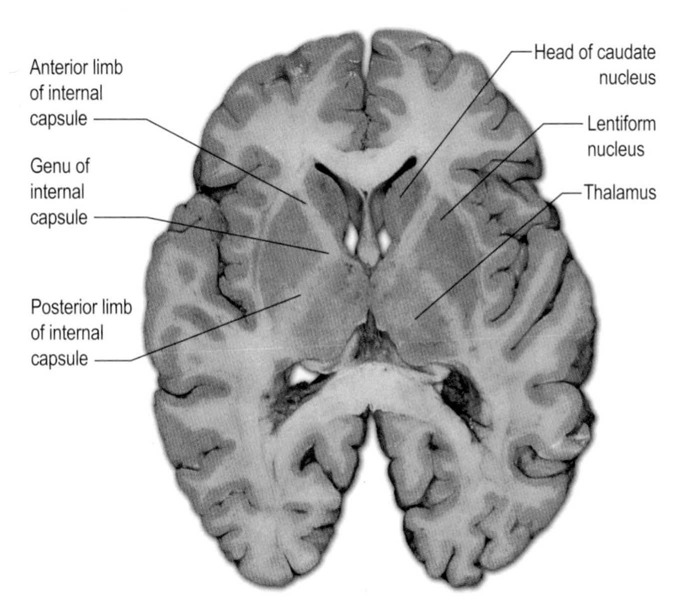

Fig. 3.22 **Axial (horizontal) section of the cerebral hemisphere showing the internal capsule.** The section passes through the cone-shaped lentiform nucleus, with its base directed laterally and its apex pointing towards the midline. The V-shaped internal capsule can be seen wrapping around the apex of the cone as the genu ('knee bend'), forming the anterior and posterior limbs. The anterior limb lies between the head of the caudate nucleus and the lentiform nucleus. The posterior limb is between the thalamus and the lentiform nucleus. From Standring: Gray's Anatomy 40th edn (2008: Churchill Livingstone) with permission.

Key Points

- The corpus striatum is the largest component of the basal ganglia and consists of the C-shaped caudate nucleus and cone-shaped lentiform nucleus.
- The lentiform nucleus has an outer part called the putamen and a pale inner portion called the globus pallidus (which itself has internal and external segments).
- The internal capsule consists of projection fibres passing through the corpus striatum. It forms a knee-bend (genu) around the apex of the lentiform nucleus and is V-shaped on axial (horizontal) sections.
- The anterior limb of the internal capsule passes between the caudate nucleus (medially) and lentiform nucleus (laterally).
- The posterior limb of the internal capsule passes between the thalamus (medially) and the lentiform nucleus (laterally).

Functional divisions

Division of the corpus striatum into the caudate and lentiform nuclei reflects their physical separation by the white matter of the internal capsule (Fig. 3.21, *left*). However, it is also possible to identify two functional zones based upon afferent and efferent connections (Fig. 3.21, *right*):

- The **striatum** (caudate nucleus and putamen) is the 'input' portion of the basal ganglia which receives projections from the overlying cerebral cortex.
- The **pallidum** (internal segment of the globus pallidus) is the 'output' portion of the basal ganglia which projects to the thalamus.

The various terms used to describe parts of the corpus striatum are illustrated in Figure 3.23; note that the **structural term**

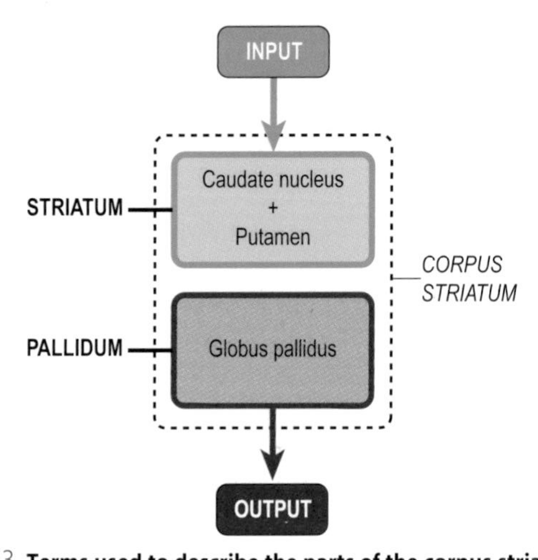

Fig. 3.23 **Terms used to describe the parts of the corpus striatum.** The striatum (caudate nucleus and putamen) is the 'input' portion of the basal ganglia which receives projections from the cerebral cortex. The pallidum (internal segment of the globus pallidus) is the 'output' portion of the basal ganglia and projects to the thalamus. The entire nuclear mass (caudate nucleus plus lentiform nucleus) is referred to as the corpus striatum.

'corpus striatum' (caudate + lentiform nuclei) is not the same as the **functional term** 'striatum' (caudate nucleus + putamen; which is the afferent or 'input' region).

Basal ganglia loops

The connections of the corpus striatum are arranged as a set of **basal ganglia loops** that arise and terminate in the frontal lobe. In each case the projections originate in the frontal cortex and project to a specific part of the striatum ('input region'). The internal connections of the basal ganglia converge on the internal pallidum ('output region') which projects in turn to the thalamus. The loop is completed as **thalamocortical neurons** project back to the cortical region of origin. Activity in the basal ganglia loops is facilitated by the neurotransmitter dopamine, which is supplied by projections from the **substantia nigra** of the midbrain.

The voluntary motor loop

The motor loop is the best understood component of the basal ganglia and is disturbed in movement disorders such as Parkinson's disease. Projections arise from the **supplementary motor area (SMA)** in the medial frontal lobe and project into the **putamen**. For this reason the putamen is regarded as the 'motor part' of the striatum. The putamen gives rise to direct and indirect connections that converge on the internal pallidum. This projects in turn to the thalamus, which completes the loop via a **thalamocortical projection** back to the SMA. **Dopamine deficiency** in Parkinson's disease leads to underactivity of the motor loop and SMA, interfering with the initiation of voluntary actions. The control of the motor loop (by the direct and indirect pathways) is discussed further in Chapter 13, in the context of Parkinson's disease.

Cognitive-executive loops

Basal ganglia loops passing through the **caudate nucleus** arise and terminate in the **prefrontal cortex**. They influence cognition and behaviour, but also contribute to the control of visual attention and voluntary gaze via projections that arise and terminate in the frontal eye fields. Over-activity in caudate-prefrontal connections has been implicated in **obsessive-compulsive disorder** (Clinical Box 3.10).

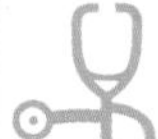

Clinical Box 3.10: Obsessive-compulsive disorder (OCD)

Obsessive-compulsive disorder is an **anxiety disorder** that affects around 2% of the population. **Obsessions** are persistent unwanted thoughts, whereas **compulsions** are irrational urges to carry out particular acts or rituals. Typical preoccupations include contamination and harm, order and symmetry, religion and sex. **Pathological doubt** is also common, leading to checking rituals, compulsive hand washing and **pathological slowness.** Neuroimaging suggests that there may be overactivity in connections between the caudate nuclei and prefrontal cortex, which appears to normalize after successful treatment using **serotonin-selective reuptake inhibitors (SSRIs)**.

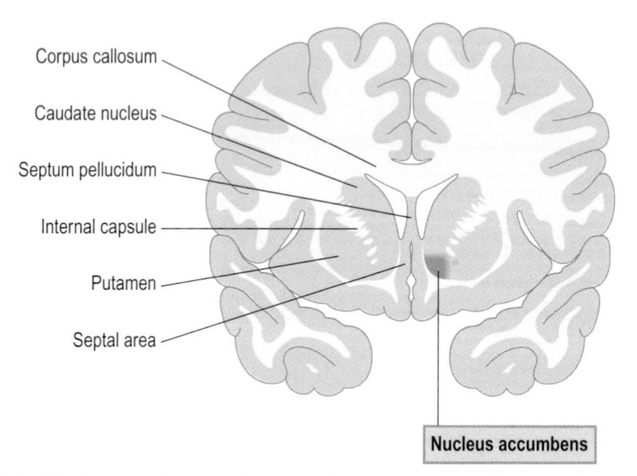

Fig. 3.24 **Coronal section through the anterior frontal lobe at the level of the nucleus accumbens (ventral striatum) and septal area.** The most anterior parts of the caudate nucleus and putamen are fused underneath the anterior limb of the internal capsule (see Fig. 3.20) to form the ventral striatum (also known as the nucleus accumbens septi).

Limbic-affective loops

Anteriorly, the caudate nucleus and putamen are fused underneath the anterior limb of the internal capsule (see Fig. 3.20) to form the **ventral striatum**. Due to its proximity to the septal area (Fig. 3.24) it is also known as the nucleus accumbens septi or **nucleus accumbens** (Latin: accumbens, leaning against). Projections taking part in the 'limbic loops' of the basal ganglia arise in the limbic lobe or amygdala and project to the ventral striatum. This region is rich in **opiate receptors** and has been implicated in motivation, reward-based learning and addictive behaviours.

Key Points

- The basal ganglia 'loops' arise and terminate in the frontal lobe and are facilitated by the neurotransmitter dopamine.
- The striatum is the 'input region' of the basal ganglia and consists of the caudate nucleus (for cognitive-executive loops) and putamen (for voluntary motor loops).
- The caudate and putamen are fused below the anterior limb of the internal capsule to form the ventral striatum. This is involved in mood, motivation, reward-based learning and addiction.
- The pallidum is the 'output region' of the basal ganglia and consists of the internal segment of the globus pallidus, which projects to the thalamus.

Thalamus and hypothalamus

The thalamus and hypothalamus are part of the **diencephalon** (Fig. 3.25). This is the portion of the cerebrum that is normally hidden from view between the cerebral hemispheres, surrounding the cavity of the third ventricle (Greek: dia, between; enkephalos, brain).

Thalamus

The thalami are a pair of large, egg-shaped masses of grey matter at the centre of the brain (Greek: thalamos, inner chamber). On a midsagittal section the medial aspect of the thalamus can be seen in the side wall of the third ventricle.

Thalamic nuclei

Almost all ascending pathways synapse in a thalamic nucleus in order to reach the cerebral cortex. The thalamus is therefore described as the 'gateway' to the cortex. It is composed of more than a dozen nuclei, separated into **anterior**, **medial** and **lateral** groups by a Y-shaped **internal medullary lamina**. This thin sheet of white matter contains a few small **intralaminar nuclei** which are involved in arousal, wakefulness and pain (see Ch. 4). The lateral nuclear group of the thalamus has dorsal and ventral tiers. The ventral tier contains **specific nuclei**, which project to discrete cortical zones such as the primary sensory and motor areas. The **non-specific nuclei** form diffuse, reciprocal connections with large regions of the cortex.

Pineal gland

The **pineal gland** is above and behind the thalamus in the roof of the third ventricle. It secretes the sleep-inducing hormone **melatonin** when light levels are low (Greek: melas, black). This helps to control sleep–wake cycles and **circadian rhythms** (Latin: circa, about; dies, day). Melatonin release is influenced by a projection from the **suprachiasmatic nucleus** of the hypothalamus, which acts as a **biological clock** that is adjusted by the amount of light falling on the retina.

Hypothalamus

The hypothalamus is a small structure which forms the lower side wall and floor of the third ventricle, just below and in front of the thalamus. It has numerous nuclei that are collectively responsible for maintaining a constant internal environment (**homeostasis**). It does this by regulating basic drives (e.g. hunger, thirst) and by co-ordinating the activity of the **endocrine** and **autonomic nervous systems**. It continuously monitors parameters such as core body temperature and blood glucose concentration and controls autonomic centres in the brain stem and spinal cord to keep them constant. It also influences hormonal release from the adjacent **pituitary gland** (Ch. 1).

> ### *Key Points*
>
> - The thalamic region (surrounding the cavity of the third ventricle) is the diencephalon. It includes the thalamus, hypothalamus and pineal gland.
> - The thalami are divided into anterior, medial and lateral nuclei by the Y-shaped internal medullary lamina. The lateral group has dorsal and ventral tiers.
> - Most ascending pathways synapse in a thalamic nucleus in order to reach the cerebral cortex. The thalamus can therefore be described as the 'gateway' to the cortex.
> - The hypothalamus occupies the lower part of the side wall and the floor of the third ventricle and controls the activities of the autonomic nervous system and endocrine system.

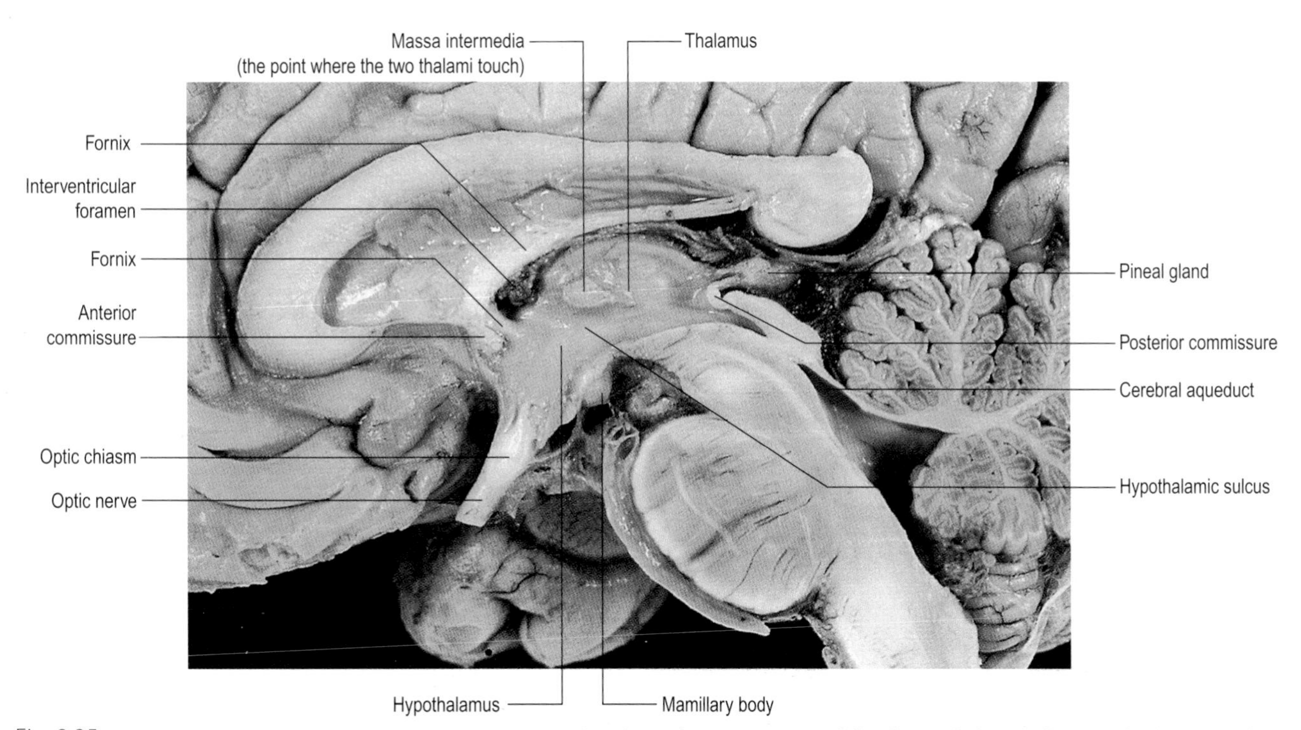

Fig. 3.25 **Midsagittal section of the cerebral hemisphere showing the major components of the diencephalon (thalamic region) surrounding the cavity of the third ventricle.** The fornix can be seen passing through the hypothalamus to reach the mamillary body in the floor of the third ventricle and forming the anterior boundary of the interventricular foramen. From Crossman: Neuroanatomy ICT 4e (Churchill Livingstone 2010) with permission.

Brain stem and cerebellum

The brain stem is composed of the midbrain, pons and medulla, which are closely related to the overlying cerebellum. Some important surface landmarks of the brain stem are illustrated in Figure 3.26.

Midbrain

The midbrain is the most rostral part of the brain stem (Figs 3.26 and 3.27). It contains the **cerebral aqueduct** which runs between the third ventricle (above) and the fourth ventricle (below). The small part of the midbrain dorsal to the aqueduct is the **tectum** or 'roof' of the midbrain (Latin: tectum, roof). The large portion in front of the aqueduct (making up half of the midbrain on each side, excluding the tectum) consists of the left and right **cerebral peduncles**.

Tectum (3.26C and 3.27B)

The tectum bears four smooth elevations or colliculi (Latin: colliculus, little hill). The **superior colliculi** (collectively: the **optic tectum**) give rise to the **tectospinal tracts** which co-ordinate head, neck and eye movements during orientation reflexes (e.g. involuntary turning towards a novel or unexpected stimulus). The **inferior colliculi** are part of a complex pathway between the cochlea and primary auditory cortex. The role of the midbrain in the control of pupil size is discussed in Clinical Box 3.11.

Cerebral peduncles (3.27B)

When viewed from the front, the cerebral peduncles resemble two stout Roman pillars, separated by the **interpeduncular fossa** (Latin: fossa, ditch). A transverse (horizontal) slice through the midbrain shows the deeply pigmented

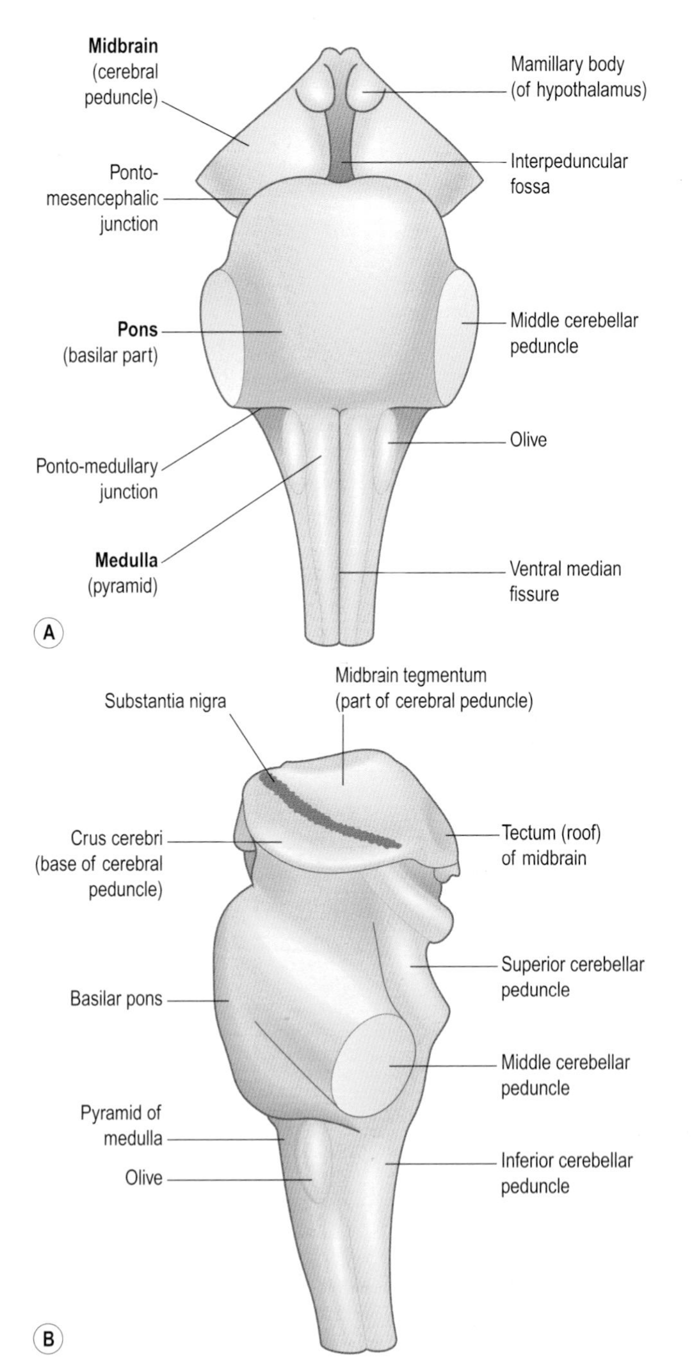

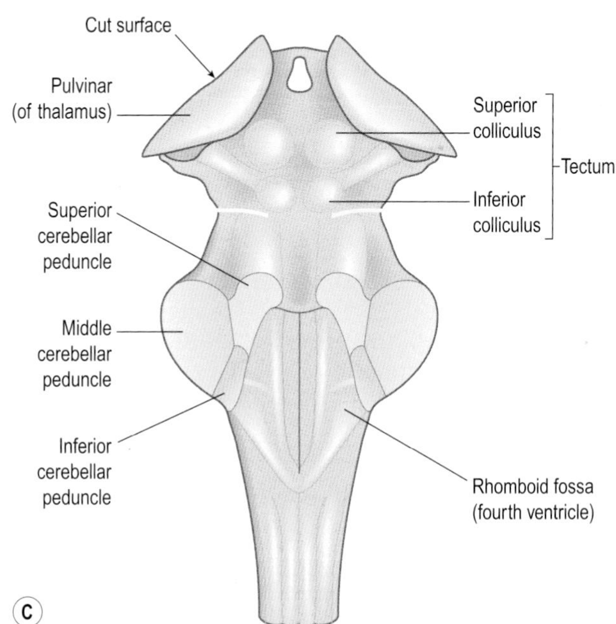

Fig. 3.26 **The brain stem, showing the main surface landmarks.** **(A)** Anterior aspect; **(B)** Lateral aspect; **(C)** Posterior aspect. The cerebellum and cerebral hemispheres have been removed.

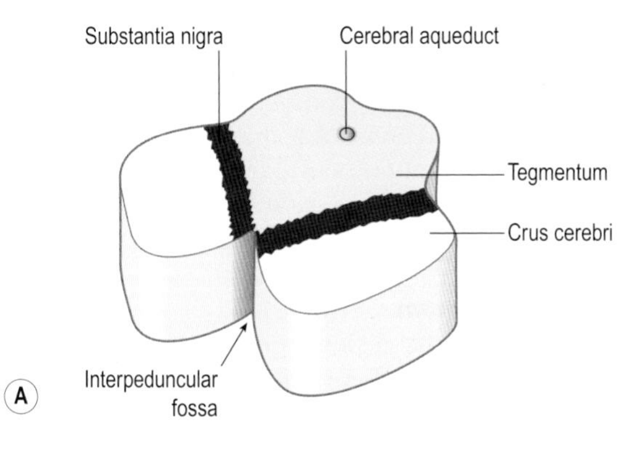

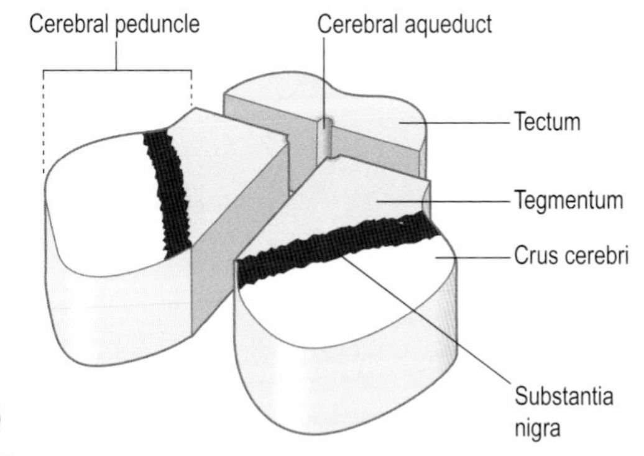

Fig. 3.27 **The midbrain. (A)** Anterolateral view of the intact midbrain separated from the rest of the brain stem; **(B)** Exploded schematic view of the midbrain illustrating the tectum and the paired cerebral peduncles. Note that the 'cerebral peduncle' makes up one half of the midbrain on each side (excluding the tectum), but the term is frequently misused to describe only the anterior part of the midbrain in which the corticospinal tract is found (the correct term for this region is the crus cerebri).

substantia nigra (Latin: nigra, black). This supplies dopamine to the basal ganglia via the **nigro-striatal tract**. The much smaller **ventral tegmental area** (which provides the ventral striatum with dopamine) is just medial to the nigra, but cannot be seen with the naked eye. The **tegmentum** is the portion of the cerebral peduncle posterior to the substantia nigra. The part in front of the nigra is the **crus cerebri** (plural: crura). The crura transmit axons of the primary motor pathway descending from the cerebral cortex to the spinal cord (the **corticospinal tract**).

Key Points

- The midbrain contains the cerebral aqueduct, which connects the third ventricle (above) with the fourth ventricle (below).
- The small portion of the midbrain dorsal (=posterior) to the cerebral aqueduct is the tectum or roof plate. It bears the superior and inferior colliculi (which are concerned with visual and auditory reflexes respectively).
- The remainder of the midbrain is made up of the cerebral peduncles. They are divided by the substantia nigra into the tegmentum (posteriorly) and crus cerebri (anteriorly).
- On each side, the crus cerebri contains the corticospinal (motor) tract. This anterior part of the midbrain (in front of the substantia nigra) is often referred to (incorrectly) as the cerebral peduncle.

Pons

The pons is the middle portion of the brain stem. When viewed from the front, it appears to bridge the cerebellar

Clinical Box 3.11: Pupillary light reflexes

The pupillary reflexes are tested clinically using a pen torch (Fig. 3.28). Illumination of one eye causes reflexive constriction of *both* pupils: via the **direct** and **indirect pupillary light reflexes**. This is mediated by projections from the retina to the **pretectal nucleus** of the midbrain, just rostral to the superior colliculus. The pretectal nucleus projects in turn to the (parasympathetic) **Edinger–Westphal nuclei** on both sides of the brain stem. Fibres from these nuclei travel with the oculomotor (III) nerves to innervate the ciliary ganglia, which supply the **sphincter pupillae** muscles (causing both pupils to constrict). The pretectal area reaches the opposite Edinger–Westphal nucleus by crossing the midline in the tiny **posterior commissure**, located just below the pineal gland (see Fig. 3.25).

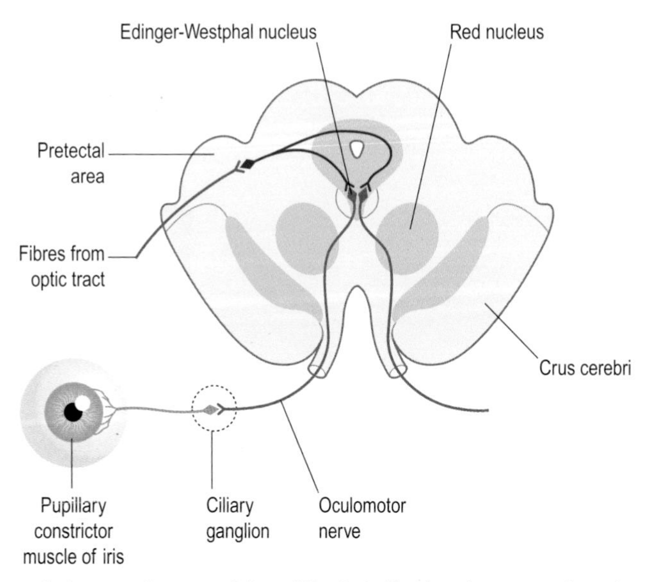

Fig. 3.28 **A transverse section through the superior part of the midbrain indicating the connections that mediate the pupillary light reflex.** From Crossman: Neuroanatomy ICT 4e (Churchill Livingstone 2010) with permission.

hemispheres (Latin: pons, bridge). The pons is divided into basal and tegmental regions.

Basilar pons

The anterior two thirds of the pons is called the **base** (or **basilar pons**). It transmits bundles of descending corticospinal tract fibres that have already passed through the internal capsule and crus cerebri (above) on their way to the spinal cord (below). It also contains the **pontine nuclei**, which give rise to axons that project to the opposite cerebellar hemisphere via the **middle cerebellar peduncle** (crossing the midline as the transverse pontine fibres).

Pontine tegmentum

The dorsal third of the pons is the **tegmentum**, the posterior surface of which forms part of the floor of the fourth ventricle. The tegmentum contains the pontine reticular formation, together with several cranial nerve nuclei and ascending tracts. The **loci coerulei** (singular: locus coeruleus) are found in the rostral pons, just beneath the floor of the fourth ventricle on each side. These pigmented nuclei (Latin: locus, place; coeruleus, dark-blue) give rise to a diffuse projection for **noradrenaline** (see Ch. 1).

Medulla oblongata

The medulla is the lowermost portion of the brain stem, which is continuous with the spinal cord at the level of the foramen magnum. It also has basal and tegmental parts.

Basilar region

The anterior medulla contains two tapering columns of white matter called the **pyramids**, which are equivalent to the 'basilar region' in the midbrain and pons. The pyramids transmit the primary motor pathway (the **corticospinal tract**) which is therefore also known as the **pyramidal tract** (Fig. 3.29). Just lateral to the pyramids in the upper medulla are the **olives** (see Fig. 3.26), which send an ascending projection to the opposite cerebellum. This **olivo-cerebellar pathway** contributes to motor learning by signalling unexpected events (e.g. dropping a ball whilst learning to juggle) and provides a 'training signal' to the cerebellum which alters synaptic strengths in such a way that the error is less likely to be repeated.

Medullary tegmentum

The tegmentum of the medulla contains the medullary reticular formation, together with cranial nerve nuclei and ascending tracts. It also includes a number of '**vital centres**' which subserve cardiorespiratory functions and airway-protective reflexes (e.g. cough, sneeze, gag).

> **Key Points**
>
> - The lower brain stem (pons and medulla) is involved in basic life support functions and contains the cardiorespiratory ('vital') centres.
> - The basal pons and pyramids of the medulla contain the primary motor fibres of the corticospinal tract (continuous with those of the crus cerebri, above).
> - The tegmental region of the brain stem contains the reticular formation, cranial nerve nuclei and ascending sensory pathways.

Cerebellum

The gross anatomy of the cerebellum has been outlined in Chapter 1. In this section its three functional divisions will be reviewed. It is important to remember that, in contrast to the cerebral hemispheres, cerebellar disease causes symptoms and signs on the same (ipsilateral) side of the body.

Functional divisions

The cerebellum has three **functional divisions**, corresponding to: (i) the **flocculonodular lobe**; (ii) the **vermis/paravermal region**; and (iii) the **cerebellar hemispheres** (Fig. 3.30). It is important to note that the

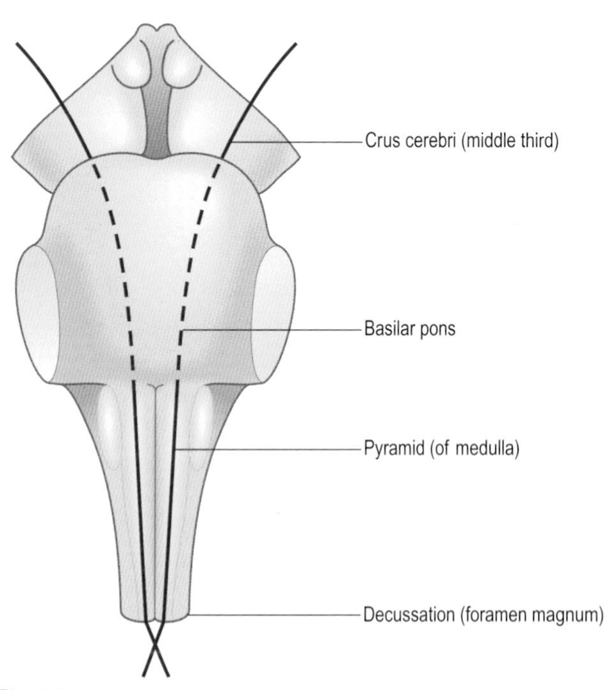

Fig. 3.29 **The course of the pyramidal (corticospinal) tract through the brain stem.** In the basilar pons (dashed lines) the corticospinal tract fibres are obscured by the transverse pontine fibres.

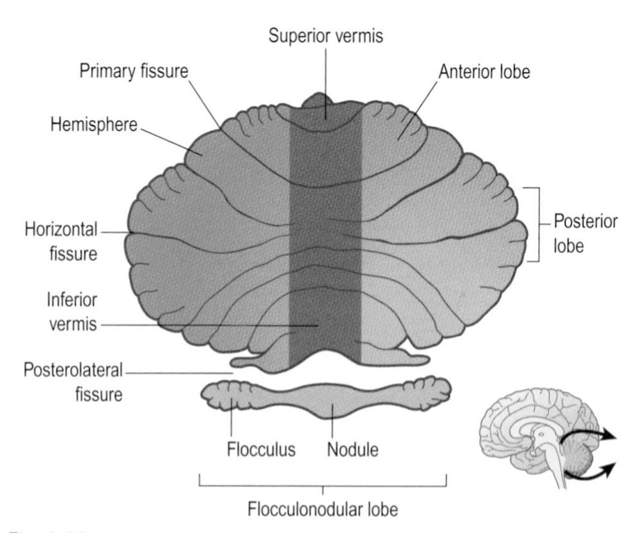

Fig. 3.30 **Functional divisions of the cerebellum.** The cerebellar cortex has been 'unfolded' and laid flat to illustrate the approximate position of the three functional sub-divisions: flocculonodular lobe (orange), vermis/paravermis (dark brown) and cerebellar hemispheres (light brown). From Crossman: Neuroanatomy ICT 4e (Churchill Livingstone 2010) with permission.

functional regions do not coincide exactly with the gross anatomical (lobar) boundaries.

Vestibulocerebellum

The vestibulocerebellum or **archicerebellum** (Greek: arkhe, beginning) is the evolutionarily most ancient division and is present in fish and amphibians. It corresponds to the flocculonodular lobe, composed of the paired **flocculi** in the hemispheres (Latin: flocculus, tuft of wool) and the **nodule** of the vermis. It is connected to the **vestibular nuclei** of the brain stem and uses information from the inner ear to help maintain balance. This is mediated by the **vestibulospinal tracts** which influence anti-gravity muscles in the trunk and limbs. It also adjusts eye movements to correct for changes in head position (the **vestibulo-ocular reflex**).

Spinocerebellum

The spinocerebellum or **paleocerebellum** (Greek: palaios, ancient) is an evolutionarily more recent division that is prominent in reptiles and birds. It corresponds to the **vermis** and **paravermal region**, incorporating much of the **anterior lobe**. The spinocerebellum receives constant sensory (proprioceptive) feedback from the spinal cord. This includes projections from the posterior columns and the **dorsal** and **ventral spinocerebellar pathways**. It contributes to the regulation of posture, muscle tone and gait.

Cerebrocerebellum

The cerebrocerebellum or **neocerebellum** is present only in mammals (Greek: neos, new) and is disproportionately large in the human brain. It incorporates most of the **cerebellar hemispheres** and **posterior** lobe, together with the **dentate nuclei** (Latin: dentus, tooth). These give rise to the main outflow of the cerebellum, via the **superior cerebellar peduncles**. Projections from the dentate nucleus synapse in the contralateral thalamus, which projects in turn to the **motor** and **premotor areas** of the frontal lobe. The neocerebellum ensures that movements are performed accurately and smoothly (e.g. finely fractionated movements of the hands). It is also involved in precision control of the larynx and tongue, which is important for speech articulation.

Role in movement control

The cerebellum acts as a **comparator**. The motor and premotor areas of the frontal lobe provide information about **intended movements** whereas the spinocerebellar tracts (and other pathways) provide information about **actual movements**. Any discrepancy between the two creates an 'error signal' that is fed back to the motor cortex, permitting continuous modification and improvement of on-going movements. Cerebellar disease therefore leads to **incoordination** (Clinical Box 3.12).

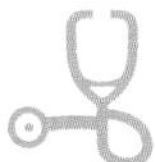

Clinical Box 3.12: Cerebellar lesions

Cerebellar disease is associated with clumsy, poorly coordinated movements, termed **cerebellar ataxia** (Greek: a-, without; taxis, order). A similar clinical picture can be caused by spinal cord or peripheral nerve disease, called **sensory ataxia**. In this case the cerebellum is prevented from functioning normally due to a lack of sensory feedback. Some clinical evidence suggests that lesions of the cerebellar hemispheres may be associated with disturbances of mood, cognition and language. This has been called the **cerebellar cognitive-affective syndrome**.

Key Points

- The cerebellum can be divided topographically into the hemispheres and vermis (with anterior, posterior and flocculonodular lobes) or into three functional divisions concerned with balance (archicerebellum), posture and tone (paleocerebellum) and coordination (neocerebellum).
- The cerebellum acts as a comparator, identifying any mismatch between intended movements and actual movements and generating an 'error signal' which is fed back to the motor cortex to enable continuous modification and improvement.
- Cerebellar lesions tend to be associated with poorly coordinated or clumsy movements (cerebellar ataxia). Unlike cerebral hemisphere lesions, the symptoms are ipsilateral.

Chapter 4
Sensory and motor pathways

CHAPTER CONTENTS

Key Points

- The spinal cord is divided into 31 segments, each with a pair of dorsal and ventral roots which unite on each side to form mixed spinal nerves.
- The dorsal root ganglia contain the cell bodies of primary afferent neurons and provide sensation to the corresponding dermatome. The ventral roots contain efferent (motor) fibres.
- The internal anatomy of the spinal cord consists of an H-shaped inner core of grey matter (arranged in dorsal and ventral horns) and an outer layer of white matter.
- The spinal white matter includes connections between cord segments, together with long tracts passing to and from the brain.

The central nervous system contains a large number of ascending and descending tracts that pass between the brain and spinal cord. However, in this chapter discussion will be restricted to the three most clinically important pathways that are routinely assessed in the neurological examination. The concept of upper and lower motor neurons will also be introduced, together with the anatomical basis of muscle tone and tendon reflexes.

Spinal segments

The spinal cord is divided into 31 segments (Fig. 4.1A), each with a pair of **dorsal (sensory) roots** and a pair of **ventral (motor) roots**. The dorsal and ventral roots unite on each side to form a mixed spinal nerve (spinal **nerve root**) (Fig. 4.1B). Each nerve root divides into a small **dorsal ramus**, which supplies the paravertebral muscles and provides cutaneous sensation to the back, and a large **ventral ramus** which innervates the limbs and trunk. The **dorsal root ganglia** at each spinal level contain the cell bodies of sensory neurons that innervate an area of skin called a **dermatome** (Fig. 4.2). They also contain the cell bodies of sensory neurons innervating muscles, tendons, ligaments and joints.

Internal anatomy of the spinal cord

The spinal cord has an H-shaped inner core of grey matter, with **dorsal** and **ventral horns**, surrounded by a thick layer of white matter. The ventral (anterior) horns contain longitudinal columns of **motor neurons** that innervate the skeletal musculature via the ventral roots; and each column supplies a functionally related group of muscles. The dorsal (posterior) horns contain **sensory neurons** that receive

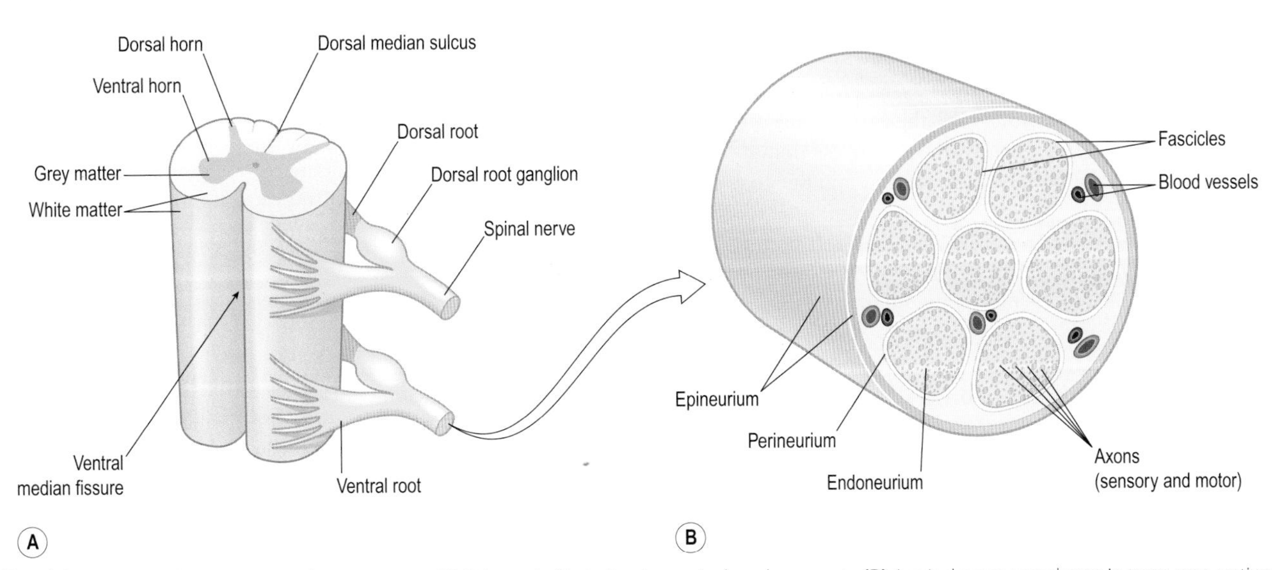

Fig. 4.1 **Spinal cord segments and nerve roots. (A)** Schematic illustrating two spinal cord segments; **(B)** A spinal nerve root shown in transverse section. The nerve root consists of sensory and motor axons arranged in bundles (fascicles) surrounded by connective tissue (endoneurium, perineurium, epineurium) and blood vessels. Modified from Fitzgerald: Clinical Neuroanatomy and Neuroscience 5e (2006) with permission.

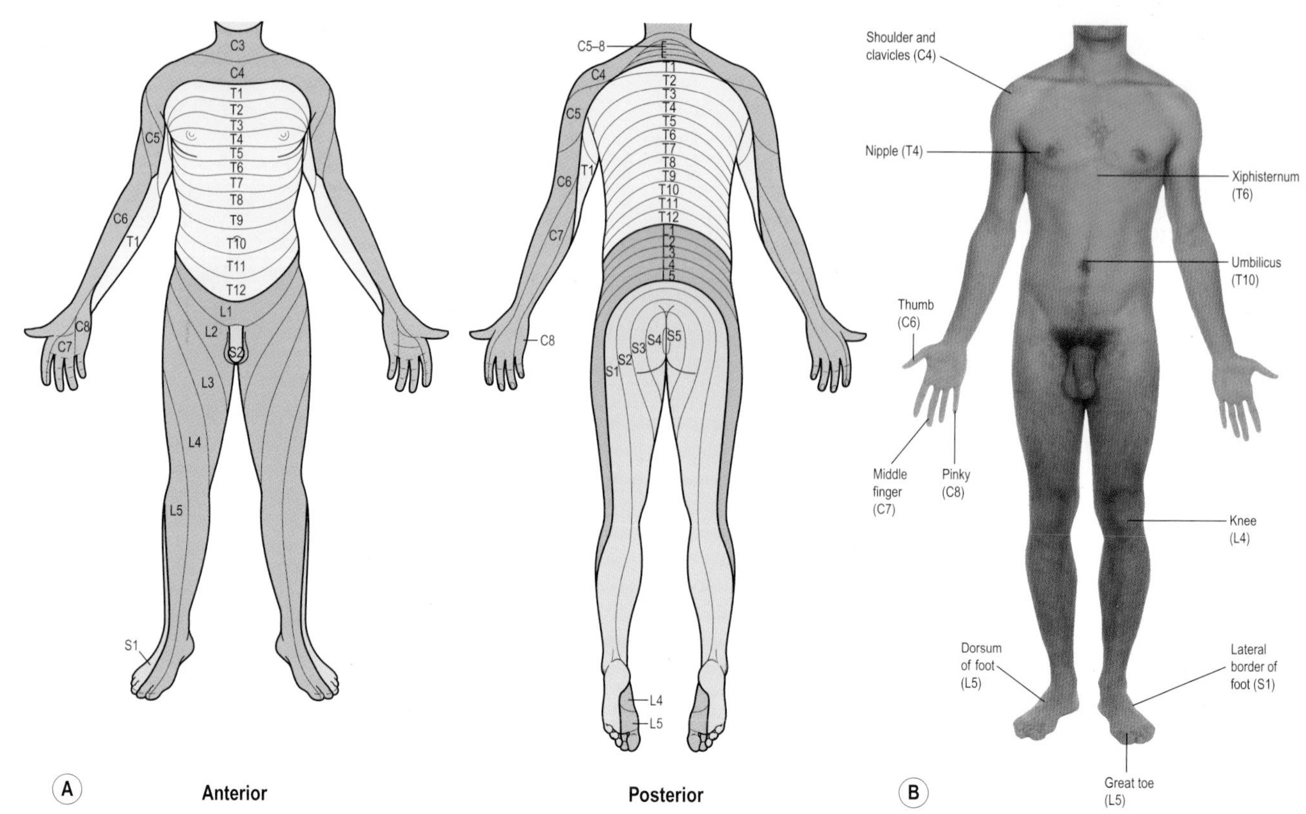

Fig. 4.2 **Dermatomes. (A)** Illustration of the complete dermatome map from anterior and posterior aspects, with the spinal root values indicated; **(B)** Photograph showing a number of key dermatome levels that it is clinically-useful to be familiar with.

afferent projections from the dorsal root ganglia. The white matter of the spinal cord includes connections between segmental levels, together with **long tracts** passing to and from the brain.

Somatic sensory pathways

Two major spinal cord pathways carry sensory information to the cerebral cortex where it can be consciously perceived. The **dorsal column pathway** is concerned with precisely localized touch and joint position sense. The **spinothalamic tract** is primarily responsible for pain and temperature sensation. Each pathway is composed of a three-neuron chain with a similar arrangement (Fig. 4.3):

- The **first-order** neurons have their cell bodies in the dorsal root ganglia, each with one process that contributes to a peripheral nerve and another that enters the spinal cord.
- The **second-order** neurons have their cell bodies in the grey matter of the brain stem or spinal cord and give rise to axons that cross the midline, before ascending to the thalamus.
- The **third-order** neurons are located in the ventral posterior (VP) nucleus of the thalamus and project to the primary somatosensory cortex, via the posterior limb of the internal capsule (see Ch. 3).

The axons of the somatic sensory pathways are arranged in a precise point-to-point or **somatotopic** fashion (Greek: soma, body; topos, place). This means that fibres innervating adjacent parts of the body surface remain side-by-side along the full length of the pathway to the brain.

Dorsal column pathway

The dorsal column pathway is mainly responsible for precisely localized touch and **proprioception** (awareness of one's own body; Latin: proprius, one's own) including **joint position sense**. It contains large myelinated axons (**A-alpha fibres**) which transmit impulses at speeds of up to 120 metres per second. Integrity of the dorsal columns is best assessed clinically using a tuning fork (Clinical Box 4.1).

Gracile and cuneate fasciculi

The dorsal columns lie between the **dorsal root entry zones**. On each side of the cord, the dorsal column contains two fasciculi. Closer to the midline, and present at all cord levels, is the **fasciculus gracilis** (Latin: gracile, slender). This transmits sensory information from the mid-thoracic (T6) level and below, including the lower limbs. The wedge-shaped **fasciculus cuneatus** (Latin: cuneus, wedge) is lateral to the gracile fasciculus but is only present in the upper half of the cord. It contains sensory fibres from above T6, including those from the upper limbs.

Pathway to the cerebral cortex (Fig. 4.4)

The **first-order neurons** of the dorsal column pathway have their cell bodies in the **dorsal root ganglia**. A central axonal process enters the dorsal column and, without crossing the midline, ascends uninterrupted to the medulla. These fibres terminate on **second-order** neurons in the **dorsal column nuclei** (the gracile and cuneate nuclei).

Axons emerge from the dorsal column nuclei and arch anteriorly and medially through the substance of the medulla as the **internal arcuate fibres** (Latin: arcuate, shaped like a bow). These axons cross the midline as the **great sensory**

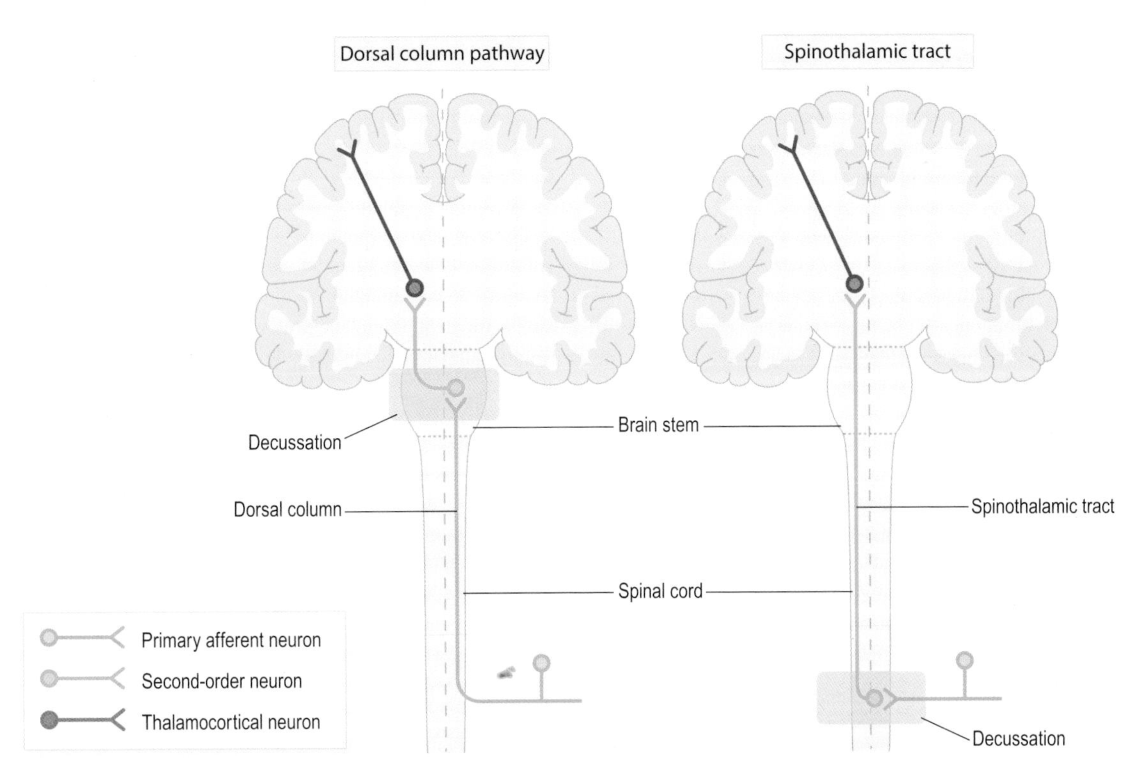

Fig. 4.3 **The general arrangement of the somatic sensory pathways.** The first-, second- and third-order neurons are coloured green, blue and red respectively. Note that in both pathways the second-order neuron has its cell body in the central nervous system (CNS) and gives rise to an axon that crosses the midline and ascends to the thalamus. The main difference between the two pathways is the location of the second neuron (which in turn determines where each pathway crosses the midline).

Clinical Box 4.1: Testing dorsal column function

Assessment of **vibration sense** is the best clinical test of the dorsal column pathway. A low-frequency (128 Hz) tuning fork is applied to bony prominences and the patient (with closed eyes) is asked to report when the vibration starts and stops. Assessment of light touch and proprioception is also possible, but less reliable: a wisp of cotton wool can be applied gently to different skin areas to assess **light touch**; whereas **joint position sense** can be tested by asking the patient (again, with closed eyes) to indicate whether the examiner is flexing or extending various joints. Another indication of impaired joint position sense is difficulty standing upright with the eyes closed, which is called **Romberg's sign**.

decussation. It is important to appreciate that in the dorsal column pathway all the second-order axons cross the midline together (in the great sensory decussation of the medulla).

Having crossed the midline, the second-order fibres turn sharply upwards and ascend to the thalamus as the **medial lemniscus**. This is a strap-like bundle which twists like a ribbon as it passes through the brain stem (Latin: lemniscus, ribbon). The medial lemniscus terminates on third-order neurons in the thalamus, which project to the **primary somatosensory cortex** in the parietal lobe.

Spinothalamic tract

The spinothalamic tract mediates pain and temperature sensations. Impulses are transmitted by small-diameter unmyelinated **c-fibres** and thinly-myelinated **A-delta** fibres which conduct impulses at relatively slow speeds of 0.5–15 metres per second. This pathway can be tested clinically using a sterile pin (Clinical Box 4.2).

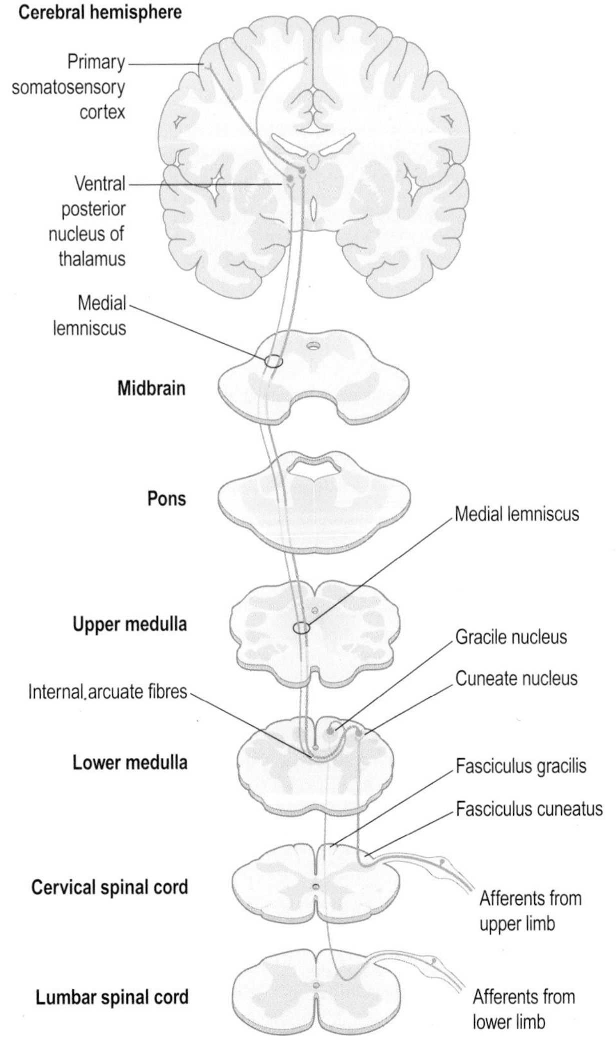

Fig. 4.4 **The dorsal column pathway.**

Clinical Box 4.2: Testing the spinothalamic tract

The best measure of spinothalamic tract integrity is appreciation of a mild **noxious stimulus**. A sterile examination pin is systematically applied to different points on the skin surface, randomly switching to the opposite (blunt) end. The patient has his or her eyes closed and is asked to say if the sensation is sharp or dull. Assessment of temperature sensitivity is impractical and is not done routinely.

Pathway to the cerebral cortex (Fig. 4.5)

The **first-order neurons** of the spinothalamic tract have their cell bodies in the **dorsal root ganglia**. The central processes enter the spinal cord where they synapse on second-order neurons in the dorsal horn.

Axons of the second-order neurons then cross the midline in the **ventral white commissure** (in the anterior spinal cord) to reach the opposite side. Having crossed over, the second-order fibres ascend in the anterolateral spinal cord as the **spinothalamic tract** and pass through the brain stem as the **spinal lemniscus**. This fibre system runs in close proximity to the medial lemniscus and also terminates on third-order neurons in the thalamus.

Finally, third-order thalamocortical fibres project to the **primary somatosensory cortex**. It is important to note that in the spinothalamic tract (in contrast to the dorsal column pathway) axons of second-order neurons can be found crossing the midline at all levels of the cord, rather than in a single sensory decussation.

The spinoreticulothalamic pathway

Some spinothalamic axons contribute to a **spinoreticular pathway** which synapses in the reticular formation of the brain stem. From here, **reticulothalamic fibres** ascend to the **intralaminar nuclei** of the thalamus before projecting on to the limbic lobe and insula, which have visceral and emotional roles including **pain perception** (Clinical Box 4.3).

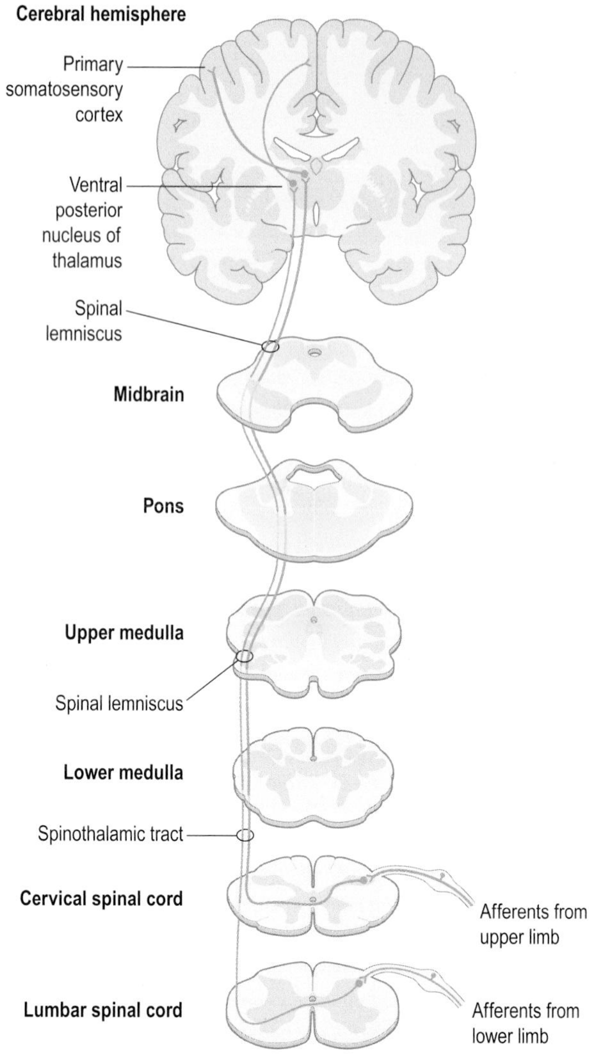

Fig. 4.5 **The spinothalamic tract.** The point at which the second order neurons cross the midline (in the anterior spinal cord) is the ventral white commissure [see text].

Key Points

- The two somatic sensory pathways have a similar organization, consisting of first-, second- and third-order neurons arranged in a linear chain.
- The first-order neurons have their cell bodies in the dorsal root ganglia and central processes that enter the spinal cord via the dorsal (sensory) root.
- Second-order neurons have their cell bodies in the CNS grey matter (brain stem or spinal cord) and give rise to axons that cross the midline, before ascending to the thalamus.
- The third-order (thalamocortical) neurons project from the ventral posterior (VP) nucleus of the thalamus to the primary somatosensory cortex in the parietal lobe.
- In the dorsal column pathway the second-order neurons are contained in the gracile and cuneate nuclei of the medulla and their axons all cross over together in the great sensory decussation.
- In the spinothalamic tract the second-order neurons are located in the dorsal horns and their axons cross the midline (at all spinal cord levels) in the ventral white commissure.

Clinical Box 4.3: Nociception versus pain

Nociception is the detection of noxious stimuli (Latin: nocēre, to harm) but its relationship to pain perception is not straightforward. For instance, soldiers injured during combat (or people involved in serious accidents) sometimes sustain devastating injuries, but feel no pain. This is termed **battleground analgesia**, which is regarded as a life-preserving anti-nociceptive mechanism. It is an example of **stimulus-induced analgesia** (another is acupuncture) and appears to rely on the release of **endogenous opiates**, which are similar to morphine. Conversely, some patients have intractable **chronic pain syndromes** with no apparent physical cause, whilst others experience pain that seems disproportionate to the degree of injury (e.g. agonising **neuropathic pain** following minor peripheral nerve damage). There is also a strong psychological element to pain perception. This is demonstrated by the **placebo effect** in which an inert substance such as a clay tablet or saline infusion can provide powerful pain relief, even in patients with serious illnesses.

Pain arising from the internal organs

The internal organs (or viscera) are insensitive to cutting and burning, but respond to stretching, twisting, inflammation and vascular compromise. Pain-related afferents from the internal organs reach the central nervous system via **visceral afferent fibres** which travel with autonomic nerves. Visceral pathology can generate three types of pain: visceral, viscerosomatic and referred.

Visceral and viscerosomatic pain

Visceral pain is diffuse, poorly localized and centred on the midline. It is often associated with autonomic features such as sweating, nausea, vomiting and pallor. In contrast, **viscerosomatic pain** is sharp and well-localized. It occurs when inflammatory exudate from a diseased organ makes contact with a somatic (body-wall) structure such as the parietal peritoneum. Abdominal pathology (e.g. appendicitis) may therefore present with diffuse visceral pain, before progressing to sharp viscerosomatic pain (Fig. 4.6).

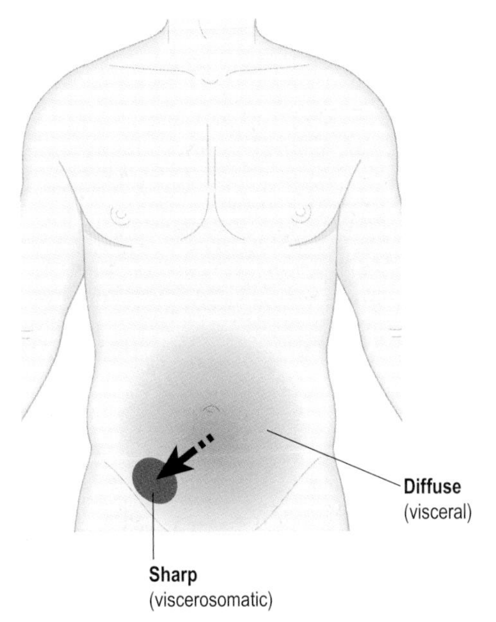

Fig. 4.6 **Visceral and viscerosomatic pain in acute appendicitis.** In the early stages of appendicitis the patient typically describes a dull, nauseating, poorly localized (visceral) pain centred on the umbilicus. As the inflammation spreads to involve the abdominal wall, a sharp (viscerosomatic) pain arises in the lower right quadrant of the abdomen, corresponding to the position of the appendix.

Referred pain

This is pain that is perceived at a distance from the affected organ (e.g. in the left arm during a myocardial infarction or in the right shoulder with inflammation of the gallbladder) (Fig. 4.7). It is thought to be due to convergence of visceral and somatic afferent fibres on **second-order spinothalamic tract neurons** so that pain of visceral origin is perceived ('misinterpreted') as somatic pain at that segmental level.

In the case of cardiac pain, visceral afferents from the heart enter the thoracic cord at T1–T5 (the origin of sympathetic innervation to the heart) and pain is referred to the corresponding dermatomes of the upper limb, with radiation to the neck and jaw. In disease of the gallbladder there may be shoulder tip (C4 dermatome) pain. This is due to the embryological descent of the liver and gallbladder from the cervical region, with retention of its original segmental nerve supply.

Sensory gating and antinociception

Sensory pathways are subject to **gating**, meaning that impulse traffic can be facilitated or inhibited by descending influences from the brain. This can occur at any synapse in a sensory pathway, including those within the dorsal horn, medulla and thalamus.

In the spinal cord, transmission of noxious signals from first-order to second-order neurons (of the spinothalamic tract) is gated in a part of the dorsal horn known as the **substantia gelatinosa**. This contains excitatory and inhibitory interneurons that influence transmission of pain-related impulses to the brain. The connections are arranged in such a way that activity in large-diameter cutaneous afferents blocks transmission in nociceptive fibres, accounting for the beneficial effect of rubbing a sore knee (Fig. 4.8).

Supraspinal influences

The **periaqueductal grey matter** (PAG) of the midbrain is involved in the supraspinal modulation of pain. Studies in non-human primates have shown that electrical stimulation of the PAG exerts a powerful **antinociceptive** (analgesic) action, blocking pain signals from the spinal cord. This is mediated by connections with the **reticular formation** and the serotonergic **raphē nuclei** of the brain stem (see Ch. 1). These **raphēspinal fibres** synapse in the substantia

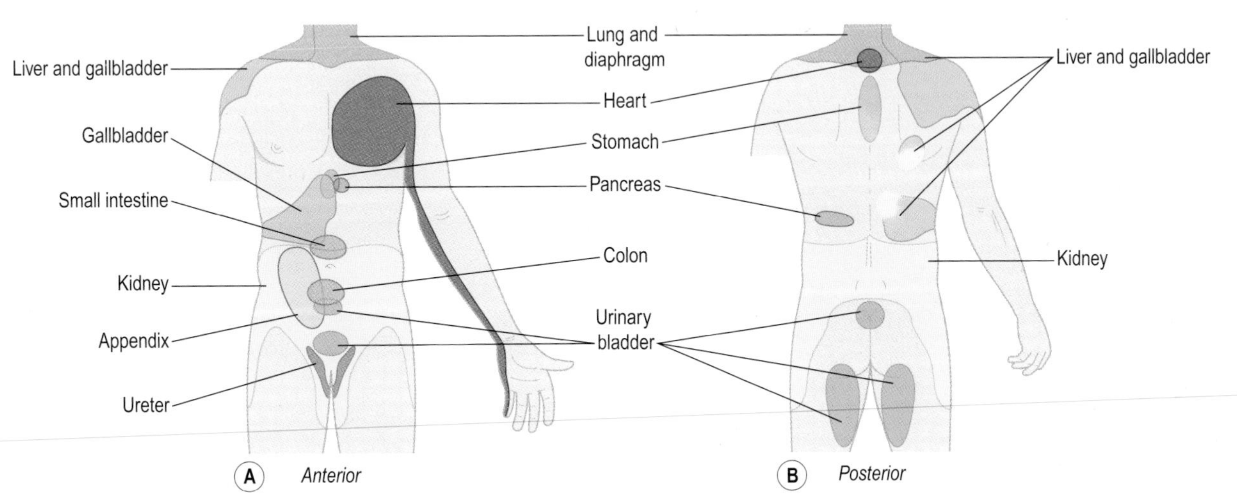

Fig. 4.7 **Common sites of referred pain viewed from (A) anterior and (B) posterior aspects.**

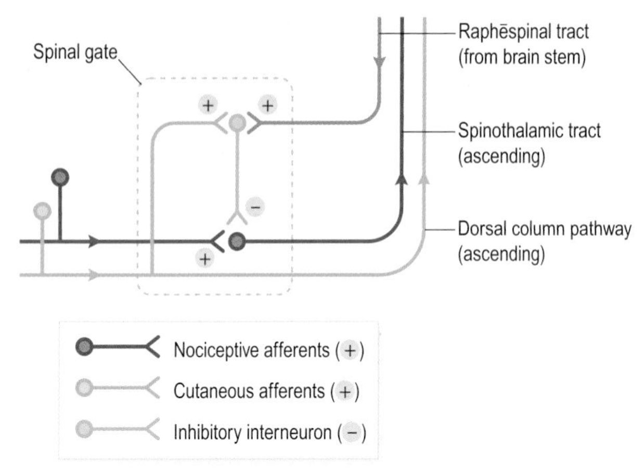

Fig. 4.8 **The concept of the spinal 'gating' mechanism.** This is a schematic to illustrate the concept that the transmission of pain-related impulses from the spinal cord to the brain can be inhibited, either by activity in large-diameter cutaneous afferents or by descending projections from the brain stem. (NB The actual synaptic connections within the substantia gelatinosa are not certain.)

gelatinosa where they inhibit synaptic transmission between first-order and second-order afferents of the spinothalamic tract (see Fig. 4.8). This partially explains why **tricyclic antidepressants** (e.g. amitriptyline) have analgesic properties, since they enhance serotonergic neurotransmission.

Trigeminothalamic pathways

In the head and neck, general somatic sensation is mediated by two analogous trigeminothalamic pathways. These transmit sensations from the territory of the **trigeminal (V) nerve** (Fig. 4.9) which is tested clinically by eliciting the corneal reflex (Fig. 4.10).

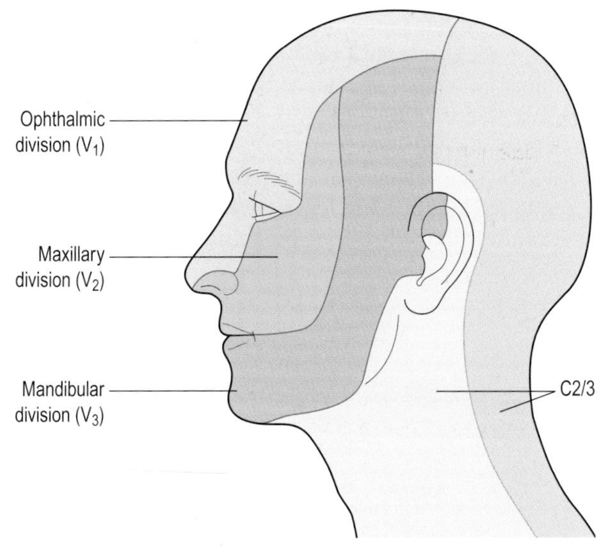

Fig. 4.9 **The three branches of the trigeminal nerve provide sensation to most of the head and neck.** The trigeminal nerve also innervates the oral and nasal cavities, paranasal air sinuses, teeth, intracranial dura and cerebral arteries.

General tactile sensation

The cell bodies of trigeminal sensory neurons are located in the **trigeminal sensory ganglion**, which is analogous to a dorsal root ganglion. The second-order neurons in the trigeminothalamic pathway are located in the **chief sensory nucleus** of the trigeminal nerve, in the pons. This gives rise to fibres that cross the midline and ascend to the thalamus in the **trigeminal lemniscus**. These axons also terminate in the ventral posterior nucleus of the thalamus, medial to those from the trunk and limbs. Third-order **thalamocortical neurons** then project to the 'face area' of the primary sensory cortex (see Ch. 3).

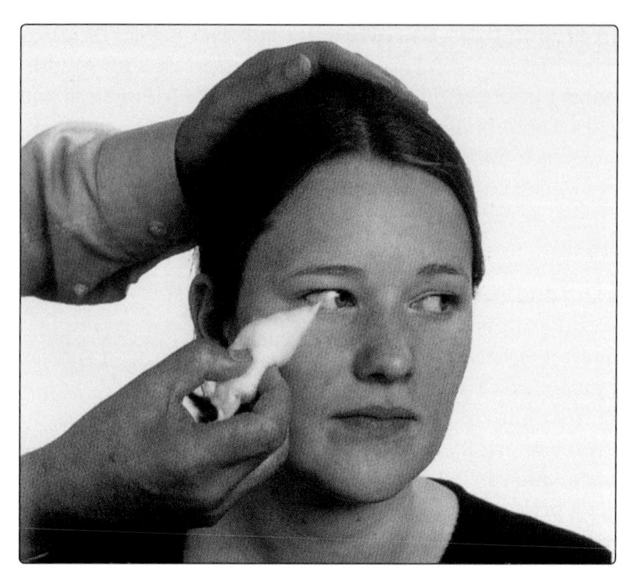

Fig. 4.10 **Testing the corneal reflex.** The cornea, which is innervated by the ophthalmic division of the trigeminal nerve, is gently touched using a wisp of cotton wool. Reflexive blinking of both eyes demonstrates that the trigeminal (sensory) and facial (motor) limbs of the reflex are intact. From Munro et al.: Macleod's Clinical Examination 10e with permission.

Pain and temperature

Pain and temperature fibres originating from the head and neck (including those mediating diverse symptoms such as headache, earache and toothache) also have their cell bodies in the trigeminal ganglion. The central processes enter the brain stem via the trigeminal nerve root (in the pons) and descend to synapse in the **spinal nucleus** of the trigeminal nerve. This is analogous to the substantia gelatinosa and is partly contained in the upper cervical cord. Axons arising from second-order neurons in the spinal nucleus cross the midline to join the trigeminal lemniscus.

Key Points

- Pain arising from the internal organs may be visceral (diffuse, central and poorly localized), viscerosomatic (sharp and well-localized) or referred.
- Referred pain is perceived at a distance from the affected organ. Impulses from visceral afferent fibres are 'misinterpreted' as somatic pain at the corresponding segmental level.
- Like other sensory projections, the central pain pathways are subject to gating. This means that supraspinal influences (from the brain) can facilitate or inhibit ascending signals.
- Pain from the head and neck region is transmitted from the territory of the trigeminal nerve via the trigeminothalamic system.
- The second-order neurons have their cell bodies in the spinal nucleus of the trigeminal nerve, which is analogous to the substantia gelatinosa in the dorsal horn of the spinal cord.

Somatic motor pathways

The control of voluntary movement is complex and incompletely understood, with contributions from several brain regions (see Ch. 3). The **prefrontal cortex**, which lies anterior to the motor and premotor areas of the frontal lobe, is involved in planning and organization of goal-directed behaviour. The **premotor cortex** is concerned with the preparation and execution of complex movement sequences, whereas the **primary motor cortex** has a more direct influence over individual muscle groups.

The **primary motor pathway** has two components. The **corticospinal tract** originates in the motor and premotor areas of the frontal lobe and projects to the spinal cord to control the limb and trunk muscles. The **corticobulbar pathway** also originates in the motor and premotor cortex but only descends as far as the brain stem, where it influences the cranial nerve motor nuclei. The primary motor pathway is also referred to as the **pyramidal motor system** (or **pyramidal tract**) because the corticospinal tract passes through the pyramids of the medulla. Interruption of the pyramidal tract causes weakness or paralysis.

Corticospinal tract

The corticospinal tract is the principal **somatic motor pathway** and the longest continuous white matter tract in the CNS. It is particularly important for finely-fractionated voluntary movements of the distal limb musculature (e.g. control of the hands). The corticospinal tract is composed of more than a million myelinated axons on each side, two thirds of which arise from the primary motor and premotor areas of the frontal lobe (Fig. 4.11).

The remaining third of fibres originate from the **primary somatosensory cortex** in the parietal lobe and synapse in the dorsal (sensory) horn of the spinal cord. This part of the corticospinal pathway is not directly involved in movement initiation, but is thought to be important for 'filtering out' the barrage of proprioceptive and other sensory information generated by complex movements. By predicting and filtering out these afferent impulses, the brain is able to increase the 'signal-to-noise' ratio and focus on more important or unexpected sensory feedback.

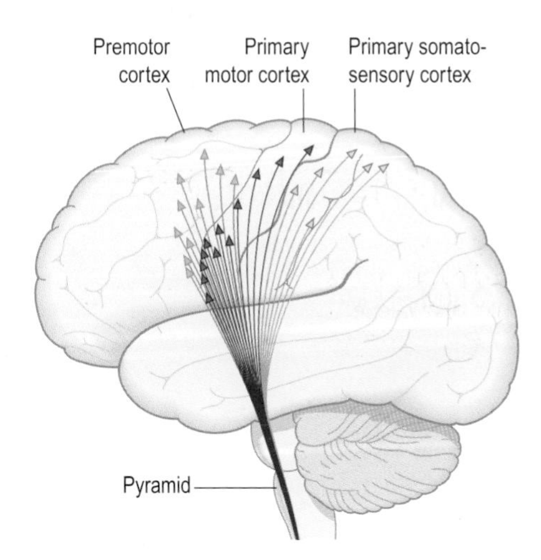

Fig. 4.11 **Origins of the primary motor (pyramidal) pathway.** This consists of the corticospinal tract (supplying the trunk and limbs) and the corticobulbar tract (for the cranial nerve motor nuclei). Modified from Fitzgerald: Clinical Neuroanatomy and Neuroscience 5e (2006) with permission.

Origin, course and destination (Fig. 4.12)

Corticospinal tract axons leave the cerebral cortex to enter the subcortical white matter, passing through the posterior limb of the **internal capsule** to reach the **crus cerebri** in the anterior midbrain.

Having traversed the crus cerebri and **basilar pons**, the corticospinal fibres enter the medulla where they occupy the anterior midline as the **pyramids**. At the lower border of the medulla, 75–90% of the pyramidal fibres decussate to enter the contralateral half of the spinal cord.

The pathway continues as the **lateral corticospinal tract**, which predominantly supplies the distal limb musculature (particularly the flexor groups). The 10–25% of uncrossed fibres are a direct continuation of the medullary pyramids. They therefore descend in the anterior part of the spinal cord on either side of the midline (as the **anterior corticospinal tract**). Many of these fibres eventually decussate and chiefly innervate the proximal and axial musculature (particularly the extensor groups).

Only a small proportion of corticospinal tract axons make direct synaptic contact with spinal motor neurons (mainly those supplying the intrinsic muscles of the hands). The majority terminate on **interneuronal pools** which influence spinal motor neurons indirectly.

Corticobulbar tract

The corticobulbar tract arises in the cerebral cortex and projects to the brain stem (the word 'bulb' is an archaic term for the lower brain stem). The projections arise mainly from

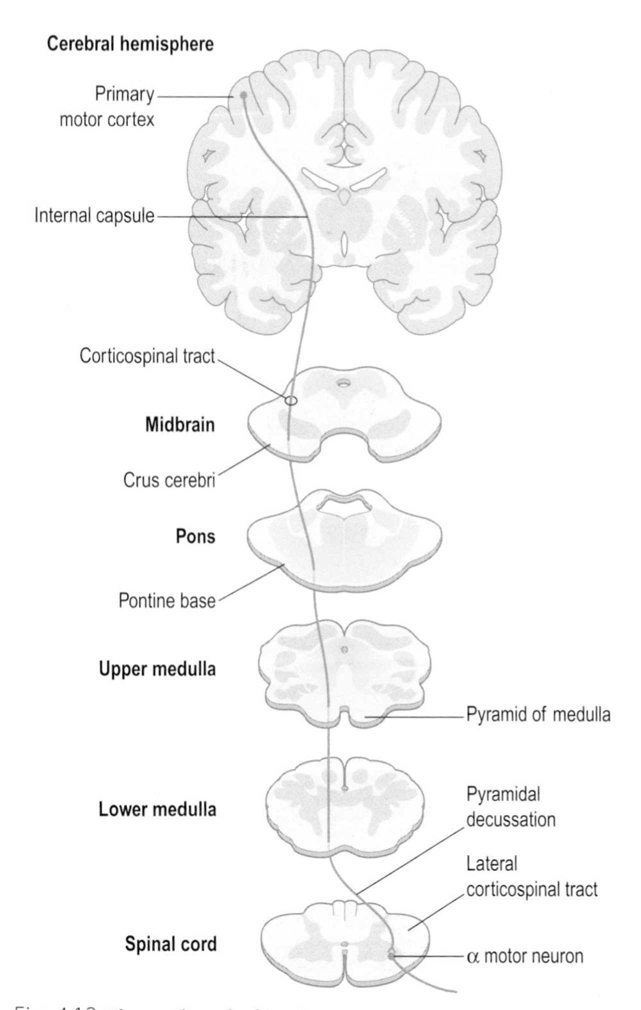

Fig. 4.12 **The corticospinal tract.**

the 'face' and 'tongue' areas of the primary motor and premotor cortices. The corticobulbar (or **corticonuclear**) projections accompany the corticospinal tract as far as the brain stem. They pass in turn through the subcortical white matter and internal capsule to reach the **crus cerebri** of the midbrain where they lie just medial to the corticospinal fibres.

Termination of corticobulbar fibres

Fibres from the corticobulbar projection part company with the corticospinal tract as they descend in the brain stem and gradually 'peel off' to reach their target nuclei. The corticobulbar tract projects directly to four **motor cranial nerve nuclei** in the pons and medulla, controlling muscles that: (i) are attached to the lower jaw, including those involved in chewing; (ii) are involved in facial expression; (iii) mediate speech, swallowing and the efferent limb of the 'gag' reflex (see Clinical Box 4.4); and (iv) control the tongue.

Voluntary eye movements are initiated by the **frontal eye fields** (see Ch. 3). These project to **vertical** and **lateral gaze centres** in the midbrain and pons, via the anterior limb of the internal capsule. The brain stem gaze centres then influence the cranial nerve nuclei innervating the extraocular muscles.

Decussation of bulbar fibres

Most of the **cranial nerve motor nuclei** receive projections from *both* cerebral hemispheres, so that damage on one side of the brain tends not to cause contralateral bulbar weakness. Exceptions are the cortical projections controlling the tongue and the lower part of the face, which arise mainly from the opposite motor cortex. This explains why isolated *lower* facial paralysis sometimes occurs after a stroke (the upper part of the face is spared since it is also controlled by the opposite cerebral hemisphere).

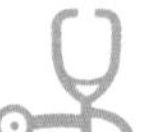

Clinical Box 4.4: The gag reflex

To test this reflex (e.g. during a routine neurological examination) a wooden tongue depressor is used to touch the **posterior pharyngeal wall** on each side. The normal response is a 'gag', with elevation of the soft palate and uvula. The afferent (sensory) limb is subserved by the **glossopharyngeal (IX) nerve** which supplies sensation to the pharynx and posterior tongue. The efferent (motor) limb is mediated by the **vagus (X) nerve** which supplies the muscles of the larynx and pharynx.

Key Points

- The primary motor (pyramidal) pathway consists of the corticospinal and corticobulbar tracts which mainly originate from the motor and premotor areas of the frontal lobe.
- The corticospinal tract descends through the internal capsule, crus cerebri of the midbrain, basilar pons and medullary pyramids.
- At the lower border of the medulla, 75–90% of corticospinal tract fibres cross the midline to enter the lateral corticospinal tract of the spinal cord.
- The corticobulbar pathway accompanies the corticospinal fibres as far as the brain stem before peeling off to innervate the cranial nerve motor nuclei (bilaterally in most cases).

Lower motor neurons

The term **lower motor neuron** is used clinically to describe the motor neurons of the spinal cord and brain stem that innervate the skeletal musculature. In contrast, the term **upper motor neuron** refers to corticospinal and corticobulbar tract neurons which have their cell bodies in the motor cortex of the frontal lobe.

Lower motor neurons of the spinal cord have their cell bodies in the anterior horns and are therefore also called **anterior horn cells**. The alternative term **alpha motoneuron** reflects their large-diameter A-alpha axons, which conduct nerve impulses at high speeds. The lower motor neuron is described as the 'final common pathway' since it is the route by which all motor activity (both voluntary and reflexive) is initiated.

Motor units and graded contraction

A **motor unit** consists of a single anterior horn cell and the squad of muscle fibres that it supplies. Motor units operate in an 'all-or-none' fashion so that muscle contraction can only be **graded** by the recruitment of whole numbers of motor units. Muscles capable of precise, finely-fractionated movements therefore have small motor units. Those that supply the intrinsic muscles of the hand typically have fewer than 10 muscle fibres, whereas the motor units of the limb-girdle and axial muscles may be composed of 1000 fibres or more.

In order to increase the force of contraction in a muscle, motor units are gradually recruited according to the **size principle**. This refers to the fact that small motor units (commanding fewer muscle fibres) are recruited before larger ones. This happens automatically since small neurons are more easily depolarized and means that movements requiring minimal force can be more finely graded.

The neuromuscular junction

The point of contact between lower motor neurons and skeletal muscle is the **neuromuscular junction (NMJ)** which is similar in structure to a synapse (Fig. 4.13). The transmitter is **acetylcholine (ACh)** which acts on nicotinic ACh receptors. The NMJ is 'fail-safe', meaning that 100% of

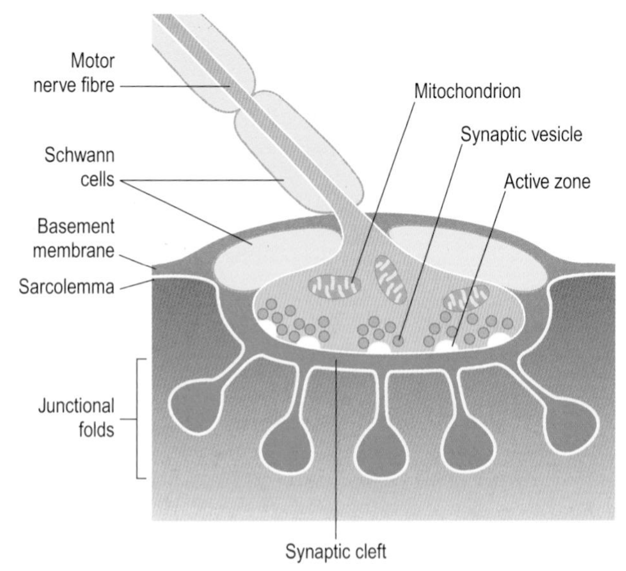

Fig. 4.13 **The neuromuscular junction (motor end plate).**

nerve impulses generated in a lower motor neuron will trigger a **muscle twitch**. Neuromuscular transmission is impaired in the autoimmune disorder **myasthenia gravis** (Clinical Box 4.5).

Clinical Box 4.5: Myasthenia gravis

This is a rare **autoimmune disease** caused by autoantibodies to the nicotinic acetylcholine receptor at the neuromuscular junction. It is characterized by **fatigable weakness**, meaning that symptoms worsen with use and improve with rest. It is more common in females and approximately three-quarters of patients have an abnormality of the **thymus gland**. This is most often **thymic hyperplasia** (increase in the size and activity of the gland) but in 10% of cases there is a benign tumour called a **thymoma**. Although myasthenia gravis cannot be cured, it can be managed using agents that (i) block degradation of acetylcholine or (ii) suppress the autoimmune response.

Key Points

- Lower motor neurons (with cell bodies in the anterior horn of the spinal cord or cranial nerve motor nuclei) represent the 'final common pathway' by which all movements are mediated.
- Axons of lower motor neurons travel in peripheral nerves and make contact with skeletal muscle at the neuromuscular junction, which uses the neurotransmitter acetylcholine.
- A lower motor neuron and the squad of muscle fibres that it innervates constitutes a motor unit. Dextrous muscles (e.g. those of the hands) have smaller motor units.
- Muscle contractions are graded by the recruitment of motor units according to the size principle: small motor neurons (commanding fewer muscle fibres) are recruited before larger ones.

Reflexes and muscle tone

A reflex is a stereotyped motor response to a particular stimulus that may vary in latency, duration or amplitude. The simplest type is **monosynaptic** and is composed of a single afferent neuron, a single efferent neuron and an intervening synapse. Some reflexes are **polysynaptic** and may extend over several spinal segments to produce more complex responses.

Muscle tone

Muscles exhibit a degree of **rest tone** which helps maintain normal posture and joint stability. This can be appreciated on clinical examination as mild resistance to passive joint flexion and extension. Rest tone is not an intrinsic property of muscle but is mediated by the **stretch reflex**. This is a simple monosynaptic reflex which enables muscles to contract automatically in response to being stretched, thereby resisting passive changes in length.

The stretch reflex

The afferent limb of the stretch reflex originates from proprioceptive organs called **muscle spindles** (Fig. 4.14). These are roughly the same size and shape as a grain of rice and are scattered throughout the skeletal musculature. They contain striated muscle within a spindle-shaped (fusiform) connective tissue capsule. Muscle fibres inside the spindle are referred to as **intrafusal**, whereas those making up the bulk of the muscle are **extrafusal**. Muscle spindles are in parallel with extrafusal fibres, so that any tension applied to the long axis of the muscle will stretch both types of fibre.

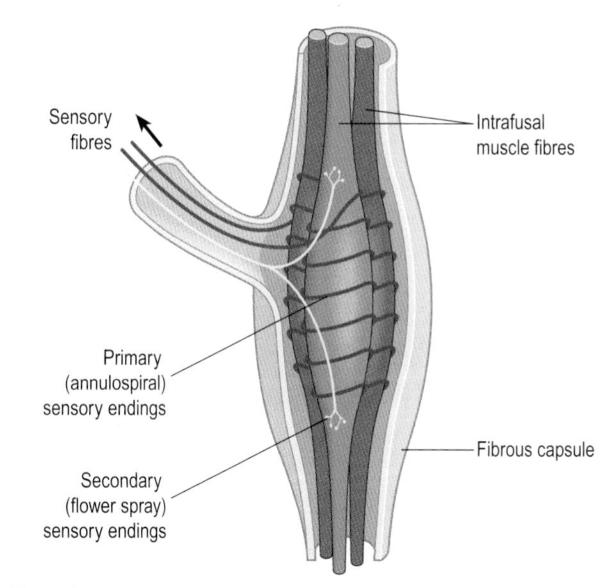

Fig. 4.14 **The muscle spindle.**

Muscle spindles are richly innervated by mechanosensitive nerve endings which terminate in the non-contractile central portion of the fibres. These nerve endings are exquisitely sensitive to changes in muscle fibre length, particularly the **rate of change of length**. A short, sharp stretch is therefore a better stimulus than sustained tension.

Afferent fibres enter the dorsal roots of the spinal nerves, then synapse directly on anterior horn cells innervating the **homonymous** (same) muscle group (Fig. 4.15). In addition, collateral fibres make synaptic connections with motor neurons supplying antagonistic muscle groups via **inhibitory interneurons**. The stretch reflex is fundamentally important in clinical neurology because it is responsible for muscle tone and tendon reflexes (Clinical Box 4.6).

The gamma loop

Intrafusal muscle fibres have a separate motor innervation that arises from **gamma motoneurons** (also located in the anterior horn). These neurons **co-activate** with alpha motoneurons to ensure that the intrafusal fibres remain under tension (do not become slack) when muscles contract, so that stretch-sensitivity is maintained during movements.

Long-latency stretch reflex

Electrical recordings from muscle show that the stretch reflex has two components. There is an early, **short-latency component** that occurs within 25–40 milliseconds, consistent with a monosynaptic reflex. A **long-latency component** can also be recorded at around 50–75 milliseconds, which probably involves the cerebral cortex. Over-activity in the 'long-loop component' of the stretch reflex may be responsible for the characteristic **rigidity** (increased muscle tone) in **Parkinson's disease** (Ch. 13).

Hypertonia and spasticity

Sensitivity of the stretch reflex is regulated by the brain to ensure normal muscle tone. Descending **reticulospinal**

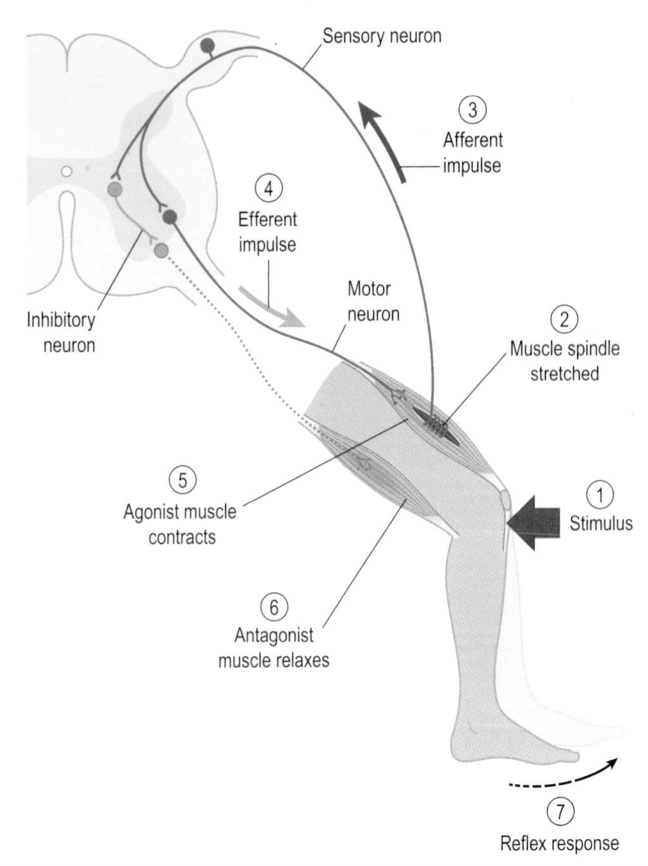

Fig. 4.15 **The stretch reflex.**

Clinical Box 4.6: Tendon reflexes

Tendon reflexes are elicited by striking a tendon with a patellar hammer. This stretches the muscle and triggers a volley of afferent impulses from its muscle spindles. **Reflexive contraction** of the muscle is combined with **reciprocal inhibition** of its antagonists, seen as a brief 'jerk' of the limb (e.g. knee extension after striking the patellar tendon). Abnormal reflexes help to localize lesions to a particular spinal root level (e.g. biceps reflex: C5/C6; patellar reflex: L3/L4). Increase in the speed or amplitude of a reflex is termed **hyperreflexia** and the response is described as **brisk**. A reduced (or absent) response is referred to as **hyporeflexia** (or **areflexia**). It is normal for reflexes to vary from person to person, but asymmetry is usually a sign of pathology.

projections (from the reticular formation of the brain stem) inhibit spinal motor neurons and 'damp down' the stretch reflex to optimize muscle tone. This influence is usually lost following an **upper motor neuron lesion** (by an uncertain mechanism) which results in hyperactivity of the stretch reflex (Clinical Box 4.7).

Spasticity

A marked increase in muscle tone is called **spasticity** (Fig. 4.16), characterized by firm resistance to passive manipulation of the limbs. It is velocity-dependent, so that rapid flexion or extension of the affected joints is met by an abrupt 'spastic catch' (similar to the resistance felt when pulling sharply on a car seatbelt). Spasticity can be overcome

Clinical Box 4.7: Upper and lower motor neuron lesions

In an **upper motor neuron** (**UMN**) lesion such as a stroke, weakness is associated with features that reflect hyperexcitability of the stretch reflex. These include hypertonia, hyperreflexia and spasticity, with clasp-knife rigidity. The typical clinical features take several days to evolve and are preceded by an initial period of **flaccid paralysis** (perhaps due to loss of descending excitatory projections from the cortex, followed by a subsequent increase in lower motor neuron sensitivity). In a **lower motor neuron** (**LMN**) lesion such as a peripheral nerve injury, there is partial or complete denervation of the affected muscles. This leads to weakness, wasting and areflexia (or flaccid paralysis in severe cases). Visible muscle twitches called **fasciculations** may also be seen, caused by random spontaneous discharge of individual motor units.

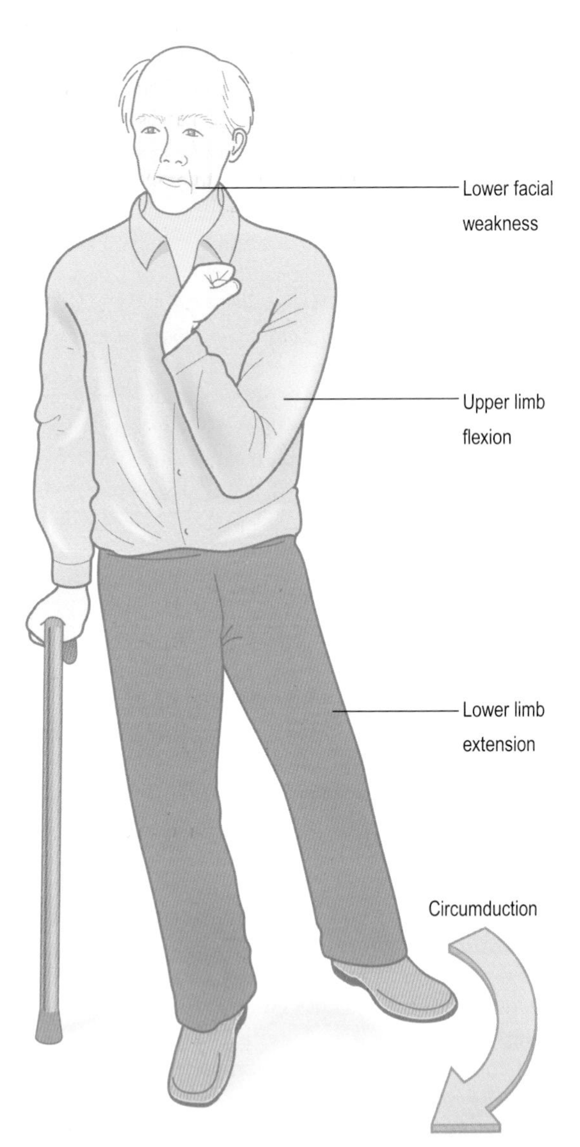

Fig. 4.16 **A typical spastic posture (or 'pyramidal pattern' of weakness).** The patient illustrated has suffered a large right hemisphere stroke leading to weakness and spasticity affecting the left side of his body. In the upper limbs, flexion dominates since the upper limb flexors are stronger than the extensors, reflecting their functional importance (e.g. for reaching and grasping). The lower limb is extended and rigid, reflecting the greater power of the extensor (antigravity) muscles.

by force so that the joint suddenly 'gives way' (the **clasp-knife phenomenon**). This is a safety mechanism that prevents tendon rupture due to excessive load. Spasticity is usually accompanied by an abnormal **plantar response** (Clinical Box 4.8). A combination of upper motor neuron features, together with lower motor neuron signs, is seen classically in **motor neuron disease** (Clinical Box 4.9).

The flexor reflex

A noxious stimulus to the sole of the foot triggers automatic limb withdrawal, mediated by the polysynaptic **flexor reflex**. Nociceptive afferents from the sole of the foot enter the lumbosacral spinal cord and divide to make collateral connections. Excitation of anterior horn cells innervating the flexor muscles of the lower limb is combined with inhibition of muscles in the extensor compartment (mediated by **inhibitory interneurons**). The flexor reflex is coupled to a **crossed extensor reflex** which causes simultaneous extension of the contralateral limb to support the body weight. The spinal cord connections mediating these reflexes provide the basic pattern for **locomotion** (alternating flexion in one limb and extension in the other).

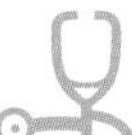

Clinical Box 4.8: The plantar response

The plantar response is a **cutaneous reflex** elicited by firmly stroking the sole of the foot. In normal adults this produces plantarflexion (downward movement) of the great toe. Dorsiflexion ('**upgoing plantars**') is an abnormal response referred to as **Babinski's sign** (Fig. 4.17). An abnormal plantar response is suggestive of an upper motor neuron lesion, but the anatomical basis is obscure. It is an example of a **primitive reflex** that is present in all healthy newborns, but usually disappears by about two years of age.

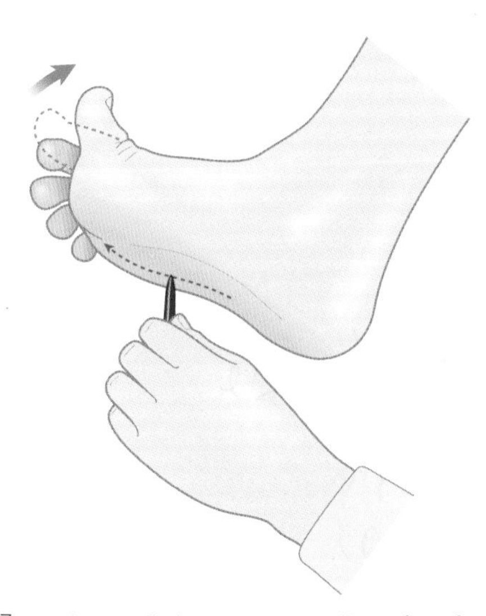

Fig. 4.17 **An abnormal plantar response ('upgoing plantars') is called Babinski's sign.** It is important to watch for the *first* movement of the great toe and not to misinterpret a withdrawal response as abnormal, particularly in patients with sensitive feet.

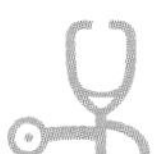

Clinical Box 4.9: Motor neuron disease

Motor neuron disease (**MND**) is a progressive and incurable neurological disorder of unknown cause, with a lifetime prevalence of around 1 in 400. It usually occurs in people over the age of 50 and two thirds of patients are male. Typical early features include clumsiness, muscle cramps and **fasciculations** in the limbs and trunk, progressing to widespread paralysis. About 25% of patients present with bulbar (cranial nerve) weakness which carries a less favourable prognosis. The characteristic examination finding is a combination of both upper and lower motor neuron signs in multiple limbs. The mean survival is around 3–4 years and death is usually due to pneumonia or respiratory failure. MND is also referred to as **amyotrophic lateral sclerosis** (**ALS**), particularly in the USA. This describes the combination of muscle wasting (amyotrophy) and degeneration of the lateral corticospinal tracts (lateral sclerosis). Dementia occurs in 5% of patients due to an overlap between the pathology of MND and **frontotemporal dementia** (Ch. 12).

Key Points

- A reflex is a stereotyped motor response to a particular stimulus that may vary in latency, duration and amplitude.
- The stretch reflex contributes to normal muscle tone. Passive stretch stimulates muscle spindles, causing reflexive contraction of the homonymous (same) muscle group together with relaxation of the antagonists.
- Activity in the stretch reflex is normally 'damped down' by a descending influence from the brain stem which helps to to prevent excessive muscle tone. This is lost in upper motor neuron lesions, resulting in hyperexcitability of the stretch reflex.
- Upper motor neuron lesions are therefore characterized by increased tone, hyperreflexia, spasticity and clasp-knife rigidity (together with loss of muscle strength).
- The features of lower motor neuron lesions reflect denervation of the muscle and include weakness, wasting and fasciculations, with depressed or absent tendon reflexes.

Chapter 5
Neurons and glial cells

CHAPTER CONTENTS

Nerve cells

The basic structure of the neuron has been outlined in Chapter 1. It was also shown how nerve cells can be classified based upon the type of information that they transmit (afferent, efferent, interneuron) or by the number of processes that they have (unipolar, bipolar, multipolar). Neuronal excitability, impulse conduction and synaptic transmission are discussed in Chapters 6 and 7.

Cortical neurons

The cerebral cortex contains more than 50 billion neurons arranged in horizontal layers or **laminae**. Although cortical neurons vary enormously in size and shape, there are two major types (discussed below).

Pyramidal and granule cells (Fig. 5.1A & B)

Pyramidal cells have large, pyramid-shaped cell bodies that range from 20–120 µm in diameter. They are excitatory neurons that have numerous apical and basal dendrites and a single axon that projects out of the cortex. Pyramidal cells are particularly prominent in motor and premotor areas. **Granule cells** (or **stellate cells**) are star-shaped multipolar neurons that have short axons and make local synaptic contacts, tending to be enriched in sensory cortices. They are much smaller than pyramidal cells, with a typical diameter of less than 20 µm, and may be excitatory or inhibitory. The cerebellar cortex also contains two main types of nerve cell: granule cells (similar to those in the cerebral cortex) and **Purkinje cells** (large efferent neurons, equivalent to cortical pyramidal cells; see Fig. 5.1C).

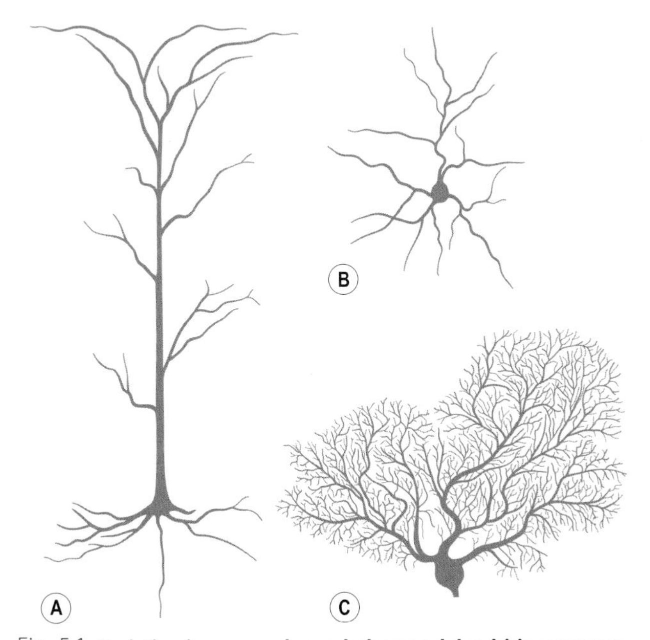

Fig. 5.1 **Variation in neuronal morphology and dendritic processes**, illustrated by **(A)** a cortical pyramidal neuron, **(B)** a granule cell and **(C)** a cerebellar Purkinje cell [not drawn to scale].

Cortical lamination

More than 90% of the cerebral cortex has a characteristic six-layered structure that appeared with the evolution of the mammalian brain (Fig. 5.2). For this reason it is referred to as **neocortex** (Greek: neos, new). Although the same six layers can be identified in all neocortical regions at some stage of development, they are not always present in the mature brain. For instance, the motor and premotor areas of the frontal neocortex are referred to as **agranular cortex** since they have lost their internal granule cell layer.

Different types of cortex

The cerebral cortex can be divided into more than fifty **Brodmann areas** based on subtle differences in the cortical structure (referred to as **cytoarchitectonics**) but there are three major cortical types (Fig. 5.3):

- The **isocortex** has a uniform six-layered structure (Greek: isos, equal) and accounts for more than 90% of the cortical surface area. This term is synonymous with **neocortex**.
- The **allocortex** is thinner and has a more primitive, three-layered structure (Greek: allos, other). It includes the archicortex (hippocampus) and paleocortex (primary olfactory areas).
- The **mesocortex** is a transitional zone between the allocortex and isocortex and has 3–6 layers. Most of the limbic lobe (cingulate and parahippocampal gyri; see Ch. 3) is composed of mesocortex.

The majority of the 'non-neocortical' regions belong to the **limbic lobe** and are primarily concerned with emotion, memory and olfaction (the sense of smell). The term **paralimbic cortex** is used to describe non-neocortical regions outside of the limbic lobe proper, including the posterior orbital cortex, anterior insula and temporal pole.

Features of the neuron

Nerve cells have many features in common with other cells, together with a number of unique structural and functional components.

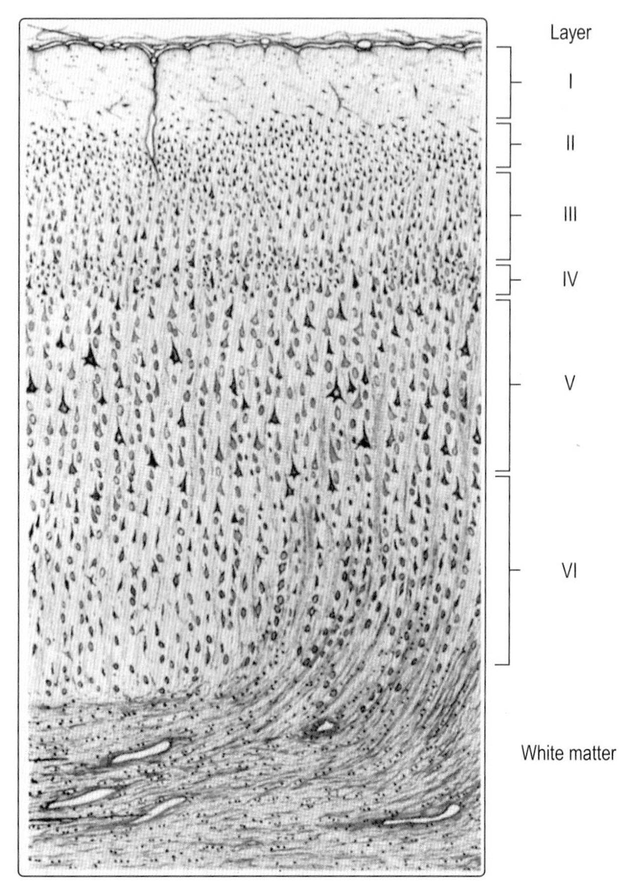

Fig. 5.2 **Structure of the cerebral cortex.** At least 90% of the cortex has six identifiable layers and is classified as neocortex. Small (granular) cells predominate in laminae that receive afferent projections, whereas large (pyramidal) cells are more numerous in layers that give rise to efferent projections. [For instance: lamina IV, the internal granule cell layer, receives projections from the thalamus; lamina V, the internal pyramidal cell layer, is the origin of projections to the brain stem and spinal cord.] From Crossman: Neuroanatomy ICT 4e (Churchill Livingstone 2010) with permission.

Isocortex (neocortex)	6 layers	90% of cerebral hemisphere (sensory, motor and association areas)
Mesocortex (periallocortex, proisocortex)	3–6 layers	Majority of limbic lobe (e.g. cingulate/parahippocampal gyri)
Allocortex	3 layers	Hippocampal formation (archicortex) Primary olfactory areas (paleocortex)

Fig. 5.3 **Different cortical types.** The two main types are isocortex (= neocortex) and allocortex. The mesocortex occupies a 'transitional zone' that lies between the six-layered isocortex and the three-layered allocortex. It has a variable number of layers and can be further subdivided into proisocortex and periallocortex, based on its similarity to the two main types.

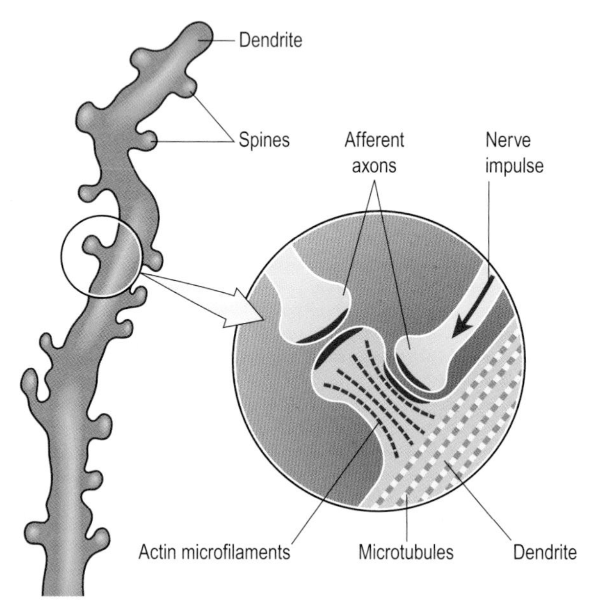

Fig. 5.4 **Dendritic spines.**

Key Points

- The two main types of cortical neuron are granular (small cells that are common in sensory areas) and pyramidal (large cells that are prominent in motor areas). The cerebellar cortex contains Purkinje cells (similar to cortical pyramidal neurons) and granule cells.
- Two major types of cortex (isocortex and allocortex) can be identified, based on microscopic differences in the pattern of lamination and cellular architecture (cytoarchitecture).
- The isocortex (= neocortex) has the same six identifiable layers and makes up 90% of the cortical mantle, including all the major sensory, motor and association areas.
- The allocortex is thinner (3-layered) and includes the hippocampus (archicortex) and primary olfactory areas (paleocortex).
- The 'transitional zone' between the allocortex and isocortex is called mesocortex. It has between 3 and 6 layers and includes the cingulate and parahippocampal gyri.
- The non-neocortical areas (allocortex and mesocortex) have visceral and emotional roles and most of these regions are contained within the limbic lobe or primary olfactory areas.

Dendritic spines

The dendrites of many neurons are studded with thousands of tiny, mushroom-shaped **dendritic spines** (Fig. 5.4). These include the **medium spiny neurons** that make up 95% of cells in the basal ganglia. In the cerebral cortex, all pyramidal cells have dendritic spines, whereas stellate cells may be spiny or smooth. Each **dendritic spine** is the site of an incoming excitatory synapse and a typical cortical pyramidal neuron has more than 10,000 spines. They are dynamic structures that can form, change shape or disappear altogether and are thought to be important in **synaptic plasticity** (Greek: plastikos, able to be moulded) and learning. Long-term memories may be mediated by the growth of new spines or the strengthening and enlargement of existing ones.

Subcellular organelles

The neuronal cell body or **soma** (Greek: soma, body) contains the same organelles found in other cell types (Fig. 5.5) but the machinery for protein synthesis and gene transcription is particularly prominent (Fig. 5.6A). The perinuclear cytoplasm or **perikaryon** (Greek: peri, around; cyton, kernel) contains a well-developed network of rough endoplasmic reticulum, often arranged in clumps called **Nissl bodies**. The Golgi apparatus is also prominent and is the site of post-translational modification and sorting of proteins including ion channels, neurotransmitter receptors and membrane ion pumps.

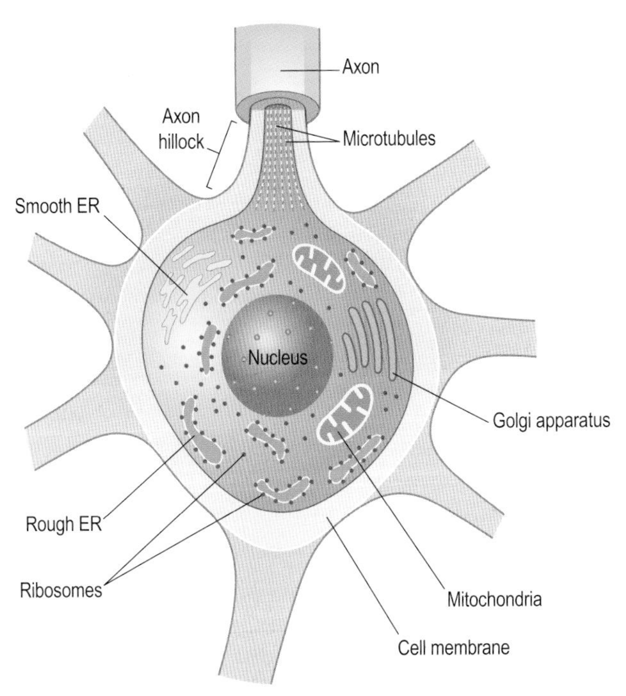

Fig. 5.5 **Some of the major subcellular organelles of the neuron.**

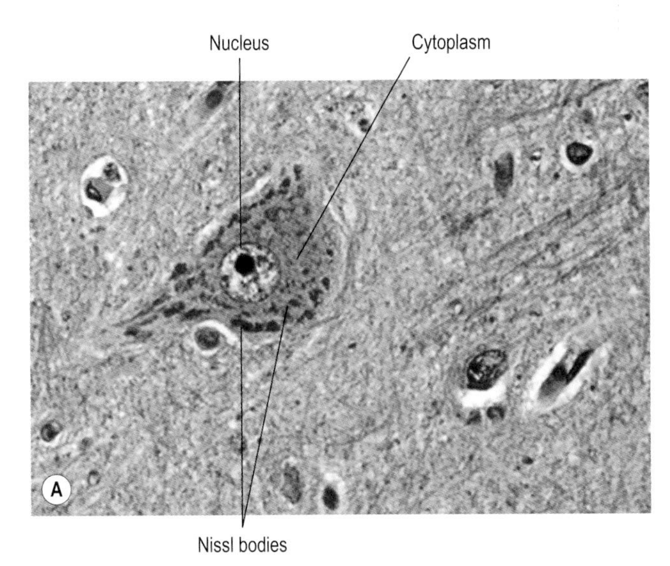

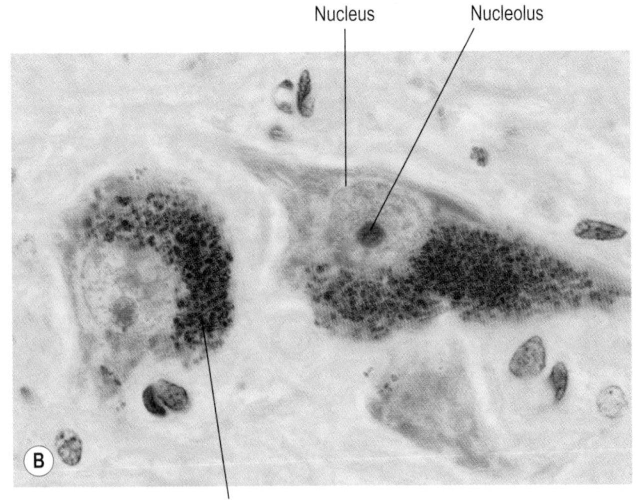

Fig. 5.6 **Cytological features of nerve cells. (A)** Micrograph showing a pyramidal motor neuron in the cerebral cortex of the frontal lobe. It has a large nucleus with a well-defined nuclear envelope and prominent central nucleolus. The cytoplasm (stained pink) contains coarse clumps of rough endoplasmic reticulum (stained blue); these structures are referred to as Nissl bodies. [Routine haematoxylin and eosin (H&E)-stained sections.] From Prayson, Richard: Neuropathology 1e (Churchill Livingstone 2005) with permission; **(B)** Micrograph of two pigmented dopaminergic neurons in the substantia nigra of the midbrain (Nissl stain). The pigment is neuromelanin and is produced as a by-product of dopamine synthesis. From Standring: Gray's Anatomy 40e (Churchill Livingstone 2008) with permission.

Lipofuscin and neuromelanin

Neurons have a high rate of membrane turnover and gradually accumulate non-digestible membrane components within lysosomal **residual bodies**. These contain golden-brown material called **lipofuscin** (pronounced: lipo-FUSKIN). This so-called 'age pigment' accumulates over time as a by-product of membrane turnover and is also abundant in the heart and liver. Catecholamine-synthesizing neurons contain the dark brown pigment **neuromelanin** (Fig. 5.6B); these include the **substantia nigra** of the midbrain and the **locus coeruleus** of the pons (see Ch. 1).

Vesicles

Neurons contain various types of membrane-bound vesicle. Neurotransmitters and neuropeptides are stored in the axon terminal (prior to release) within **synaptic vesicles** (see Ch. 7). **Coated vesicles** are derived from internalization of membrane constituents and macromolecules that have been taken up from the extracellular fluid by receptor-mediated endocytosis.

The neuronal cytoskeleton

All cells have a **cytoskeleton** composed of an internal framework of fibrillar proteins, that gives each cell its characteristic shape. This molecular scaffold is particularly important in **process-bearing cells** such as neurons and glia, which have a complex structure. The cytoskeleton is also involved in the transport of materials between intracellular compartments (see below). The main components include microtubules, neurofilaments and microfilaments (Fig. 5.7).

Microtubules

Microtubules are tubular polymeric proteins that are composed of repeating subunits of **alpha** and **beta tubulin**. They are 24 nm in diameter and up to 1 mm in length. Some microtubules are stable, whereas others are dynamic and can grow or shrink by the addition or removal of tubulin subunits. Microtubules are polarized. The part that is closest to the neuronal cell body is arbitrarily termed the minus (−) end and that which is nearer to the axon terminal is designated the plus (+) end. Microtubules are stabilized by binding to a range of **microtubule associated proteins (MAPs)**. These include the phosphoprotein **tau** which accumulates in various degenerative conditions including **Alzheimer's disease** (Ch. 12).

Neurofilaments

Neurofilaments are twisted protein strands of approximately 10 nm diameter and variable length. They are part of the large family of **intermediate filaments**. There are three neurofilament subunits or chains that differ in molecular weight: **light** (**NF-L**), **medium** (**NF-M**) and **heavy** (**NF-H**). These subunits form dimers, each with the NF-L subunit. After dimerisation they assemble in pairs to form

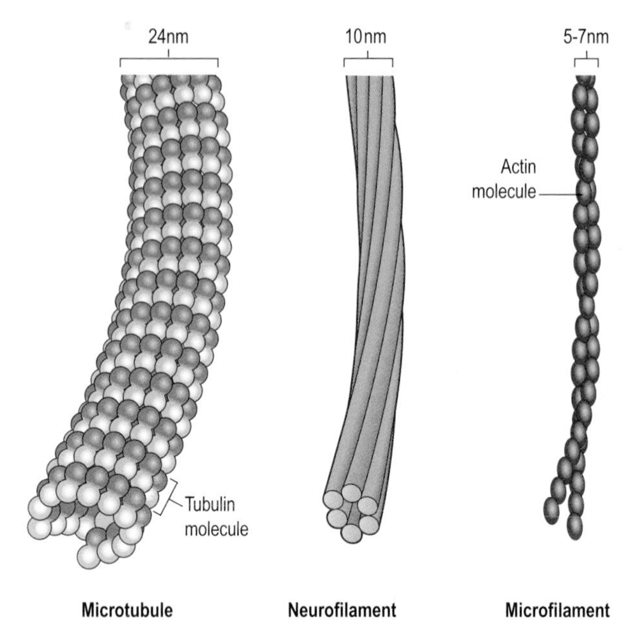

Fig. 5.7 **Components of the neuronal cytoskeleton.**

biochemically stable tetramers. Neurofilaments have negatively charged side-arms that limit their packing density and are arranged at right angles to the long axis of the axon, helping to determine its calibre.

Microfilaments

The neuron also contains a network of microfilaments that is particularly well-developed immediately beneath the plasma membrane as the **cortical cytoskeleton**. Microfilaments are a family of double-stranded fibrillar proteins that are around 5–7 nm in diameter and up to 800 nm in length. One of the most important members is the contractile protein **actin**. The cortical cytoskeleton interacts with membrane-associated and integral membrane proteins (e.g. receptors and ion channels) and helps to create localized 'domains' within the plasma membrane. In addition, the cortical cytoskeleton is anchored to the extracellular matrix via transmembrane **linkage proteins**.

Axonal transport

The biological machinery for protein synthesis (in the neuronal cell body) may be quite a distance from the axon terminal. For this reason, the neuron has a **fast axonal transport** mechanism for membrane-bound materials and organelles:

- **Anterograde** fast axonal transport carries mitochondria and vesicles (e.g. enzymes for neurotransmitter synthesis) towards the axon terminal. The maximum speed is 40 cm per day.
- **Retrograde** fast axonal transport carries worn-out mitochondria and membrane components towards the cell body (for degradation or recycling). The maximum speed is 20 cm per day.

Fast axonal transport is mediated by a group of molecular **motor proteins** called **kinesins** (for anterograde transport) and **dyneins** (for retrograde transport). These proteins are ATPases that carry vesicle-bound cargo along microtubule tracks that run the length of the axon. Retrograde axonal transport is involved in some central nervous system viral infections (Clinical Box 5.1).

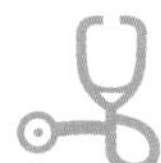

Clinical Box 5.1: Axonal transport and viral infections

Retrograde fast axonal transport is exploited by the **herpes viruses**, a large group that includes the pathogenic agents responsible for cold sores **(herpes simplex virus I, HSV1)**, genital herpes **(herpes simplex virus II, HSV2)**, chicken pox and shingles **(varicella-zoster virus, VZV)**. Herpes viruses travel along the axon (Greek: herpein, to creep) to reach the **cell body** of **primary sensory neurons** in spinal or cranial ganglia, where they may lie dormant for many years. Reactivation may occur at any time, but is more likely during periods of stress or immunocompromise, causing outbreaks in the sensory territory of the affected nerve. The **rabies virus** also uses retrograde axonal transport to reach the cell body following a bite from an infected animal.

Small molecular components and soluble enzymes that are not membrane-bound move towards the axon terminal via **slow anterograde axonal transport**. This is also referred to as **axoplasmic flow** and proceeds at a rate of 1–5 mm per day. The mechanism is not clear.

Key Points

- The dendrites of many neurons are studded with microscopic spines which receive excitatory synapses. A typical cortical pyramidal neuron may have 10,000 dendritic spines.
- The neuronal cell body contains the same range of organelles found in other cells, but the apparatus for gene transcription and protein synthesis is especially prominent.
- The neuronal cytoskeleton is important in maintaining the shape of the cell and the calibre of neuronal processes. It contains microtubules, neurofilaments and actin microfilaments.
- Fast anterograde axonal transport is mediated by kinesins (maximum speed 40 cm/day) and retrograde transport is mediated by dyneins (maximum speed 20 cm/day).
- The herpes viruses travel along axons via the retrograde fast axonal transport system to reach the neuronal cell body where they may lie dormant for many years.

Astrocytes

Astrocytes are process-bearing cells with a stellate morphology (Greek: astron, star) and are the main support cells of the central nervous system (CNS). Astrocytic processes have specialized structures called **end-feet** that make contact with neurons and capillaries (Fig. 5.8A).

Astrocyte functions

Astrocytes contribute to **homeostasis**, helping to maintain a constant internal environment for neurons (e.g. by removing excess potassium ions and glutamate from the extracellular fluid). They are also involved in the response to injury, releasing cytokines and growth factors and multiplying to form a **glial scar** (see Ch. 8). Some other key roles are discussed in more detail below.

The blood–brain barrier (Fig. 5.8B)

Endothelial cells in CNS capillaries have **tight junctions** that restrict solute exchange between the brain and bloodstream.

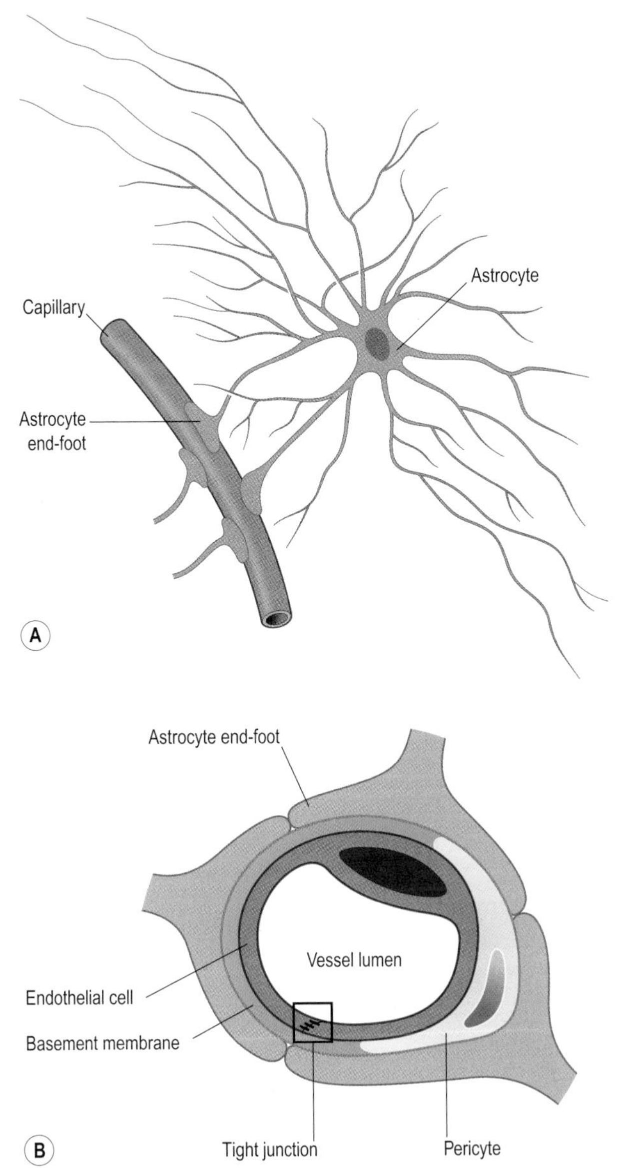

Fig. 5.8 **Astrocytes and the blood–brain barrier. (A)** Illustration of an astrocyte and its relationship to a cerebral capillary. Note the astrocytic end-feet making contact with the blood vessel; **(B)** Astrocytic end-feet are responsible for initiating the structural features of the blood–brain barrier, including the presence of tight junctions between capillary endothelial cells. In this figure a capillary is seen in cross-section, surrounded by three astrocytic end-feet.

This is normally referred to as the **blood–brain barrier (BBB)**, but is more accurately described as a blood–CNS barrier since it is also present in the spinal cord and retina. A similar arrangement in the choroid plexuses of the ventricles creates a blood–CSF barrier.

The blood–brain barrier is maintained by astrocytes via an **inductive interaction** between perivascular end-feet and CNS capillaries. Cerebral capillaries also lack fenestrations and contain few pinocytotic vesicles, so that transcellular flux is similarly limited. The blood–brain barrier effectively blocks charged or polar molecules, but lipid-soluble substances (including many centrally-active drugs and **anaesthetic agents**) pass relatively freely.

The existence of the blood–brain barrier requires that the brain has a number of carrier-mediated transport mechanisms for the uptake of essential nutrients. Glucose is imported by a specific **glucose transporter (GLUT-1)** which is present on the surface of endothelial cells. **Large neutral amino acids** such as phenylalanine also have a specific transporter protein, and drugs used in the treatment of **Parkinson's disease** gain access to the brain via the same transporter (Ch. 13).

Clinical Box 5.2: Hepatic encephalopathy

This is a neurological syndrome caused by **liver failure**. In the early stages it is characterized by mild personality change and confusion, progressing to delirium, seizures and coma. It is thought to be caused by the build-up of **nitrogenous waste products** such as ammonia that are normally detoxified by the liver. The main pathological changes occur in astrocytes rather than neurons and the clinical features of hepatic encephalopathy are thought to represent **secondary neuronal dysfunction** due to loss of normal metabolic support from astrocytes.

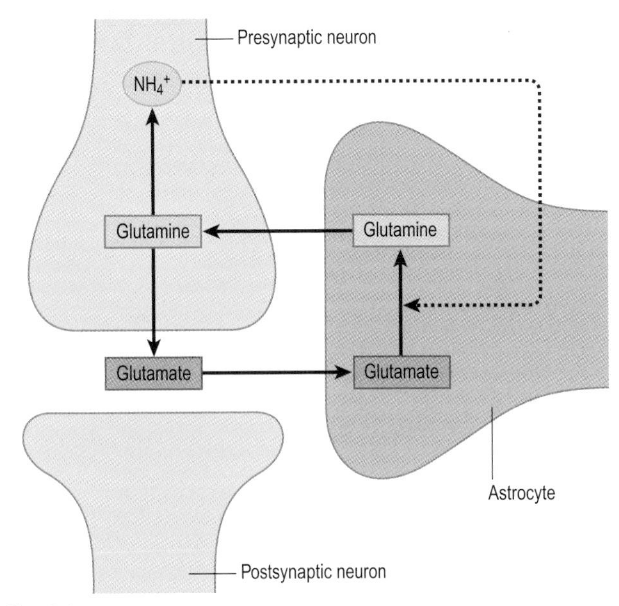

Fig. 5.9 **The glutamate–glutamine shuttle.** See text.

Energy metabolism

Astrocytes are intimately involved in brain energy metabolism. In addition to storing a modest amount of **glycogen** they also take up glucose and pre-digest it to **lactate** (via the glycolytic pathway). The lactate is then exported to the extracellular compartment where it is taken up by neurons as their principal source of energy.

Following activity at an excitatory (glutamatergic) synapse, **perisynaptic astrocytes** take up some of the released glutamate via specific transporters. These membrane pumps import sodium ions (Na^+) together with glutamate, thereby increasing the sodium ion concentration in the perisynaptic astrocytes. This in turn stimulates the **sodium–potassium exchange pump (Na^+/K^+-ATPase)** which promotes glycolysis. More lactate is thus produced, which can be made available to the metabolically active neurons. This is an example of **metabolic coupling** between neurons and astrocytes, which is relevant in certain neurological conditions (Clinical Box 5.2).

The glutamate–glutamine shuttle (Fig. 5.9)

One of the roles of astrocytes is to help clear glutamate from the extracellular space. Astrocytes metabolize glutamate to

glutamine by the enzyme **glutamine synthetase**. This consumes ammonia, which provides the amine group ($-NH_2$) of glutamine and serves an important metabolic role by detoxifying this **nitrogenous waste product**. Glutamine is released into the extracellular fluid where it is taken up by neurons and hydrolysed by the mitochondrial enzyme **glutaminase**, converting it back to glutamate.

Key Points

- Astrocytes are process-bearing cells with a stellate morphology and 'end-feet' that make contact with neurons and capillaries.
- The numerous roles of astrocytes include: (i) reuptake of excitatory transmitters and potassium; (ii) reactive gliosis in response to disease; and (iii) maintenance of the blood–brain barrier (or blood-CNS barrier).
- Due to the presence of the blood–CNS barrier, specific transport mechanisms exist for the uptake of essential nutrients such as glucose and amino acids.
- The main energy substrate of the brain is glucose, which is metabolized by astrocytes to form lactate before being taken up by neurons.

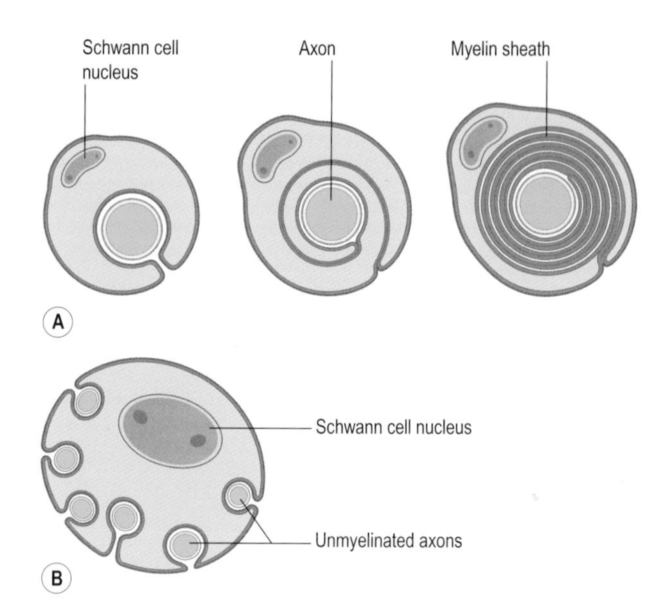

Fig. 5.11 **Myelination. (A)** In the peripheral nervous system, Schwann cells myelinate axons by investing them with up to 300 concentric layers of plasma membrane. The intervening cytoplasm between the layers is gradually 'squeezed out'; **(B)** Unmyelinated fibres do not have a myelin sheath, but are associated with and enveloped by Schwann cells, which provide trophic support.

Oligodendrocytes and Schwann cells

Oligodendrocytes are small, rounded cells with relatively few cytoplasmic processes (Greek: oligo, few). They are numerous in the CNS white matter and are responsible for investing central axons with a lipid-rich **myelin sheath**. Each oligodendrocyte makes contact with up to a dozen neighbouring axons and provides a single segment of myelin to each (Fig. 5.10). In the peripheral nervous system, **Schwann cells** are responsible for myelination, but each cell makes contact with only one axon and provides a single segment of myelin. Both types of cell secrete growth factors and provide trophic support to the axons that they invest.

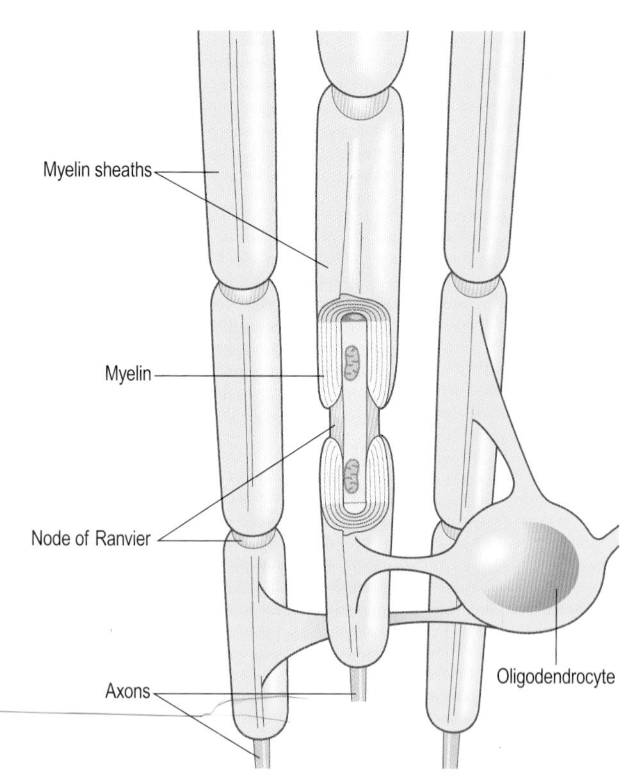

Fig. 5.10 **Oligodendrocytes make contact with up to a dozen neighbouring axons, providing a single segment of myelin to each.** The gap between myelinated segments is the node of Ranvier.

Myelination

Myelin consists of multiple concentric layers of glial cell membrane (Figs 5.11A and 5.12). A small amount of cytoplasm is initially present between the layers but this is gradually squeezed out as the myelin is **compacted** and the lipid bilayers fuse. Axons are myelinated in 1 mm segments interrupted by microscopic gaps called **nodes of Ranvier**, at which point the axon is in direct contact with the extracellular fluid. The myelinated segments are called **internodes** (Latin: inter-, between). Some small-diameter axons do not have a myelin sheath, but are contained within an infolding of Schwann cell membrane, along with several other non-myelinated axons (see Fig. 5.11B).

Composition of myelin

CNS myelin is rich in **myelin basic protein (MBP)** and **proteolipid protein (PLP)**. The major protein component of peripheral myelin (around 80%) is **myelin protein zero (P0)**. This is a member of the immunoglobulin superfamily and is essential for compaction of adjacent myelin lamellae which enables axons to be tightly wrapped. Another component is **peripheral myelin protein 22 (PMP-22)** which has been implicated in some heritable forms of peripheral neuropathy (Clinical Box 5.3).

Saltatory conduction

Myelination significantly increases **axonal conduction velocity**. This is because the nerve impulse 'jumps' from node to node (Latin: saltare, to leap) rather than spreading continuously along the axonal membrane (see Ch. 6). Focal disruption of the myelin sheath can lead to failure of impulse conduction in the denuded axon segments (termed **conduction block**) in part because of a paucity of

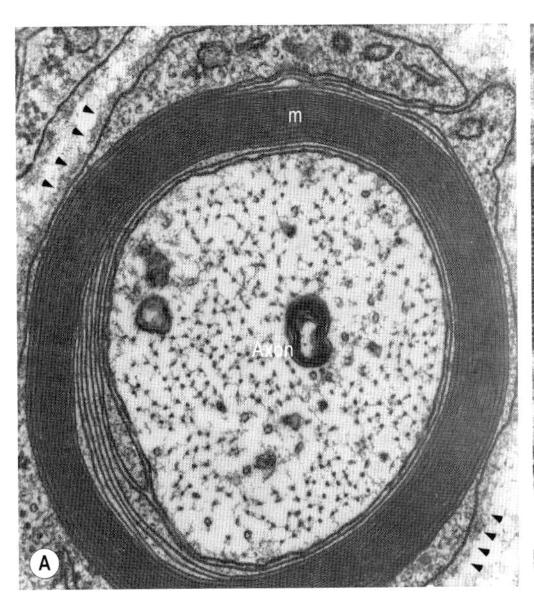

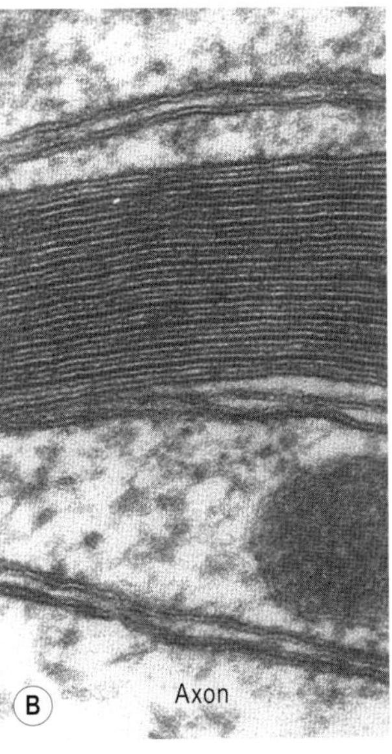

Fig. 5.12 **Electron micrograph illustrating the ultrastructure of the myelin sheath. (A)** An axon is shown in transverse section, together with its myelin sheath [labelled "m"] composed of multiple individual layers of cell membrane [arrowheads]; **(B)** Examination of the myelin sheath at higher magnification shows dark (major dense) lines between paler (intraperiod) lines. The dark lines result from fusion of the inner layers of plasma membrane after the intervening cytoplasm has been squeezed out. The pale lines represent apposition of the outer faces of the plasma membrane, which are less closely packed due to the presence of glycoproteins which project from the external surface of the plasma membrane. From SS Scherer (1997) Molecular genetics of demyelination: New wrinkles on an old membrane. Neuron 18: 13–16 with permission.

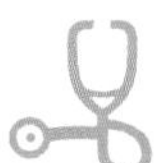

Clinical Box 5.3: Inherited peripheral neuropathy

The most common inherited peripheral neuropathy is **hereditary motor and sensory neuropathy (HMSN)**. This term encompasses a large group of peripheral nerve disorders that were previously referred to as **Charcot–Marie–Tooth disease (CMT)**. The characteristic features are distal weakness and wasting, depressed reflexes, high-arched feet (pes cavus) and mild sensory loss. The peripheral nerves are often palpably thickened. **HMSN type 1A** is caused by an autosomal dominant mutation of the ***PMP-22*** gene on chromosome 17. It is usually due to gene duplication (70% of cases) and presents early (in the teens). **Hereditary neuropathy with liability to pressure palsies (HNPP)** is a milder neuropathy that presents in the second or third decade of life and is brought on by pressure or trauma to an affected nerve. Multiple individual named nerves may therefore be affected **(mononeuritis multiplex)**. HNPP is also inherited in an autosomal dominant manner but is caused by deletion rather than duplication of the *PMP-22* gene.

voltage-gated sodium ion channels between the nodes of Ranvier. Conduction block is a feature of demyelinating conditions such as **multiple sclerosis** (Ch. 14).

Key Points

- Myelin is composed of multiple concentric layers of glial plasma membrane (oligodendrocytes in the CNS, Schwann cells in the PNS) wrapped around axons. The purpose of myelination is to increase axonal conduction velocity.
- Axons are myelinated in short segments that are interrupted by microscopic nodes of Ranvier. The myelinated segments (internodes) are around 1 mm in length.
- Central myelin is rich in myelin basic protein and proteolipid protein. The main constituent of peripheral myelin is protein zero which is responsible for compaction of myelin lamellae.
- Peripheral myelin also contains PMP-22 which has been implicated in a number of hereditary peripheral neuropathies.

Other glial cells

The most important types of glial cell other than astrocytes and oligodendrocytes are **microglia** and **ependymal cells**, which are discussed in more detail below. Others include:

- **Bergmann glia** of the cerebellum.
- **Pituicytes**, in the posterior lobe of the pituitary gland.
- **Müller cells** of the retina.
- **Satellite cells**, within spinal and cranial nerve ganglia.
- **Olfactory ensheathing cells**, located in the olfactory bulb.

Many of these cells are related to astrocytes and have similar roles. **Olfactory ensheathing cells (OECs)** are of particular interest because they permit new axons to grow into the mature CNS, which only normally occurs in the olfactory bulb. These cells therefore provide some hope of encouraging axonal regrowth in the CNS after brain or spinal cord injury.

Microglia

Microglia are relatively small cells (Greek: micro, small) with rod-shaped nuclei (Fig. 5.13) and are the resident **phagocytes**

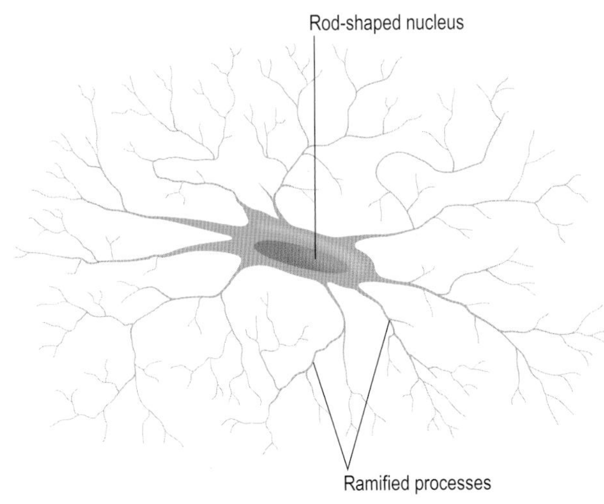

Fig. 5.13 **Microglia are the resident macrophages (scavengers) of the central nervous system.** They are sometimes called 'rod cells' because of the elongated shape of the nucleus.

of the CNS. At rest they exist in a quiescent state and are described as ramified (entwined within the feltwork of axons and dendrites). In response to tissue damage and inflammation they transform into **activated microglia** which migrate to the site of injury and internalize particulate materials and microorganisms. Microglia are discussed further in Chapter 8 in the context of brain inflammation and gliosis.

Ependymal cells

Ependymal cells form a continuous epithelial sheet (the **ependyma**) that lines the ventricles and the central canal of the spinal cord. These cells are of glial lineage, but have many epithelial characteristics including a basement membrane, cell–cell junctions and motile cilia. The **choroid plexus** of each ventricle (which is responsible for the secretion of cerebrospinal fluid as an ultrafiltrate of plasma) is composed of a capillary network covered by a sheet of modified ependymal cells. These cells are connected by tight junctions, which represents a blood–CSF barrier.

> *Key Points*
>
> - The nervous system contains a large number of glial cell types in addition to astrocytes and oligodendrocytes, including microglia and ependymal cells.
> - Microglia are the resident professional phagocytes and immunocompetent cells of the CNS and are of monocyte–macrophage lineage. They exist both in ramified (quiescent) and activated states.
> - Ependymal cells are also of glial lineage, but have epithelial characteristics. They form a continuous sheet lining the ventricles, choroid plexuses and the central canal of the spinal cord.

Glial tumours

Intracerebral tumours can be classified as **primary** (arising within the brain) or **secondary** (metastatic tumours that have spread from another site). Secondary tumours are more common and often originate from the lung, breast or bowel. **Primary CNS tumours** are further classified as extrinsic or intrinsic (Fig. 5.14). **Extrinsic tumours** derive from the coverings of the CNS. They tend to be benign and slow-growing and include meningiomas (derived from the meninges) and peripheral nerve sheath tumours. **Intrinsic tumours** of the brain and spinal cord are of neuroepithelial lineage and usually show evidence of glial differentiation; for this reason they are referred to as glial tumours or **gliomas**.

Glial tumours are thought to arise from **stem cells** (which normally give rise to new neurons or glia) that have accumulated mutations enabling them to proliferate in an uncontrolled manner and to diffusely infiltrate brain tissue. The typical MRI appearances of a malignant glial tumour are shown in Fig. 5.15.

General features of gliomas

Glial tumours are relatively uncommon, with a lifetime risk of less than 1 in 200, but tend to be highly malignant and carry a poor prognosis. The presenting features are discussed in Clinical Box 5.4.

Classification and grading

Tumour type (e.g. astrocytoma, oligodendroglioma, etc.) is determined by examining a tissue sample under the microscope. Classification is based on the growth pattern and microscopic appearance of the cells, often supplemented by **immunohistochemistry** (antibody labelling) to identify proteins that are typically expressed in certain types of tumour.

Tumours are also given a **histological grade** (from I to IV) that attempts to quantify their malignant potential (degree of biological aggressiveness) (Fig. 5.17). Grading is based on **tumour architecture** (pattern of growth), **atypical cytology** (cells and nuclei with abnormal structural features) and **proliferation rate** (speed of growth). Grade I and II tumours are termed **benign** (or **low grade**) whereas grade III and IV tumours are designated **malignant** (or **high grade**). In general, the prognosis is less favourable as the histological grade increases. The most common (and also the most aggressive) form of glial tumour is **glioblastoma** (grade IV) in which the median survival is less than 12 months.

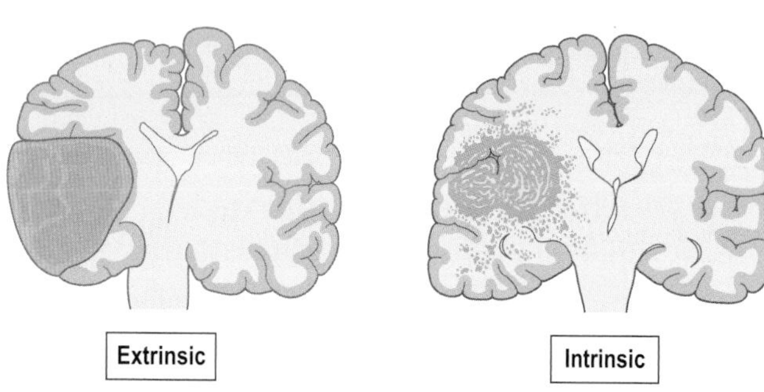

Fig. 5.14 **Primary central nervous system (CNS) tumours can be classified as extrinsic or intrinsic.** Extrinsic tumours arise from the coverings of the CNS and are usually separate from the underlying brain or spinal cord. Intrinsic tumours arise within the CNS itself and tend to be diffusely infiltrative.

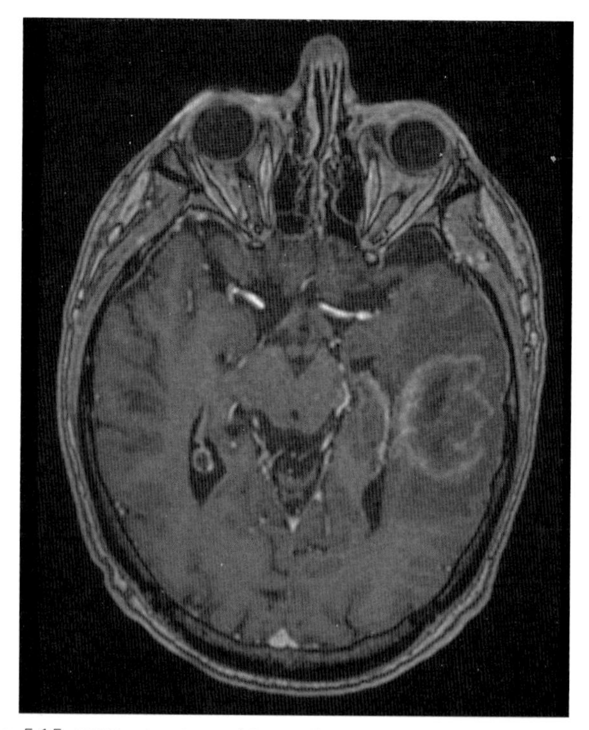

Fig. 5.15 **MRI in a patient with a malignant astrocytic tumour (glioblastoma).** This is an axial, T1-weighted MRI scan showing an irregular, poorly circumscribed intrinsic brain lesion diffusely infiltrating the temporal lobe. The patient has been injected with the intravenous contrast agent gadolinium and the tumour shows a peripheral rim of enhancement (it is described as 'ring enhancing'). The darker area surrounding the mass corresponds to peritumoural oedema (swelling). These appearances are typical of a glioblastoma, the most common malignant glial tumour. Courtesy of Dr Andrew MacKinnon.

Clinical Box 5.4: Clinical features of brain tumours

Brain tumours act as **space-occupying lesions** within the cranial cavity and cause **raised intracranial pressure** (Ch. 9). This typically presents with **headaches** that tend to be worse in the morning and are exacerbated by coughing, stooping or straining. There may also be nausea, vomiting or transient visual obscurations. Some patients present with **seizures** or **focal neurological deficits**. There is often **papilloedema**, defined as bilateral swelling of the optic discs due to raised intracranial pressure (Fig. 5.16). Drowsiness is an ominous sign that occurs in the later stages and may precede rapid neurological deterioration.

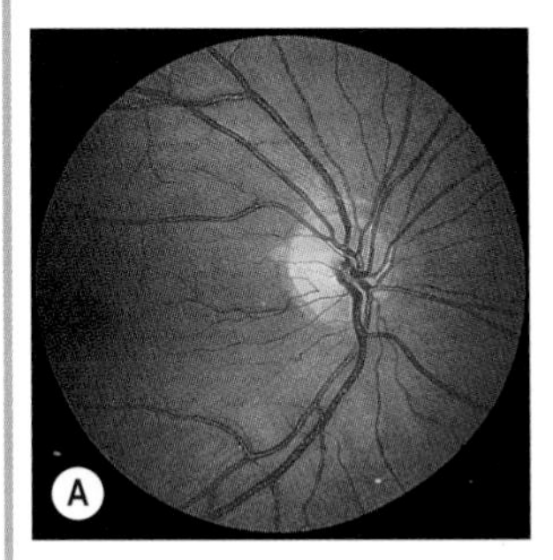

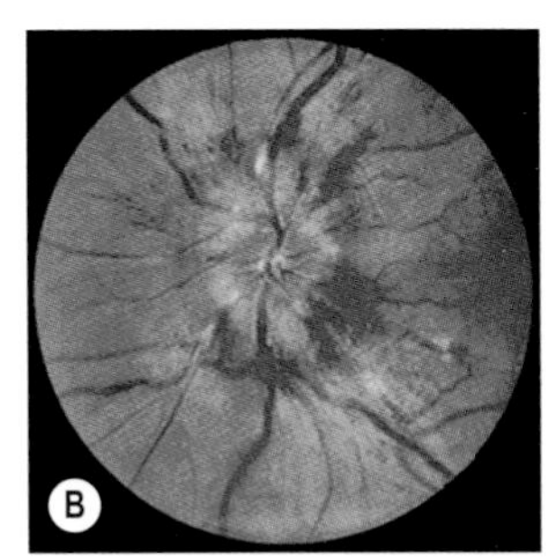

Fig. 5.16 **Papilloedema. (A)** Normal appearance of the retina and optic disc; **(B)** Swelling of the optic nerve head (optic disc) in a patient with raised intracranial pressure. From Munro: Macleod's Clinical Examination 12e (Churchill Livingstone 2009) with permission.

Molecular genetics

The most useful molecular test in gliomas is assessment of **1p19q status** in oligodendroglial tumours. At least 70% of oligodendrogliomas have a combined loss of chromosomal arms **1p** and **19q**. This is found in less than 5% of astrocytic tumours and around 40% of mixed oligo-astrocytomas. The presence of **1p19q codeletion** in an oligodendroglioma is an independent prognostic indicator and predicts a robust response to chemotherapy. Studies show that 100% of patients with 1p19q co-deletion show a good response to **PCV chemotherapy** (procarbazine, CCNU, vincristine).

Another useful molecular signature is mutation in one of the two isoforms of the Kreb's cycle enzyme **isocitrate dehydrogenase** (**IDH1**/**IDH2**). This is present in 80% of low-grade astrocytic and oligodendroglial tumours and predicts a more favourable outcome. In **glioblastoma**, the presence of a particular molecular genetic change predicts response to chemotherapy (Clinical Box 5.5).

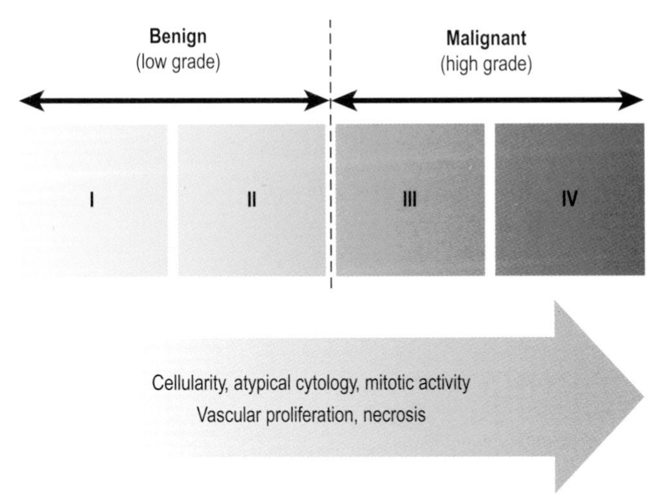

Fig. 5.17 **World Health Organization (WHO) grading of glial tumours.**

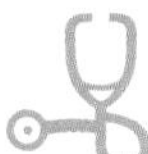

Clinical Box 5.5: MGMT status in glioblastoma

In glioblastoma, the most common and malignant form of primary brain tumour, a molecular test can be used to predict response to the alkylating chemotherapeutic drug **temozolomide**. Like most anti-cancer drugs, this acts by causing widespread DNA damage in an attempt to trigger **programmed cell death** (Ch. 8) in rapidly dividing tumour cells. Many alkylating agents work by adding **methyl groups (–CH_3)** to guanine residues, which is reversed by the DNA repair protein **methyl-guanyl-methyltransferase (MGMT)**. Activity of MGMT therefore antagonizes temozolomide and reduces its efficacy. In some tumours the ***MGMT*** gene is inactivated ('silenced') by methylation of its promoter region and this group responds best to temozolomide. ***MGMT*** **silencing** can be detected by **methylation-specific PCR** (polymerase chain reaction) using a small amount of tumour DNA extracted from a biopsy specimen. The result can then be used to select patients who will benefit from temozolomide.

Management of gliomas

Glial tumours are managed primarily by surgical resection. Oral corticosteroids (**dexamethasone**) help to relieve **cerebral oedema** and raised **intracranial pressure**, whereas **anti-epileptic drugs** can be used to control **seizures**. Surgery usually has one of two main aims:

- **Debulking** is removal of a large portion of the tumour. This is the most common operation in high-grade gliomas, which relieves raised intracranial pressure and provides diagnostic material.
- **Brain biopsy** is a less radical procedure that enables a tissue diagnosis to be made (by examination under the microscope). It may also be undertaken to exclude lesions with similar clinical and radiological features.

Complete removal of glial tumours is usually not possible (even with extensive resection) due to their highly infiltrative nature. Surgery may also be limited by involvement of **eloquent** (language or motor) areas. The role of radiotherapy and chemotherapy is relatively limited in primary brain tumours, but may prolong survival by a few months in high-grade gliomas.

Key Points

- Secondary (metastatic) tumours are more common than primary brain tumours and most frequently arise from the lung, breast or bowel.
- Primary CNS tumours can be classified as extrinsic (e.g. meningiomas) or intrinsic (e.g. gliomas).
- Tumours are assigned a histological grade on the WHO scale. Grade I and II tumours are benign (low grade); grade III and IV tumours are malignant (high grade or 'cancerous').
- Gliomas are managed primarily by surgery, supplemented by chemotherapy or radiotherapy. Complete resection is rarely possible because of the diffusely infiltrative growth pattern.
- The most common and aggressive type of glial tumour is glioblastoma (WHO grade IV) accounting for 50% of cases. The median survival time (even with optimal treatment) is less than 12 months.
- 1p19q loss in oligodendroglioma (present in at least 70% of cases) predicts an excellent response to chemotherapy and a significantly longer median survival.

Chapter 6
Electrical signalling in neurons

CHAPTER CONTENTS

Neurons are **excitable cells**, meaning that they respond to stimulation and can generate nerve impulses. These travel along axons at speeds of up to 120 metres per second, which permits rapid, long-distance communication between different parts of the nervous system. This chapter will examine the electrical properties of neurons and the cellular basis of excitability and axonal conduction.

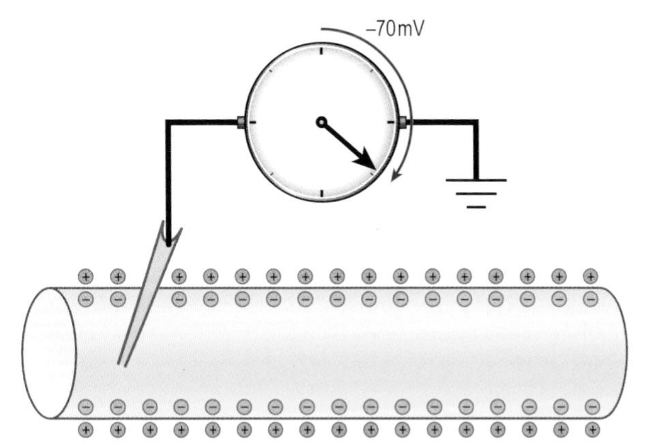

Fig. 6.1 **The resting membrane potential.** The potential difference across the cell membrane of a typical neuron is around –70 millivolts (negative on the inside).

The neuron at rest

There is a small difference in **electrical potential** across the plasma membrane of all living cells, the inside usually being slightly negative compared to the outside. This potential difference is referred to as the **membrane potential** of the cell. It is due to a slight excess of negative charge on the inner face of the plasma membrane and is measured in millivolts (mV). The **resting membrane potential** can be recorded with an intracellular microelectrode and its value is typically around –70 mV in nerve cells (Fig. 6.1).

The neuronal membrane is therefore said to be **polarized** at rest. An increase in polarization (so that the interior of the cell becomes even more negative) is referred to as **hyperpolarization**. Loss of normal polarity (so that the membrane potential moves closer to zero) is termed **depolarization**. It is important to understand that the uneven charge distribution responsible for the membrane potential is restricted to the immediate vicinity of the cell membrane. This means that there is a very small excess of negative charge on the inner face of the membrane, balanced by an equal amount of positive charge on the outer face. By contrast, the comparatively vast volumes of intracellular and extracellular fluid are electrically neutral.

Origin of the resting membrane potential

The resting membrane potential of –70 mV is mainly due to the efflux of positively charged potassium ions (K^+). These diffuse out of the cell via **leak channels**, leaving the inner face of the membrane slightly electronegative. The **driving force** for potassium efflux is passive diffusion, since the concentration of potassium inside the cell is 30 to 40 times higher than that of the extracellular fluid. Permeability to other ions is much less at rest, so the resting membrane potential is mainly determined by the potassium gradient. The sodium gradient is more important for changes that occur when the cell is stimulated (discussed below).

The sodium pump

The transmembrane gradients for sodium and potassium are maintained in the long term by the **sodium-potassium exchange pump** ('sodium pump') which works continuously in the background (Fig. 6.2). The sodium pump is a membrane-bound protein that hydrolyses adenosine triphosphate (ATP) and uses the energy released to move ions across the plasma membrane against their concentration gradients. In each cycle the sodium-potassium pump (or **Na^+/**

Key Points

- The neuronal membrane is polarized, with a resting membrane potential of –70 mV (negative on the inside) due to a slight excess of negative charge on the inner face of the membrane.
- An increase in the membrane potential (so that it becomes more negative) is called hyperpolarization. Movement of the membrane potential closer to zero is depolarization.
- The resting membrane potential is mainly due to efflux of potassium (K^+) ions via leak channels. This depends on the steep concentration gradient for potassium (35× higher on the inside).
- Sodium is more concentrated in the extracellular fluid and the sodium gradient (12× higher on the outside) is more important for depolarizing the cell during a nerve impulse.
- The sodium and potassium gradients are maintained in the long term by the sodium-potassium pump, which is responsible for two thirds of the basal energy expenditure in the brain.

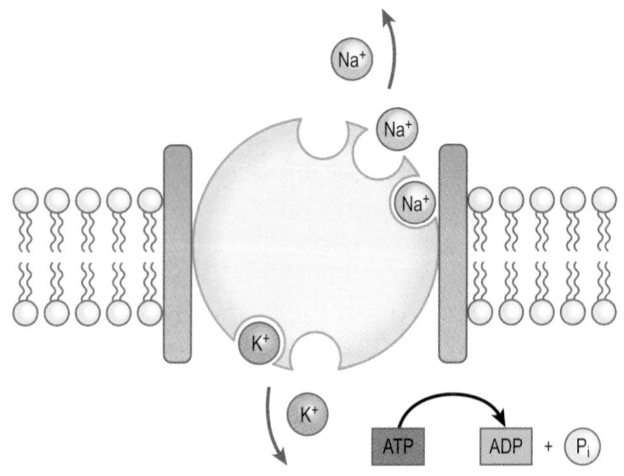

Fig. 6.2 **The sodium-potassium exchange pump.** Na^+/K^+-ATPase ('the sodium pump') is responsible for maintaining the intracellular and extracellular sodium and potassium gradients in the long term.

K^+-ATPase) transfers three sodium ions out of the cell and moves two potassium ions into the cell, consuming a single molecule of ATP in the process. In this way, the intracellular potassium concentration is maintained at approximately 140 mM compared to the extracellular concentration of around 3–5.5 mM, representing a potassium gradient of around 35 : 1 (higher on the inside). In contrast, the sodium ion concentration is around 12 mM on the inside and 140 mM on the outside, which equates to a 12 : 1 gradient for sodium ions (higher on the outside).

The sodium pump accounts for two thirds of the basal energy expenditure in nerve cells. It also contributes to the excess of negative charge on the inner face of the plasma membrane since it expels three positively charged ions in each cycle but only imports two. It is therefore described as **electrogenic** and the resting membrane potential is 3–5 mV more negative than predicted from passive ion flow.

Ionic basis of the resting membrane potential

Consider the hypothetical membrane-bound cell depicted in Figure 6.3A. It contains a concentrated solution of potassium salt and is immersed in saline (a solution of sodium chloride). It is important to emphasize that although only potassium (K^+) is illustrated in the figure, the intracellular and extracellular fluids contain many different positive and negative ions and are electrically neutral overall.

Now suppose that the cell membrane is *exclusively* permeable to potassium. Since the intracellular concentration is much higher, potassium will passively diffuse out of the cell down its steep concentration gradient (Fig. 6.3B). A slight excess of negative charge will therefore build up on the inner face of the membrane, since each potassium ion that leaves the cell carries a single positive charge. However, this generates a growing **electrical field** that acts in the opposite direction to the concentration gradient and tends to attract potassium back inside the cell. The net efflux of potassium ions is therefore gradually reduced as the opposing electrical field builds up.

Ultimately the rate of potassium efflux (down its concentration gradient) is exactly counterbalanced by potassium influx (down the electrical gradient) and there is no *net* movement of potassium ions into or out of the cell (Fig. 6.3C). At this **equilibrium point** the membrane potential is stable and will be slightly more negative on the inside.

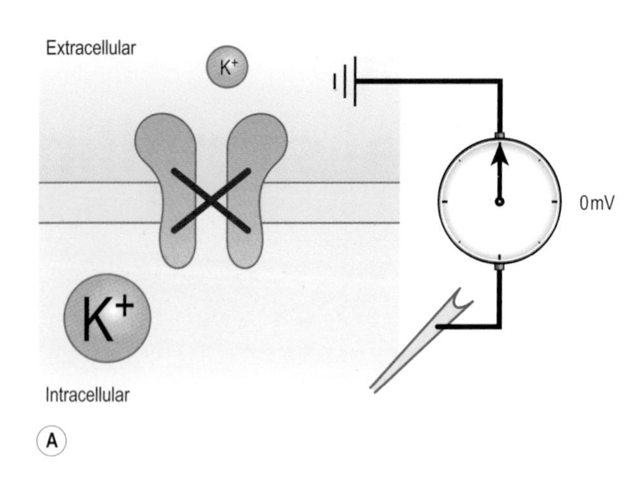

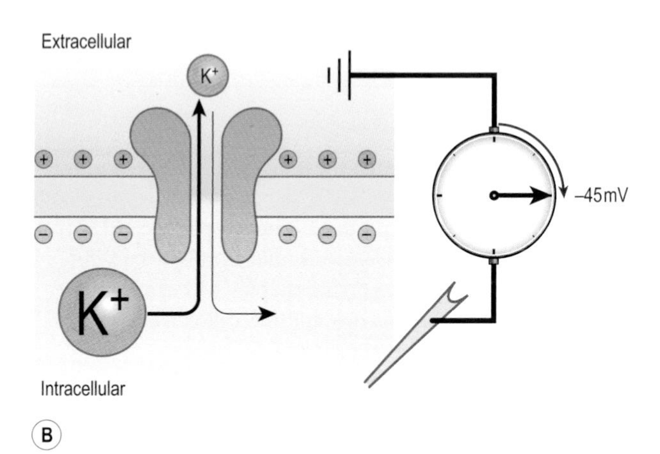

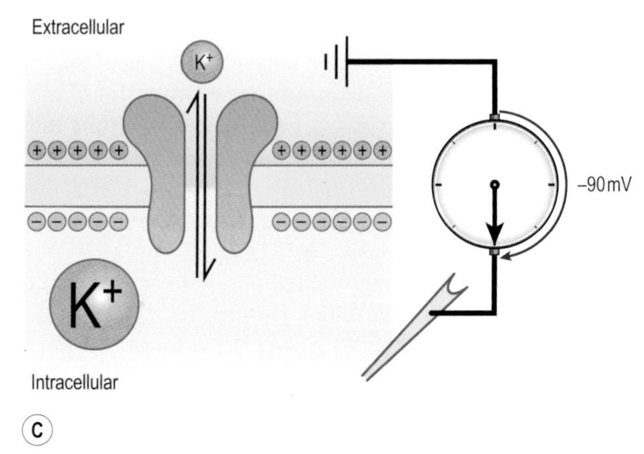

Fig. 6.3 **The ionic basis of the resting membrane potential.** See text for explanation.

The potential difference across the membrane at this point is the **equilibrium potential** for potassium and is around –90 mV. It should be emphasized that this process is very rapid (the equilibrium point is reached almost instantaneously).

The absolute number of ions moving across the cell membrane to establish the equilibrium potential is a few tens of millions, which is a negligible fraction of the total number of potassium ions inside the cell. The intracellular potassium concentration is therefore unchanged.

Calculating the equilibrium potential

Under normal physiological conditions, such as constant body temperature, the equilibrium potential for a particular ion is

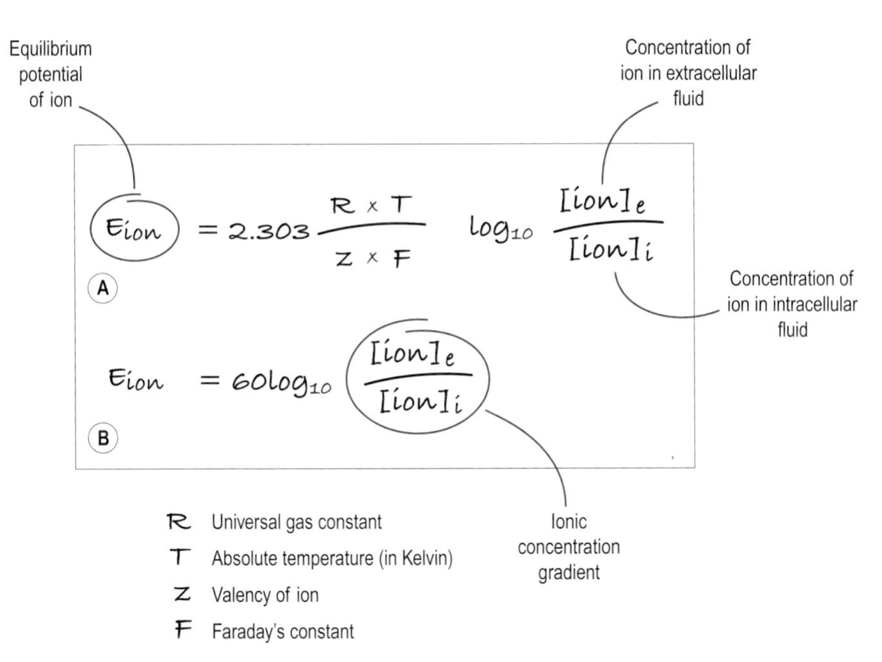

Fig. 6.4 **The Nernst equation. (A)** This equation is used to calculate the equilibrium potential for any particular ion, taking into account variables such as temperature and ionic charge; **(B)** This shows exactly the same expression, but the numerical part of the equation has been simplified. Once this has been done, it is clear that the main determinant of the equilibrium potential for a particular ion is the concentration gradient (in other words: the difference in ionic concentration between the inside and outside of the cell).

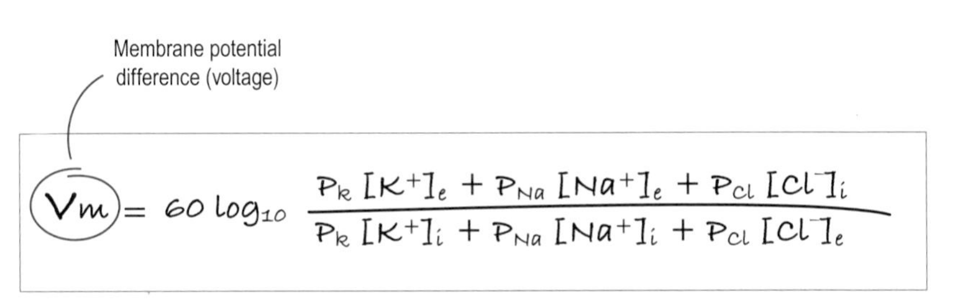

Fig. 6.5 **The Goldman equation.** This equation combines the equilibrium potentials for each of the main ions (determined from the Nernst equation) in a single expression. The relative permeability of each ionic species is also factored in (e.g. if the membrane were mostly permeable to one particular ion, then the membrane potential would be closer to the equilibrium potential for that ion; if there were two main ionic species of equal permeability, the membrane potential would be halfway between the two equilibrium potentials).

mainly determined by the concentration difference between the inside and outside of the cell. Its value is given by the **Nernst equation** (Fig. 6.4). This takes into account the size of the transmembrane gradient together with a number of physical and chemical factors including the absolute temperature (measured in Kelvin) and the charge carried by the ion.

Effect of membrane permeability

The value of the membrane potential at a particular moment depends mainly on the **relative permeability** to sodium, potassium and chloride ions. This changes when **ion channels** open or close.

The resting membrane potential (–70 mV) is close to the equilibrium potential for potassium (–90 mV) because the neuronal membrane is normally 50–100 times more permeable to potassium than to other ions. If the sodium permeability were to increase suddenly – as it does when a nerve impulse is generated – then the membrane potential would move towards the equilibrium potential for sodium (+60 mV). Note that the value of the sodium equilibrium potential is positive. This is because positively charged sodium ions (Na^+) are more concentrated in the extracellular fluid and therefore diffuse into the cell, making the inner face of the plasma membrane positive with respect to the extracellular fluid. If a membrane were equally permeable to sodium and potassium ions, then the membrane potential would be halfway between –90 mV and +60 mV (i.e. –15 mV).

The value of the resting membrane potential in a typical neuron (–70 mV) reflects the fact that the membrane is predominantly permeable to potassium and slightly permeable to sodium, therefore the membrane potential is close to, but a little less negative than, the potassium equilibrium potential.

The resting membrane potential can be calculated by considering the equilibrium potentials for sodium, potassium and chloride ions and factoring in the membrane permeability for each. This information is combined in the **Goldman equation** (Fig. 6.5) which gives a predicted membrane potential that closely matches recordings from intracellular electrodes.

The reversal potential

Increasing permeability to a particular ion causes the membrane potential to shift towards the equilibrium potential for that ion. Depending on the starting value of the membrane potential, this may therefore depolarize or hyperpolarize the cell. If the membrane potential is already the same as the equilibrium potential for that particular ion, then opening more ion channels will not alter its value. This

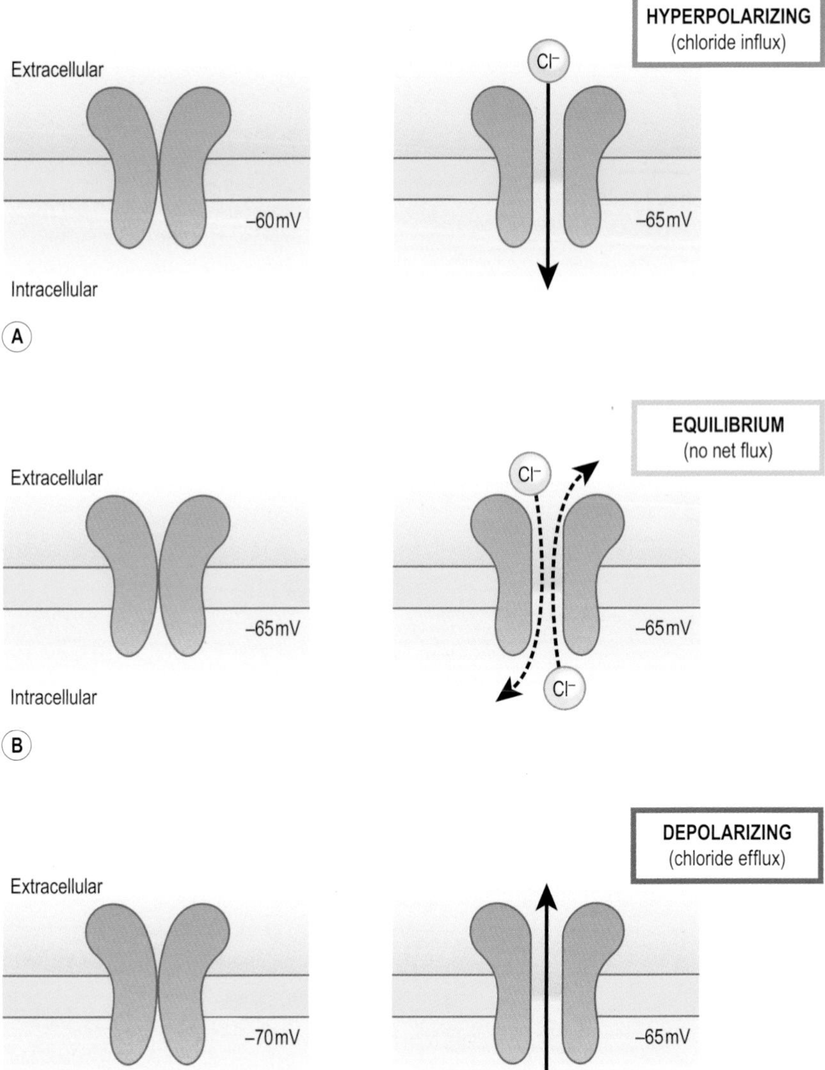

Fig. 6.6 **The reversal potential.** The net direction of ion flux through a membrane channel depends on the initial membrane potential of the cell and the reversal potential of the particular ion. Increasing ion conductance by opening additional channels may therefore **(A)** hyperpolarize the cell; **(B)** have no net effect on the membrane potential; or **(C)** depolarize the cell [see text for explanation].

concept is illustrated in Figure 6.6 with reference to the **chloride channel**, which has an equilibrium potential of –65 mV.

Figure 6.6A shows the effect of opening additional chloride channels in a membrane that is initially polarized to a value of –60 mV. In this case the membrane is **hyperpolarized** (from –60 mV to –65 mV). In Figure 6.6B the cell membrane is already at the equilibrium potential for chloride (–65 mV) when the additional chloride channels are opened, so there is no change in membrane voltage (no net ion flux). In Figure 6.6C, the cell membrane starts at a value of –70 mV, which is more negative than the chloride equilibrium potential. Therefore, as the chloride conductance is increased the membrane is **depolarized** (from –70 mV, towards –65 mV).

The point at which the direction of net current flow reverses is called the **reversal potential** and is the same as the equilibrium potential. The rate of net current flow for a particular ion is proportional to the difference between the membrane potential and the equilibrium potential for that ion. This is referred to as the **driving force**. If the membrane potential is the same as the reversal potential, then the driving force is zero.

Key Points

- The equilibrium potential for a particular ion is the stable membrane potential at which point the opposing electrical and concentration gradients are balanced and there is no net ion flux.
- It is mainly determined by the ionic concentration difference between the inside and outside of the cell and is calculated using the Nernst equation.
- The potassium equilibrium potential is –90 mV since the intracellular potassium concentration is higher and potassium tends to leak out of the cell, leaving the inside slightly negative.
- In the case of sodium, the equilibrium potential is +60 mV. The value is positive because sodium is more concentrated in the extracellular fluid and therefore diffuses into the cell.
- Increasing permeability to a particular ion (by opening ion channels) causes the membrane potential to shift towards the equilibrium potential for that particular ion.
- The value of the membrane potential at a particular moment therefore depends on the relative permeability of sodium, potassium and chloride ions, combined in the Goldman equation.
- The normal resting membrane potential (–70 mV) is close to the equilibrium potential for potassium since the membrane is predominantly permeable to this ion at rest.

Excitability

Local depolarization of the cell membrane in response to a stimulus is called a **graded potential**. It is described as 'graded' because its size and duration are proportional to the stimulus responsible for it. The amplitude of graded potentials ranges from 5–20 mV and the duration may be anything from one millisecond to several seconds. When generated by sensory receptor cells in the peripheral nervous system, they are called **receptor potentials**. Graded potentials are unsuitable for long-distance communication as they are not able to travel very far along the axon before dissipating.

If a graded potential is sufficiently strong it may trigger an **action potential**. This is a stereotyped sequence of electrical changes in the neuronal membrane that is able to propagate along the full length of the axon without decrement. The action potential (or **nerve impulse**) depends on the presence of specific ion channels in the cell membrane.

Types of ion channel

The neuronal membrane is composed of a **lipid bilayer**. This is a natural barrier to charged species, but water molecules are able to cross freely by passing through channels called **aquaporins**. The plasma membrane also contains specific **ion channels**. These are large, transmembrane proteins, usually made up of multiple subunits surrounding an aqueous pore (Fig. 6.7).

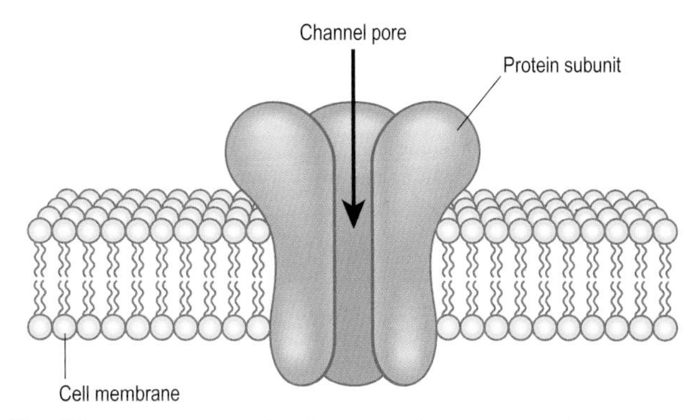

Fig. 6.7 **Basic structure of an ion channel.** Multiple, membrane-spanning protein subunits are arranged around a central, aqueous pore. The channel may open or close in response to the binding of extracellular ligands or changes in the membrane voltage.

Gated channels

There are two types of 'gated' ion channel. **Ligand-gated** channels open in the presence of a particular signalling molecule, such as a neurotransmitter or peptide, which acts at a binding site on the extracellular aspect of the channel. This type of channel is discussed further in Chapter 7 in the context of synaptic transmission. **Voltage-gated** ion channels open and close in response to changes in the membrane potential and are involved in the generation and propagation of action potentials. The presence of a **selectivity filter** means that a channel only allows certain types of ion to pass (by exploiting the physical and chemical properties of amino acids lining the channel pore).

Channel kinetics

It is possible to study the behaviour of individual ion channels using the **patch-clamp technique** in which a single channel is extracted from a living cell, together with a small patch of the surrounding membrane. This is achieved by applying suction to microscopic pipettes. Recordings from single ion channels show that during gating, the pore is not simply 'open' or 'closed' but rapidly alternates between the two conformational states in a stochastic (probabilistic) manner, spending more time in either the open or the closed configuration.

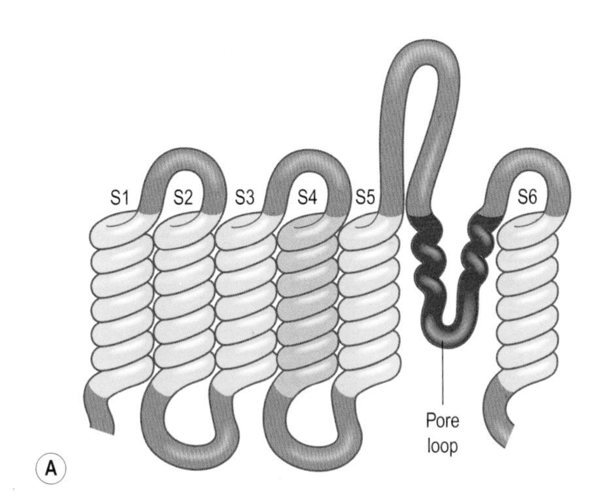

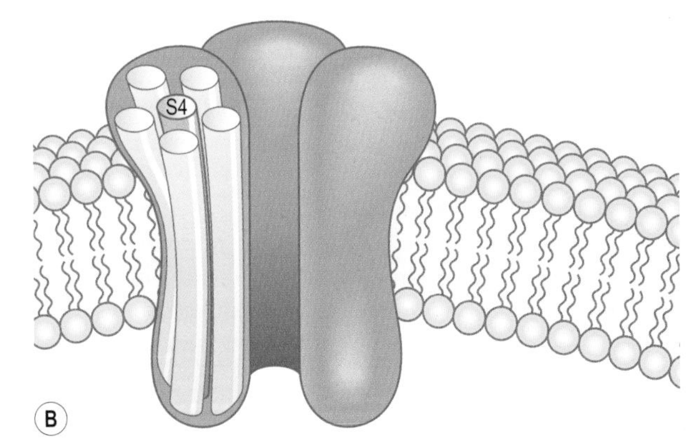

Fig. 6.8 **Structure of voltage-gated ion channels. (A)** The channel subunits are composed of six membrane-spanning alpha-helices (S1–S6) together with a pore loop that is responsible for ion selectivity. The charged domain (S4) acts as a voltage sensor; **(B)** The voltage-gated sodium channel consists of a single large protein with four repeating motifs (each with six membrane-spanning domains and a pore loop). The potassium channel has a similar structure (once assembled) but is composed of four separate subunits arranged as a tetramer.

Voltage-gated channel structure

Voltage-gated ion channels are **integral membrane proteins**. They have a similar molecular structure that includes a repeating motif with six membrane-spanning alpha helices (Fig. 6.8A). There is also a **pore loop** that contributes to the selectivity filter and a charged domain that acts as a **voltage sensor**. During depolarization the inner face of the cell membrane becomes more positive and the voltage sensor (which carries a positive charge) is thrust upwards through the membrane by electrostatic repulsion. This movement induces a **conformational change** in the channel complex which opens the pore. Conductance changes steeply, increasing 150-fold with a 10 mV shift in membrane potential.

Sodium and potassium channels

The **voltage-gated sodium channel** is composed of a single large protein with four repeating motifs labelled I, II,

III and IV. Each motif contains the six membrane-spanning regions, a pore loop and a voltage sensor. In contrast, the **voltage-gated potassium channel** is composed of four separate subunits, each with the characteristic motif. Once assembled, the overall molecular structure of sodium and potassium channels is therefore similar (Fig. 6.8B). The sodium channel also has an **inactivation gate**. This closes when the neuronal membrane is fully depolarized and only opens again ('resets') once the cell has repolarized.

Key Points

- Neurons are excitable cells, meaning that they can respond to stimulation and generate nerve impulses (action potentials).
- Excitability depends on the presence of voltage-gated sodium and potassium channels in the neuronal membrane. These have a common motif with six membrane-spanning alpha helices.
- Voltage-gated ion channels have an aqueous pore with a selectivity filter that only permits certain types of ion to pass. A voltage sensor enables the channel to open or close in response to changes in the membrane potential.
- The structures of the voltage-gated sodium and potassium channels are similar, but the sodium channel also has an inactivation gate. When this is closed, the channel becomes unresponsive until the membrane is repolarized.

The action potential

The electrical changes that occur during an action potential are illustrated in Figure 6.9. The membrane first **depolarizes** rapidly from its normal resting value of –70 mV with a slight **overshoot** to a positive value of around +30 mV. The normal membrane polarity is thus briefly reversed. The membrane very quickly **repolarizes** to its normal (negative) value and there is a slight **undershoot**, before eventually returning to baseline. The timescale is about 1–2 milliseconds.

Properties of the action potential

An action potential may be initiated in the **neuronal cell body** (where excitatory and inhibitory influences from other nerve cells have been integrated) or in **sensory nerve endings** in response to a sufficiently strong **graded potential** (triggered by mechanical, thermal or other forms of stimulation).

Nerve impulse generation

To trigger an action potential, a stimulus must be large enough to depolarize the neuronal membrane to a particular **threshold** value (typically –55 mV). Once this point has been reached a full action potential will occur. It is not possible for an action potential to vary in magnitude like a graded potential: a full action potential either occurs or does not occur. This is referred to as the '**all or none**' **law**. Since each action potential depolarizes the adjacent membrane to threshold, the nerve impulse propagates along the full length of the axon like a row of falling dominoes (Fig. 6.10).

Frequency coding

Given that the amplitude of the action potential does not vary, the intensity of a stimulus is encoded by the frequency of nerve impulse traffic. The signal is said to be **frequency-modulated** (as in an FM radio) rather than **amplitude-modulated**. Neurons vary greatly in their discharge frequency, but since each action potential lasts 1–2 milliseconds, the maximum theoretical rate of impulse generation is 500–1000 Hz (1 Hz = one per second).

Refractory periods

Once a nerve impulse has been generated, a second action potential cannot occur until the membrane has recovered:

- The **absolute refractory period** is the interval in which it is not possible to trigger a second action potential, regardless of stimulus strength.
- The **relative refractory period** is the interval in which a second action potential can be generated, but only with a stronger stimulus than usual.

The absolute refractory period is due to inactivation of the **voltage-gated sodium channels** (Fig. 6.11). Another action potential is not possible until the sodium channel **inactivation gate** reopens (which does not happen until the membrane has repolarized). The relative refractory period is due to the **after-hyperpolarization** (undershoot) that follows the action potential, when the membrane is more negative than it was at rest; a larger than usual excitatory stimulus is therefore needed to overcome this and depolarize the membrane to threshold. Most **local anaesthetic agents** inhibit voltage-gated sodium channels and prolong the refractory period in sensory neurons (Clinical Box 6.1).

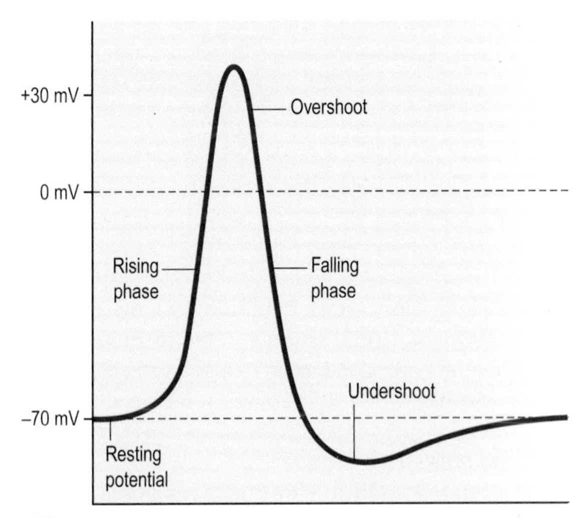

Fig. 6.9 **The action potential.**

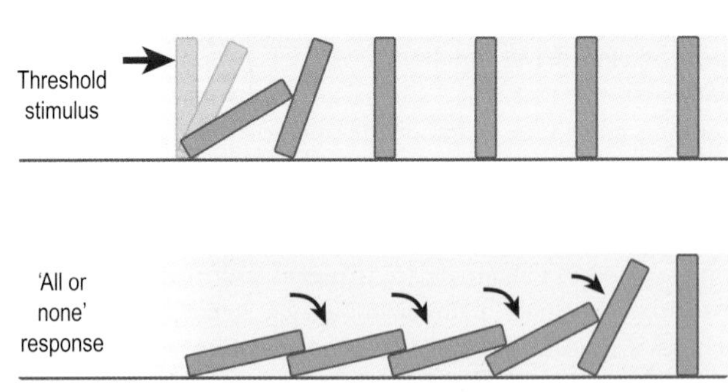

Fig. 6.10 **Nerve impulse propagation is similar to a row of falling dominoes.** The dominoes will only fall if the minimum effective (threshold) stimulus has been applied, but once the threshold has been reached, all dominoes will fall. Application of even greater (suprathreshold) stimuli has exactly the same effect.

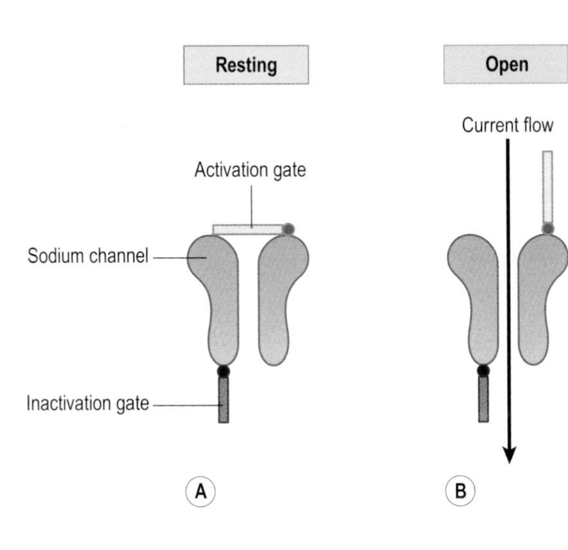

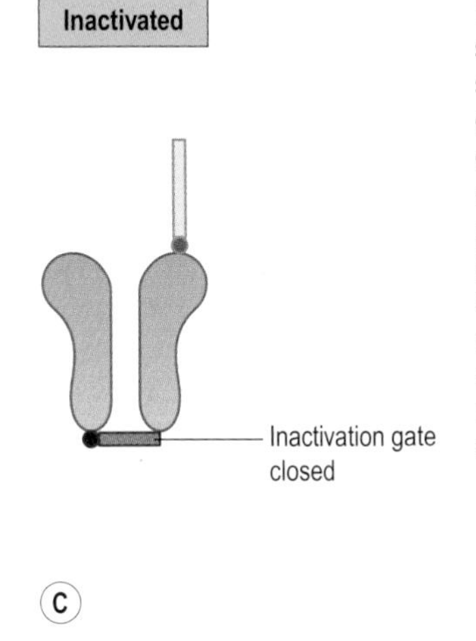

Fig. 6.11 **The voltage-gated sodium channel exists in three states.** **(A)** At rest, the activation gate is closed and the inactivation gate is open; **(B)** During the depolarizing phase of the action potential both gates are open; **(C)** Once the inactivation gate has closed it is not possible to generate another action potential until the sodium channels have reset, corresponding to the absolute refractory period.

Clinical Box 6.1: Local anaesthesia

Local anaesthetics such as **lignocaine** (or lidocaine) are cocaine derivatives that work by blocking the voltage-gated sodium channel, preventing the generation of action potentials. The binding site for lignocaine is inside the channel pore so it can only act on open channels (preferentially blocking active nerve cells). These agents are used to provide **regional analgesia** for minor procedures such as dental surgery. The local anaesthetic agent can be injected into soft tissues such as the gums (**infiltration anaesthesia**) or a specific nerve can be targeted (**nerve block**). Injection of local anaesthetic into the extradural (epidural) space surrounding the spinal cord can be used to provide pain relief during childbirth (**epidural anaesthesia**).

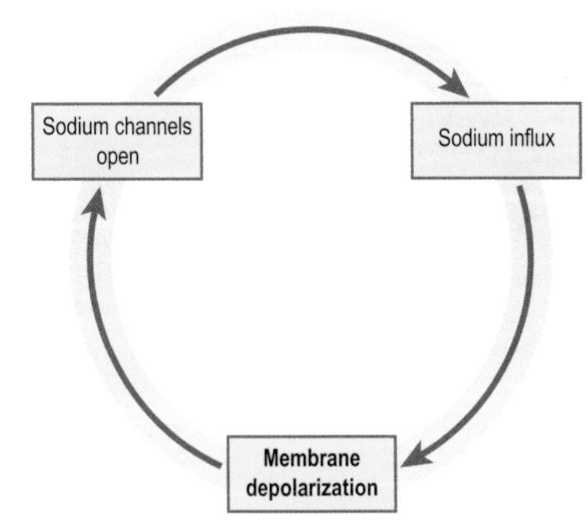

Fig. 6.12 **The Hodgkin cycle.**

Key Points

- An action potential is a stereotyped sequence of electrical changes in the neuronal membrane, with rapid depolarization followed by immediate repolarization.
- After repolarization the membrane potential is slightly more negative than it was at rest, which is referred to as the undershoot or after-hyperpolarization.
- The action potential is an 'all or none' phenomenon. This means that once the membrane has been depolarized to threshold (around −55 mV) a full action potential will occur.
- Since the amplitude of the action potential does not vary, stimulus strength is represented in the nervous system using frequency coding.
- Once a nerve impulse has been generated, a second action potential cannot occur until the membrane has recovered. This is the refractory period.
- The absolute refractory period coincides with inactivation of voltage-gated sodium channels which makes it impossible to generate another nerve impulse.
- The relative refractory period is due to the after-hyperpolarization that follows the action potential, which must be overcome in order to depolarize the neuron to threshold.

Ionic basis of the action potential

The action potential is mediated by voltage-gated sodium and potassium channels. Depolarization of the neuronal membrane causes both types of ion channel to open, but sodium channels open earlier.

Depolarization (Na^+ influx)

Sodium channels open rapidly and are responsible for the **depolarizing phase** of the action potential in which there is brisk sodium influx. A **threshold stimulus** is one that is just strong enough to open the minimum number of channels necessary to set up a 'positive feedback loop' in the neuronal membrane, referred to as the **Hodgkin cycle** (Fig. 6.12). Once this critical threshold is reached, the membrane depolarization caused by inflowing sodium ions triggers more voltage-gated sodium ions to open, leading to a self-reinforcing cycle. Sodium influx drives the membrane potential towards zero, before overshooting to a positive value (+30 mV) which approaches the equilibrium potential for sodium (+60 mV). At this point the sodium channels close and inactivate.

Repolarization (K^+ efflux)

Potassium channels are also stimulated by depolarization, but open about one millisecond later and are responsible for the **repolarizing phase** of the action potential. Potassium channels open just as the sodium channels are closing. At this point the net current flow is reversed as potassium ions rush out of the cell, driving the membrane potential back towards the potassium equilibrium potential of –90 mV. Since these channels return the membrane potential to its normal negative value (termed 'rectification') and open after a short delay, they are called **delayed rectifiers**.

Summary of ionic events

The ionic events responsible for the different phases of the action potential can be summarized as follows (Fig. 6.13):

- **At rest:** voltage-gated Na^+ and K^+ channels are closed but responsive.
- **Depolarization (rising) phase:** Na^+ channels open; K^+ channels remain closed.
- **Maximum depolarization (overshoot):** Na^+ channels inactivate; K^+ channels open.
- **Repolarization (falling) phase:** K^+ channels remain open, Na^+ channels remain inactivated.
- **At rest:** Na^+ channels reset; both channels closed but responsive.

The **after-hyperpolarization** that follows an action potential (corresponding to the relative refractory period) occurs because some of the delayed rectifiers are still open and the membrane is therefore more permeable to potassium than it was at rest. This means that the membrane potential is closer to the equilibrium potential for potassium (closer to –90 mV). As the remainder of the voltage-gated potassium channels close the membrane returns to its resting value of –70 mV.

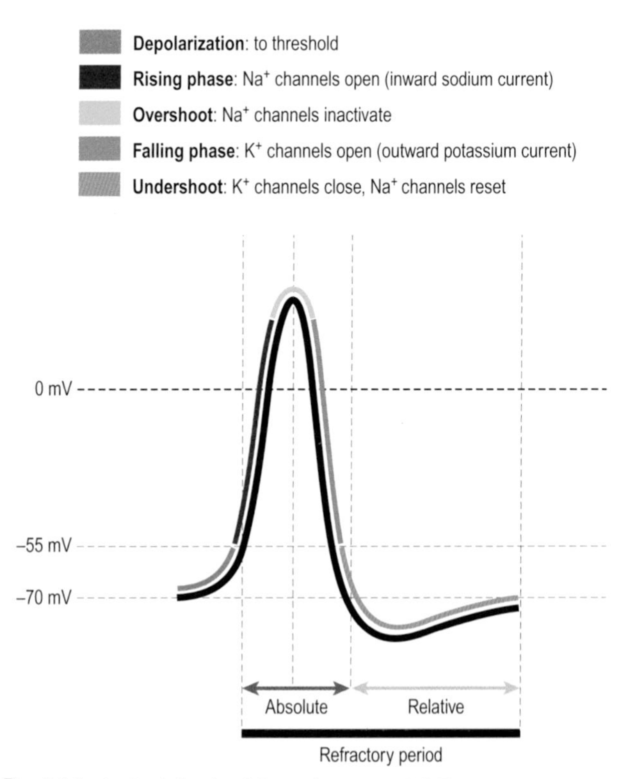

Fig. 6.13 **The ionic basis of the action potential.** The ionic events responsible for each part of the action potential are shown. The absolute and relative refractory periods are also indicated.

> ### *Key Points*
>
> - The action potential is mediated by voltage-gated sodium and potassium channels.
> - Threshold depolarization causes the sodium channels to open first, followed by the potassium channels (after a millisecond delay).
> - The depolarizing phase of the action potential is due to a rapid influx of sodium ions. At maximal depolarization the sodium channels close and inactivate. The potassium channels then open.
> - The repolarizing phase of the action potential is due to a rapid efflux of potassium ions. Once the membrane has repolarized the sodium channel inactivation gate is reopened ('reset').

Axonal conduction

A fundamental property of the nerve impulse is the ability to travel along the full length of an axon without decrement. Although each action potential is a discrete 'all or none' event, localized to a small patch of the axonal membrane, the inward sodium current generates a threshold depolarization (and a new action potential) in the adjacent membrane. The impulse therefore propagates along the nerve fibre as a succession of separate action potentials, rather like a Mexican wave.

Passive current flow

Each action potential is associated with a brisk influx of positively charged sodium ions which enter the cell via voltage-gated channels. This creates an **electrotonic wave** of positive charge that enters the nerve fibre in the region of action potential generation and then spreads passively along the axon (in both directions). The electrotonic wave travels quickly, but rapidly dissipates as positive charge 'leaks out' across the plasma membrane, particularly in fibres that do not have a myelin sheath (Fig 6.14A).

Depolarization is therefore maximal in the part of the membrane where the action potential was initiated, falling rapidly on either side of this point as the distance increases. This can be plotted as an **exponential decay curve** and expressed mathematically as the **length constant** (lambda) of the axon (Fig. 6.14B). The length constant is defined as the distance along the axon at which the voltage change has decayed to 37% of its maximum value.

One advantage of myelination is to reduce current leakage across the axonal membrane: in other words to increase **membrane resistance**. This enables the fast-moving electrotonic wave to spread further before dissipating and to trigger the next action potential as far along the axon as possible, thereby increasing conduction speed.

Conduction in unmyelinated fibres

In fibres that lack a myelin sheath, the nerve impulse propagates gradually from one end of an axon to the other, like a slow-burning fuse (often travelling at speeds below 1.5 metres per second). As each action potential is generated, the electrotonic wave spreads passively along the axon for a short distance and generates a new action potential in the adjacent patch of membrane (Fig. 6.15). The impulse always continues in the forward direction since the more proximal or 'upstream' part of the axon (which has just generated an action potential) is refractory. By the time it has recovered, the nerve impulse has passed.

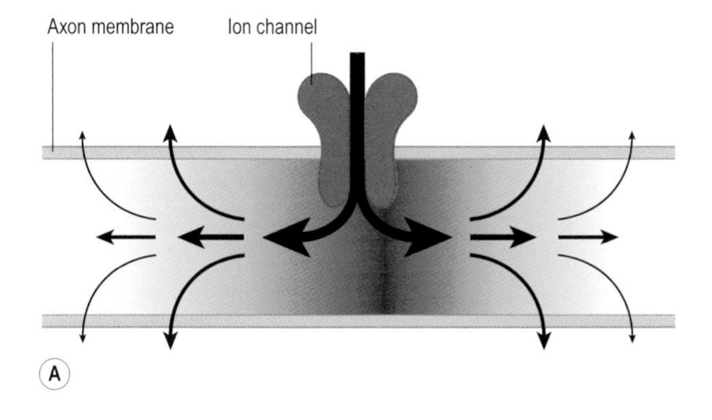

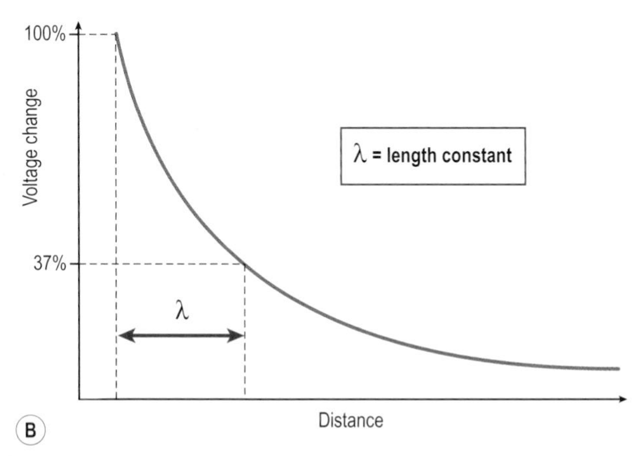

Fig. 6.14 **The electrotonic wave and length constant. (A)** At the point of action potential generation, the inflowing (depolarizing) current spreads in both directions for a variable distance along the axon but quickly dissipates by passive leakage through the axonal plasma membrane; **(B)** The length constant (lambda) quantifies the rate of current leakage across the membrane and reflects the distance that an electrotonic wave is able to travel along an axon before dissipating.

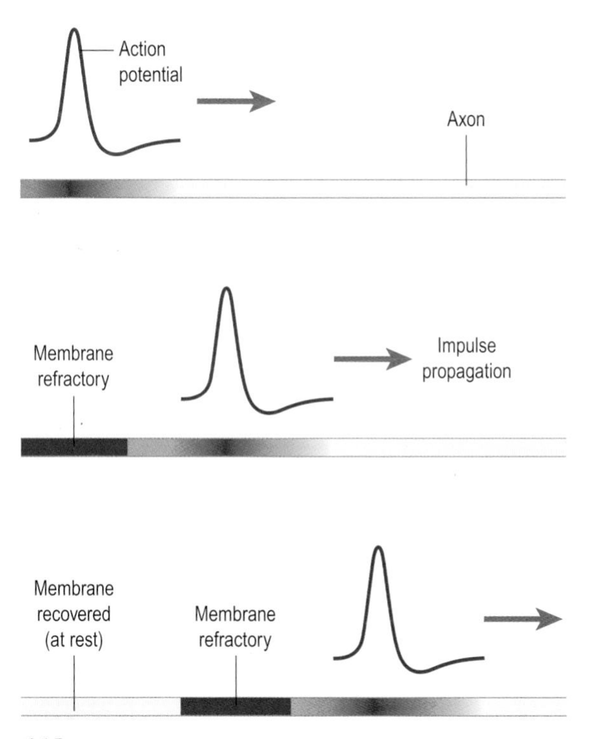

Fig. 6.15 **Continuous propagation.** In unmyelinated fibres the nerve impulse spreads gradually and continuously along the full length of the axon, like a slow-burning fuse (travelling at 0.5–2.0 metres per second). At each point the action potential brings the adjacent membrane to threshold and triggers a new action potential.

Antidromic conduction

Axons are capable of transmitting a nerve impulse in either direction, but this does not normally happen because the action potential is always initiated at one end or the other. Impulse propagation in the 'normal' direction (for instance, away from the CNS in the case of motor neurons) is referred to as **orthodromic conduction** (Greek: orthos, correct).

A nerve fibre can be made to transmit an impulse in the opposite direction in an experimental setting (or during clinical investigation of peripheral nerve disease) by using an electrical stimulator. This is termed **antidromic conduction** (Greek: anti-, opposite) which is like setting off a row of dominoes from the 'wrong' end. Similarly, artificial stimulation half way along an axon would generate two simultaneous waves of conduction away from the trigger-point (one orthodromic, another antidromic).

Axonal conduction velocity

A simple approach to increasing axonal conduction velocity is to use larger-diameter fibres. For instance, the **giant axon of the squid** (which is involved in an escape reflex) is up to 1 mm in diameter and is able to conduct impulses at more than 30 metres per second. This is because fibres with a greater cross-sectional area have lower internal resistance to current flow and this allows the electrotonic wave to reach and depolarize a more distant patch of membrane before dissipating (i.e. the length constant is increased).

In the vertebrate (including human) nervous system, rapid axonal conduction is achieved more efficiently by investing axons with multiple layers of lipid-enriched plasma membrane, creating a fatty **myelin sheath** (see Ch. 5). The insulating effect of myelin (reducing current leakage across the membrane and extending the reach of the electrotonic wave) has already been discussed. Myelin also increases conduction speed by reducing membrane capacitance (discussed below).

Myelination and membrane capacitance

Capacitance is the ability to store electrical charge. The type of capacitor found in electrical devices consists of a thin layer of insulting material called the **dielectric**, sandwiched between parallel metal plates. The positive and negative charges are 'stored' by the plates on either side of the dielectric. A good capacitor has a thin dielectric so that the opposing charges are close together, since the strength of attraction between them (and amount of charge that can be stored) is inversely proportional to the separation.

The cell membrane acts as a **biological capacitor**, storing positive and negative charges on either side of a thin phospholipid membrane. This has a limiting effect on axonal conduction speed, because it takes some time for the negative charge to be displaced from the inner face of the membrane during depolarization. The time course of depolarization is exponential and can be expressed mathematically as the **time constant** (tau), meaning the time taken to reach 63% of the maximum depolarization. Adding a myelin sheath reduces the membrane capacitance and therefore lowers the time constant. This means that membrane depolarization (hence impulse propagation) is quicker.

The reason that myelination lowers total membrane capacitance is that the countless layers of cell membrane act like hundreds of miniature capacitors connected in series – and when capacitors are arranged in this way (rather than in parallel) the total charge stored is significantly reduced. This

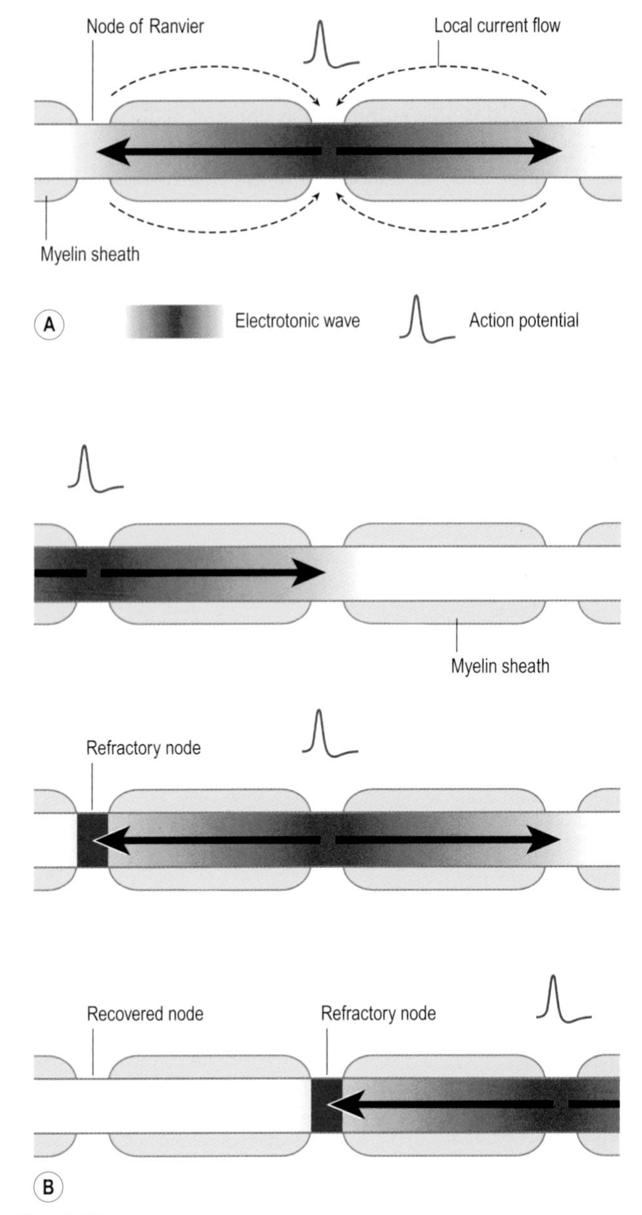

Fig. 6.16 **Conduction in myelinated fibres. (A)** When an action potential is triggered at a node of Ranvier, an inward sodium current (electrotonic wave) enters the axon and flows rapidly in both directions, triggering local current flow in the surrounding extracellular fluid; **(B)** Illustration of a nerve impulse moving from left to right along a single myelinated axon by causing a threshold depolarization at three successive nodes of Ranvier. Due to the presence of the myelin sheath, the electrotonic wave is able to reach the next node of Ranvier before dissipating and trigger a new action potential there. The previous node is always refractory, ensuring one-way propagation of the impulse.

is similar to capacitors connected in series in an electrical circuit. For instance: wrapping an axon in one hundred layers of cell membrane is like having 100 capacitors connected in series, thereby reducing the total amount of electrical charge stored to 1/100th of its original value.

Conduction in myelinated fibres

In myelinated fibres, each action potential arises at a **node of Ranvier**. This is a small gap between adjacent myelinated segments where the axon is in direct contact with the extracellular fluid. The myelinated segments are called

Key Points

- Each action potential is associated with a brisk influx of positively charged ions (the electrotonic wave) which enter the cell via voltage-gated ion channels.
- Exponential decay of the electrotonic wave is represented by the length constant of the axon: the distance at which the voltage change has fallen to 37% of its maximum value.
- Insulation of the axon with a myelin sheath reduces current leakage across the membrane. This increases the length constant and therefore improves axonal conduction velocity.
- The cell membrane acts as a biological capacitor, storing negative charge on the inner face of the membrane. This takes time to discharge during the depolarizing phase of the action potential, represented by the time constant.
- Myelination reduces the time constant (and therefore increases conduction velocity) by lowering the membrane capacitance.

internodes (Latin: inter-, between) and are about 1 mm long. Figure 6.16A illustrates the sodium current flowing into the axon at a node of Ranvier and the **electrotonic wave** spreading away from the node in both directions, reaching the two adjacent nodes (both 'upstream' and 'downstream' of the active node). Note also that **local circuit currents** are generated in the extracellular fluid in response to the ion flow.

Figure 6.16B illustrates the process of **nerve impulse propagation** along a myelinated axon. This is referred to as **saltatory conduction** since the action potential 'jumps' from node to node (Latin: saltere, to leap). As discussed above, myelination (i) lowers membrane capacitance (decreasing the time constant) and (ii) reduces current leakage (increasing the length constant). In this way the electrotonic wave depolarizes the membrane very quickly and is easily able to reach the next node of Ranvier before dissipating, triggering a new action potential there.

As in continuous conduction, the more proximal node will always be refractory, therefore the nerve impulse can only ever move forward. Saltatory conduction can be compared to setting off a line of fire crackers that are spaced a little distance apart: the heat from each cracker being just sufficient to trigger an explosion in the next, always moving forward since at each point the previous one is spent. A margin of error or **safety factor** prevents signal failure part way along the axon. Saltatory conduction is not only rapid but also efficient, since voltage-gated sodium channels are only required at the nodes of Ranvier.

Key Points

- In myelinated axons, action potentials are only generated at nodes of Ranvier (and effectively 'jump' from node to node) so very few voltage-gated ion channels are required between nodes.
- Although the electrotonic wave generated at each node spreads along the axon in both directions, impulse conduction always proceeds in the forward direction since the proximal node is refractory.
- A margin of error (safety factor) is built in to ensure that conduction does not fail part way along the internode.

Chapter 7
Synaptic transmission

CHAPTER CONTENTS

General principles

The majority of synapses in the brain and spinal cord are chemical, meaning that the communication between nerve cells is mediated by a **neurotransmitter** substance. Electrical synapses are much less common and can be used to synchronize activity in a group of neurons.

Electrical synapses

Electrical synapses are also known as **gap junctions** and are direct points of contact between the cytoplasm of adjacent neurons (Greek: sunapsis, point of contact). This allows very rapid two-way communication and synchronization of electrical discharges.

A gap junction is composed of around 100 intercellular channels called **connexons** that are inserted into the plasma membranes of adjacent cells (Fig. 7.1). Each connexon is composed of a hexagonal array of proteins called **connexins**, surrounding an aqueous channel that is 2 nm wide. The pores in adjacent cell membranes are aligned to form a 'tunnel' between the two cells. These can be opened or closed by a conformational change in the constituent proteins, regulated by phosphorylation state.

Gap junctions represent a low-resistance pathway that allows charged particles and small molecules to flow freely in either direction and couples the electrical activity of adjoining cells. Groups of cells linked by gap junctions form an **electrical syncytium** which can generate large, synchronized discharges. This happens in certain brain stem nuclei that control breathing and may contribute to the generation of abnormally synchronized discharges in some forms of **epilepsy** (Ch. 11).

Chemical synapses

Most central nervous system synapses are chemical. The general structure and arrangement is similar to that of the **neuromuscular junction** (see Ch. 4) and a great deal of information about central synapses has been derived from experiments at the point of contact between nerve and muscle.

General structure (Fig. 7.2)

At a chemical synapse the plasma membranes of the two nerve cells are in close proximity, separated by a narrow **synaptic cleft**. The axon terminal of the **presynaptic neuron** contains membrane-bound **synaptic vesicles** that are loaded with neurotransmitter; it also contains numerous mitochondria to provide energy for neurotransmission.

Peptide transmitters are synthesized in the cell body and pre-loaded into vesicles which are delivered to the axon terminal by **fast axonal transport** (see Ch. 5). Other transmitters are synthesized within the axon terminal and are loaded into synaptic vesicles by transport pumps in the vesicle membrane. Some are synthesized within the vesicle itself.

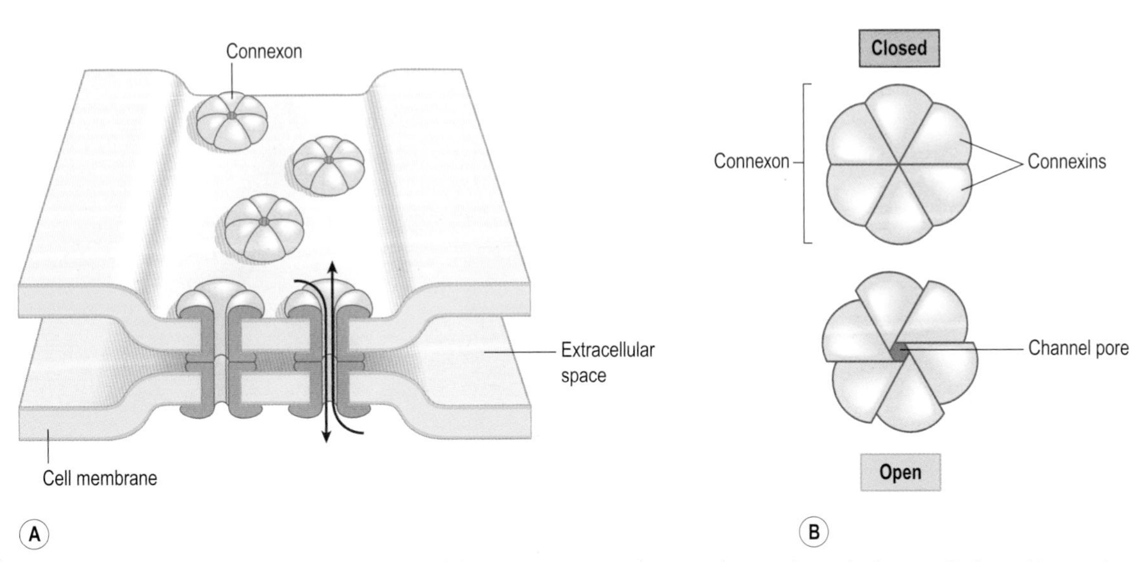

Fig. 7.1 **Electrical synapses. (A)** Gap junctions are points of direct communication between the cytoplasm of adjacent cells, formed by protein complexes called connexons; **(B)** Each connexon is composed of six connexin subunits, surrounding a central pore.

Excitatory and inhibitory synapses (Fig. 7.3)

Synapses can be excitatory or inhibitory. If the presynaptic neuron releases an excitatory transmitter (most commonly **glutamate**) then the membrane of the postsynaptic cell will be depolarized. This is referred to as an **excitatory post-synaptic potential** (**EPSP**) and is typically associated with an inward **sodium current**. If the presynaptic neuron releases an inhibitory neurotransmitter (the most common of which is **gamma-aminobutyric acid** or **GABA**) then the postsynaptic membrane will be hyperpolarized (inhibited). This is an **inhibitory postsynaptic potential** (**IPSP**) and is often associated with an inward **chloride current** (or an outward potassium current). EPSPs and IPSPs are **graded potentials** of a few millivolts that only influence the local membrane and then rapidly decay (see Ch. 6).

Release of neurotransmitter (Fig. 7.4)

Once loaded with neurotransmitter, synaptic vesicles are **docked** at the presynaptic membrane awaiting release. Docking takes place at **active zones.** These consist of multi-protein complexes that tether the synaptic vesicle to the presynaptic membrane and contain high concentrations of **voltage-gated calcium channels**. This leads to brisk calcium influx in response to axon terminal depolarization, since the concentration of calcium is 10,000 times higher in the extracellular fluid. The focal rise in free calcium causes a number of synaptic vesicles to fuse with the presynaptic membrane, emptying their contents into the synaptic cleft by **exocytosis.**

Release is said to be 'packeted' (or **quantized**) since the total amount of transmitter entering the synaptic cleft is a whole-number multiple of the amount stored in a single vesicle. Transmitter release is regulated by presynaptic **autoreceptors** which exert negative feedback.

Mechanism of membrane fusion

The mechanism by which synaptic vesicles fuse with the presynaptic membrane is complex and relies on a group of

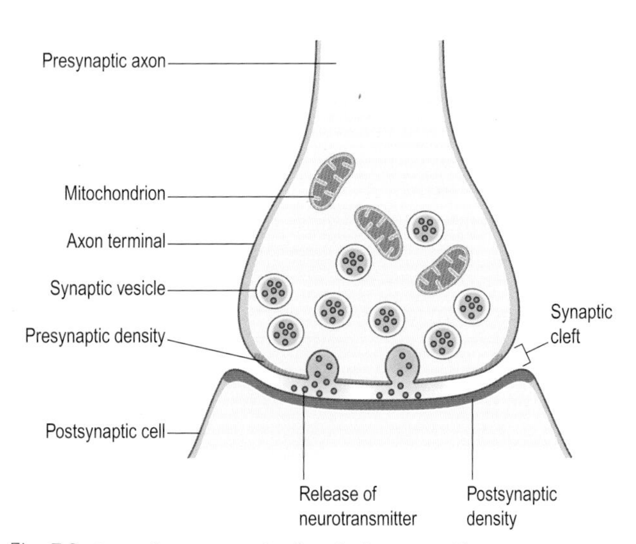

Fig. 7.2 **General structure of a chemical synapse.** The arrangement is similar to that of the neuromuscular junction between nerve fibres and skeletal muscle.

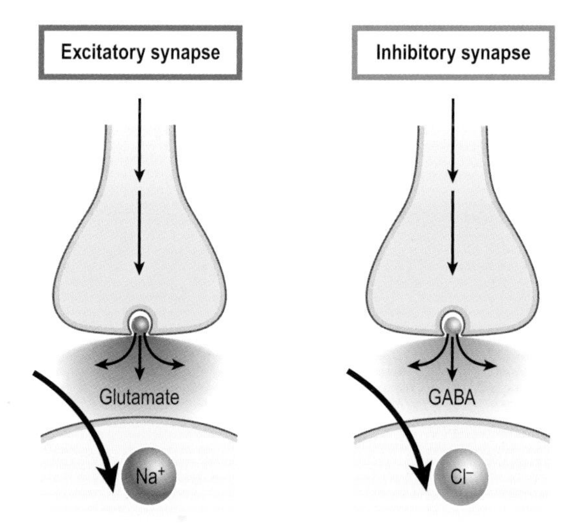

Fig. 7.3 **Excitatory and inhibitory synapses.** Most excitatory synapses in the central nervous system utilize glutamate as a neurotransmitter (or aspartate, which acts at the same receptors); the main inhibitory transmitter in the brain and spinal cord is gamma-aminobutyric acid (GABA).

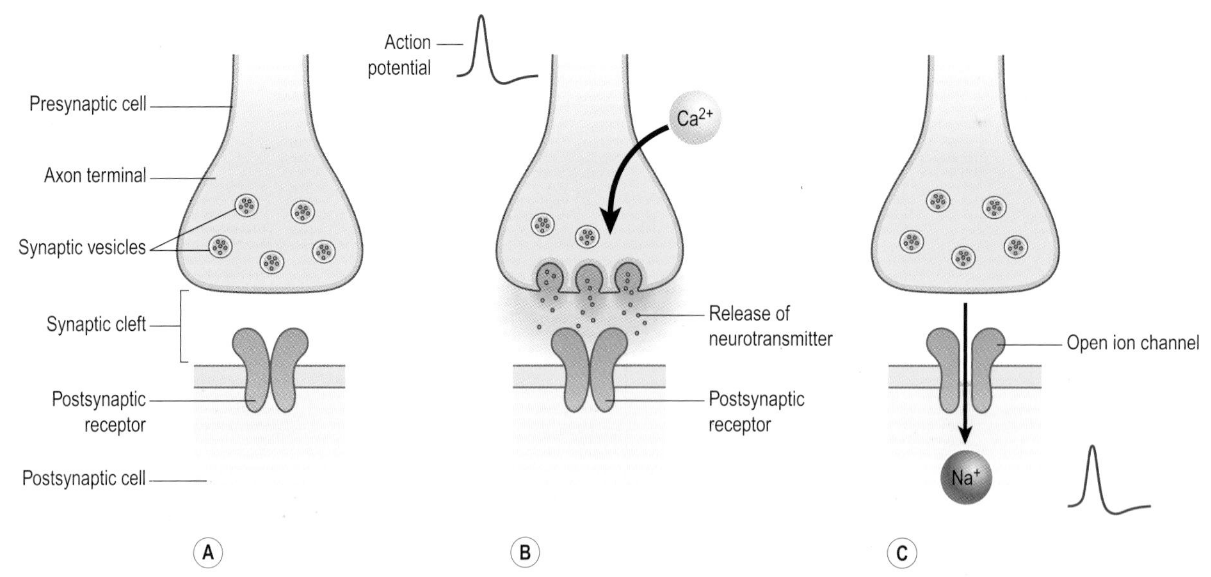

Fig. 7.4 **Neurotransmission. (A)** Neurotransmitter molecules are stored in the presynaptic element within membrane-bound synaptic vesicles; **(B)** Arrival of an action potential at the axon terminal triggers calcium influx via voltage-gated calcium channels which causes the vesicles to fuse with the presynaptic membrane and discharge their contents into the synaptic cleft; **(C)** The transmitter diffuses across the synaptic cleft and interacts with receptors on the postsynaptic membrane, leading to ion fluxes that will either inhibit or (as in this case) excite the postsynaptic neuron.

proteins belonging to the **SNARE (SNAP receptor) family**. The vesicle and presynaptic membranes 'kiss' and the interaction between complimentary proteins creates a small **fusion pore**. This quickly expands as the lipid membranes unite to form a large opening through which the contents of the vesicle are discharged into the synaptic cleft. After exocytosis the vesicle membrane thus becomes part of the presynaptic membrane. However, a similar amount of membrane is reclaimed from the axon terminal to make new vesicles, so there is no net increase in the size of the axon terminal.

Transmitter inactivation

To ensure that neurotransmission is a discrete event, the transmitter substance must be quickly removed from the synaptic cleft. In the case of acetylcholine this is achieved by **enzymatic degradation** (by acetylcholinesterase) but in most cases the transmitter molecule is reclaimed by the presynaptic neuron via membrane-bound **reuptake proteins** and recycled into new synaptic vesicles. Postsynaptic cells (and surrounding glia) also take up and metabolize neurotransmitters.

The entire process of synaptic transmission, from the arrival of the nerve impulse at the presynaptic element to the generation of a new nerve impulse in the postsynaptic cell, incurs a **synaptic delay** which may be up to five milliseconds. Chemical synapses are thus much slower than electrical synapses. However, each synaptic station in a neural pathway provides an opportunity for impulse traffic to be modulated or filtered.

Key points

- The majority of CNS synapses are chemical, meaning that communication is mediated by a neurotransmitter substance. This incurs a synaptic delay of up to five milliseconds.
- Electrical synapses (gap junctions) are much less common, but are faster and allow electrical synchronization of activity among groups of neurons.
- Chemical synapses can be excitatory or inhibitory. The most common excitatory transmitter in the CNS is glutamate, whilst the most common inhibitory transmitter is GABA.
- Transmitter is stored in synaptic vesicles which are 'docked' at active zones in the presynaptic membrane. Membrane fusion (and exocytosis) is triggered by a rise in intracellular calcium.
- Neurotransmitter diffuses across the synaptic cleft (between the presynaptic and postsynaptic cells) and interacts with specific receptors in the postsynaptic membrane.
- Transmitters are inactivated by enzymic destruction (e.g. in the case of acetylcholine) or by specific reuptake proteins on presynaptic cells, postsynaptic cells or perisynaptic glia.

Neurotransmitters

Approximately 50 to 100 substances are known (or suspected) to be neurotransmitters in the central nervous system. The reason that many of these chemicals are referred to as suspected or putative transmitters is that it is surprisingly difficult to prove that a substance is acting as a neurotransmitter, particularly in the human brain. This is because nervous tissue is densely packed with neurons, glial cells and blood vessels, surrounded by extracellular fluid in which there are numerous transmitters, peptides and hormones – and because synaptic events are fleeting and occur on a microscopic scale.

A number of criteria must be satisfied to establish that a substance is a neurotransmitter. It must be demonstrated that the candidate molecule: (i) is synthesized in the presynaptic neuron; (ii) is present within the axon terminal; and (iii) is released in a calcium-dependent manner upon depolarization of the presynaptic cell. It must also be shown that exogenous application of the substance has the same effect on the target cell as depolarizing the presynaptic cell. Relatively few molecules have satisfied these strict criteria unequivocally.

Classical neurotransmitters

Classical, small molecule neurotransmitters are stored in **clear-cored vesicles** that are approximately 50 nm in diameter. The first to be identified was **acetylcholine (ACh)** and it remains the best understood. Acetylcholine is found at the neuromuscular junction and throughout the autonomic nervous system. It differs from other types of neurotransmitter and has a distinct chemical structure, biosynthesis and mechanism of inactivation (Fig. 7.5). Acetylcholine is synthesized in axon terminals from two metabolites that are present in all cells: acetyl-coA and choline. This is achieved by the enzyme **choline acetyltransferase (ChAT)** which is only present in cholinergic neurons. The remaining small molecule neurotransmitters are divided into **amino acids** and **biogenic amines**.

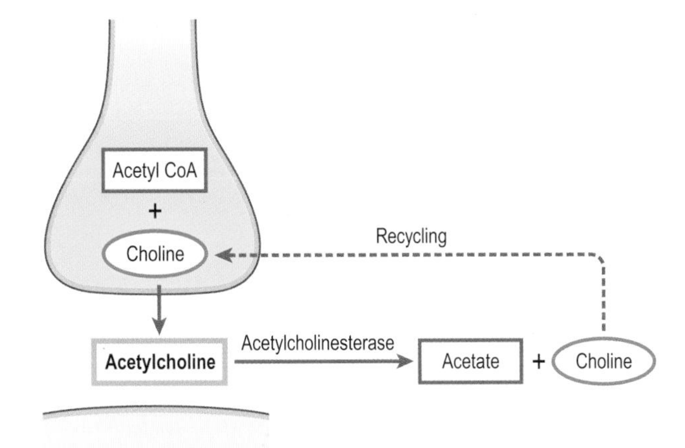

Fig. 7.5 **Acetylcholine synthesis, release and degradation.**

Amino acid transmitters

The majority of fast neurotransmission in the central nervous system involves amino acid neurotransmitters. The principal excitatory transmitter of the CNS is **glutamate** (together with the related amino acid **aspartate**, which acts at the same receptors). The main inhibitory transmitter of the brain and spinal cord is **gamma-aminobutyric acid (GABA)**. It is synthesized from **glutamic acid** by the enzyme **glutamic acid decarboxylase (GAD)** which removes one of its two carboxylic acid groups (Fig. 7.6). Another amino acid, **glycine**, is an important inhibitory transmitter in the spinal cord.

Biogenic amines

This group of neurotransmitters includes **noradrenaline** (norepinephrine), **adrenaline** (epinephrine) and **dopamine**. These transmitters are produced from the amino acid **tyrosine** by decarboxylation (removal of the carboxylic acid group) leaving a single amino group ($-NH_2$) to form a **monoamine**. They are classified as **catecholamines** due to

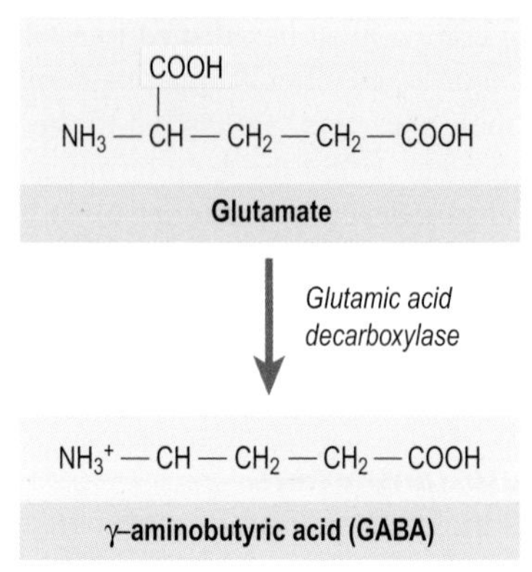

Fig. 7.6 **Synthesis of GABA.**

the presence of a **catechol** ring, which is composed of six carbon atoms. The common biosynthetic pathway for the catecholamines is illustrated in Figure 7.7.

Inactivation of catecholamines is achieved via reuptake into axon terminals. After reuptake, the catecholamines face one of two fates: (i) recycling into new synaptic vesicles; or (ii) degradation by the enzymes **catechol-O-methyltransferase** (**COMT**) or **monoamine oxidase** (**MAO**).

Serotonin (**5-hydroxytryptamine, 5-HT**) is also a biogenic amine, but contains an indole group which has a bicyclic (or two-ring) structure rather than a single catechol ring. It is therefore classified as an **indolamine**. Serotonin is synthesized from the amino acid **tryptophan** and its pathway for biosynthesis and degradation is separate from that of the catecholamines (Fig. 7.8).

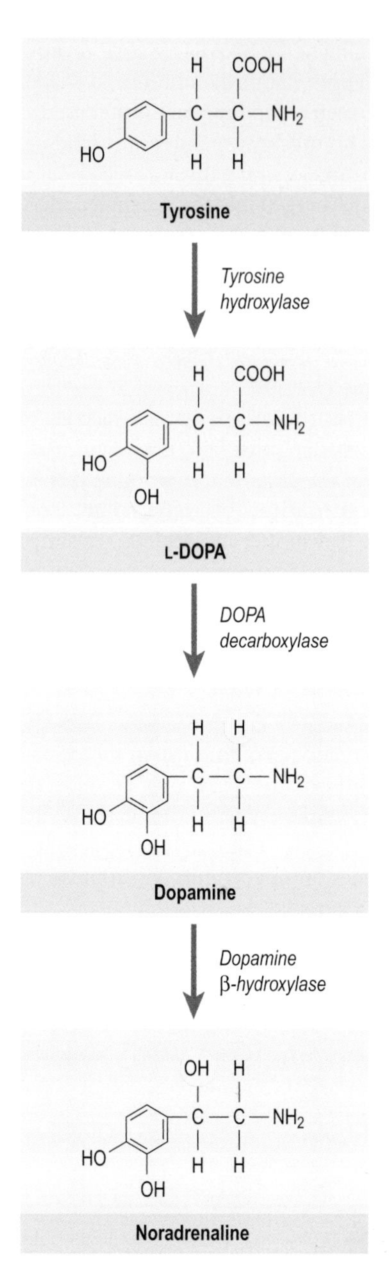

Fig. 7.7 **Synthesis of catecholamines.**

Key Points

- Classical small-molecule neurotransmitters are stored in small, clear-cored vesicles and are released into the synaptic cleft on depolarisation of the presynaptic membrane.
- The main small-molecule neurotransmitters are (i) acetylcholine, (ii) the amino acid transmitters (glutamate, aspartate, GABA, glycine) and (iii) the biogenic amines.
- The catecholamines (noradrenaline, adrenaline, dopamine) are all synthesized from tyrosine and have a common biosynthetic pathway and mechanisms for metabolism/disposal.
- Serotonin (5-hydroxytryptamine, 5-HT) is an indolamine that is synthesized from tryptophan and its pathway for synthesis and degradation is separate from that of the catecholamines.

Other signalling molecules

A number of other molecules are present in the synaptic cleft and are often co-released with a classical transmitter. The most important of these are the **neuropeptides** and **nitric oxide** gas.

Neuropeptides

More than 40 neuromodulator peptides (varying from 3–40 amino acids in length) have been identified in the central nervous system. They are stored within large, **dense-cored vesicles** that are over 100 nm in diameter. Peptides have a longer-term, neuromodulatory effect on the target cell by interacting with **metabotropic** (**G-protein-coupled**) **receptors** (discussed below). Their actions are thus mediated by second messenger molecules and may lead to lasting changes in gene expression.

Three groups of neuromodulator peptides are part of the endogenous nociceptive (pain) and analgesic system of the brain: **enkephalins**, **endorphins** and **dynorphins**. The enkephalins (**met-enkephalin** and **leu-enkephalin**) have incredibly potent pain-relieving properties: more than 100 times stronger than morphine. The endorphins and dynorphins are referred to as **opioid peptides** because they share the same endogenous receptors with opiates such as morphine and heroin (diamorphine) and have similar effects including pain relief and euphoria.

Nitric oxide

A small number of gaseous molecules have been shown to act as central neurotransmitters. The best known is **nitric oxide** (**NO**) which is synthesized from the amino acid L-arginine by the enzyme **nitric oxide synthase** (**NOS**). Unlike small molecule transmitters and neuropeptides, nitric oxide is a volatile gas which cannot be stored in synaptic vesicles and must therefore be synthesized as required. Its action is relatively brief (less than ten seconds) since it is rapidly inactivated to form inert nitrates and nitrites.

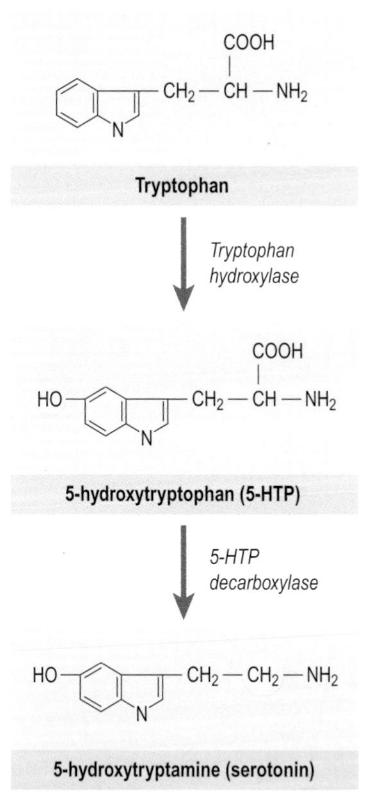

Fig. 7.8 **Synthesis of serotonin.**

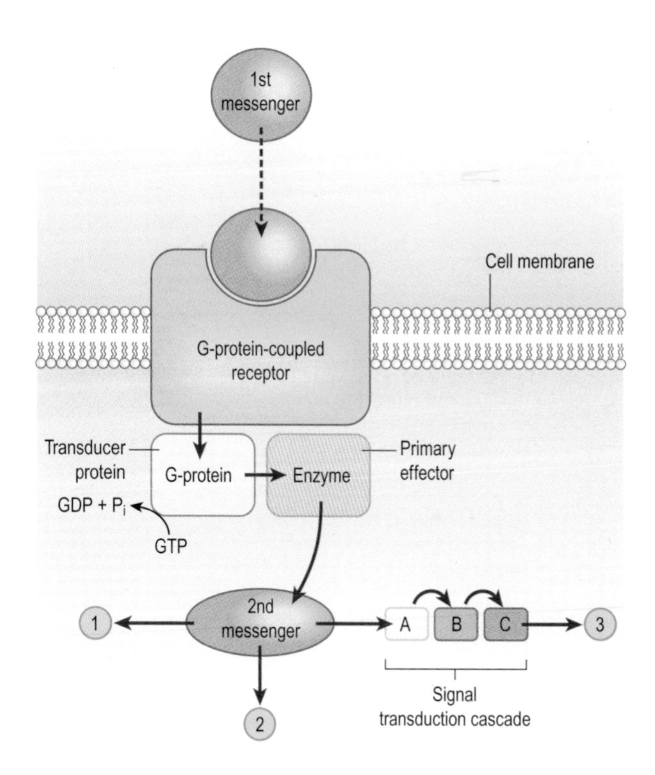

Fig. 7.9 **Metabotropic (G-protein-coupled) receptors interact with second-messenger cascades in the neuronal cytoplasm, rather than directly opening or closing ion channels.** This can have complex and long-lasting effects on the cell, including changes in gene expression.

Nitric oxide is unusual in other respects, including the ability to diffuse freely away from the point of origin, permeate cell membranes and influence neighbouring cells. Nitric oxide produced in a postsynaptic cell can therefore diffuse backwards across the synapse to the presynaptic element and act as a **retrograde messenger** (Latin: retro, backwards). The mechanism of action is by modulation of intracellular second messenger cascades, increasing the cytosolic concentration of cyclic GMP.

Key Points

- The central nervous system contains numerous neuromodulator peptides (that are often co-released with classical transmitters) which act on G-protein-coupled receptors.
- Neuropeptides have longer-lasting effects on the neuron, acting via second messenger cascades, alterations in cytosolic calcium and changes in gene expression.
- Nitric oxide gas also acts as a neurotransmitter and has the unique property of diffusing backwards across the synapse (to act as a retrograde messenger).

Postsynaptic receptors

The majority of fast neurotransmission is mediated by glutamate and GABA, which act at a number of postsynaptic receptors. The effect on the target cell depends on the receptor expressed (or its subunit composition). For this reason, the same transmitter may excite one cell, but inhibit another.

Types of receptor

The process by which a transmitter alters the electrical properties of the postsynaptic cell is called **transduction**. It is mediated by postsynaptic receptors of two types: **ionotropic** and **metabotropic**.

Ionotropic receptors

These are **ligand-gated ion channels**, meaning that the receptor site is part of the ion channel protein or closely linked to it via an adaptor protein. The neurotransmitter binds to its receptor on the extracellular aspect of the ion channel, initiating a conformational change that opens the channel pore. Direct gating of ion channels permits very fast neurotransmission and is associated exclusively with small-molecule transmitters like glutamate and GABA.

Metabotropic receptors

These channels are linked to **GTP-binding proteins** (**G-proteins**) which influence the cell via **effector proteins** which may be ion channels, enzymes or elements within an **intracellular cascade** (Fig. 7.9). For instance, receptor binding may activate an enzyme that alters the phosphorylation state of the target: activation of **kinases** leads to phosphorylation (addition of phosphate group) whereas **phosphatases** have the opposite effect. If the target is an ion channel, alteration of the phosphorylation state may open or close it (Fig. 7.10). Alternatively, intracellular cascades may lead to changes in **second messengers** such as cyclic AMP (cAMP, the concentration of which is controlled by the enzyme adenylate cyclase) or cytosolic free calcium levels. In some cases there are long-term changes in **gene expression** caused by activation of nuclear **transcription factors**. Metabotropic receptors are therefore responsible for long-term neuromodulation rather than fast neurotransmission.

Glutamate receptors

Glutamate is synthesized and stored in perisynaptic glia and in the neuronal axon terminal. It acts both at ionotropic and

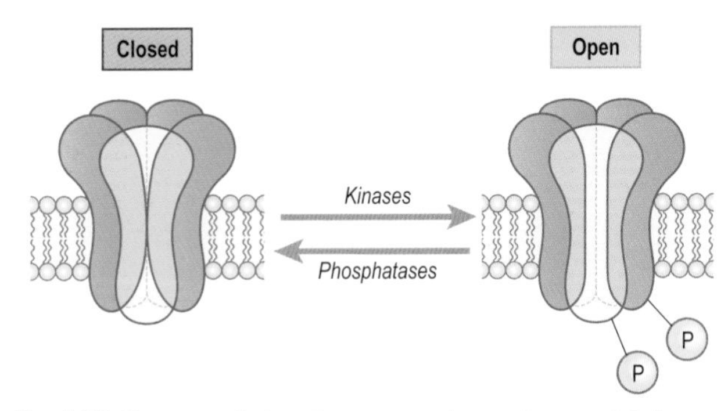

Fig. 7.10 **Kinases and phosphatases may be used to regulate ion channels by adding and removing phosphate groups (P).**

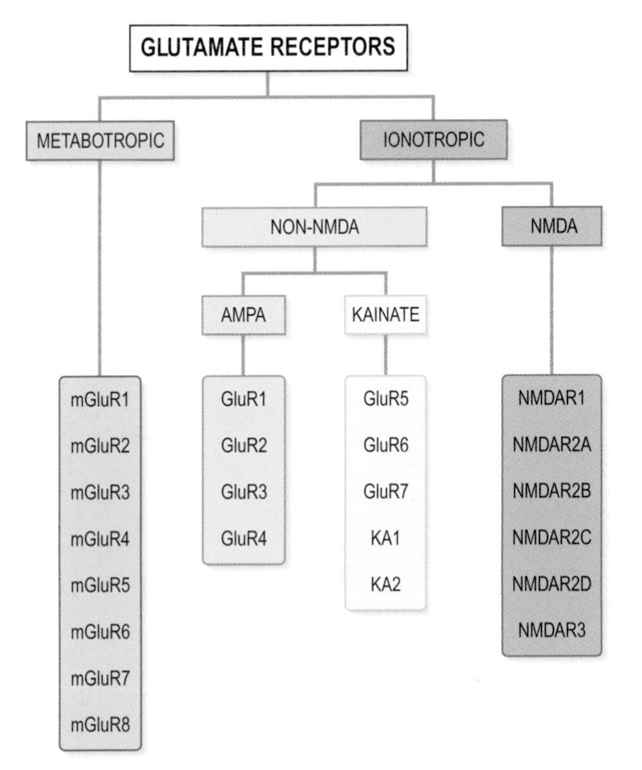

Fig. 7.11 **Classification of glutamate receptors.** The figure shows the various subunits from which individual receptors of each type can be assembled, in various combinations. Ionotropic receptors are tetrameric, whereas metabotropic receptors form heterodimers. Most AMPA receptors incorporate the GluR2 subunit which makes them impermeable to calcium; those lacking the GluR2 subunit behave more like NMDA receptors and take part in learning, memory and excitotoxicity.

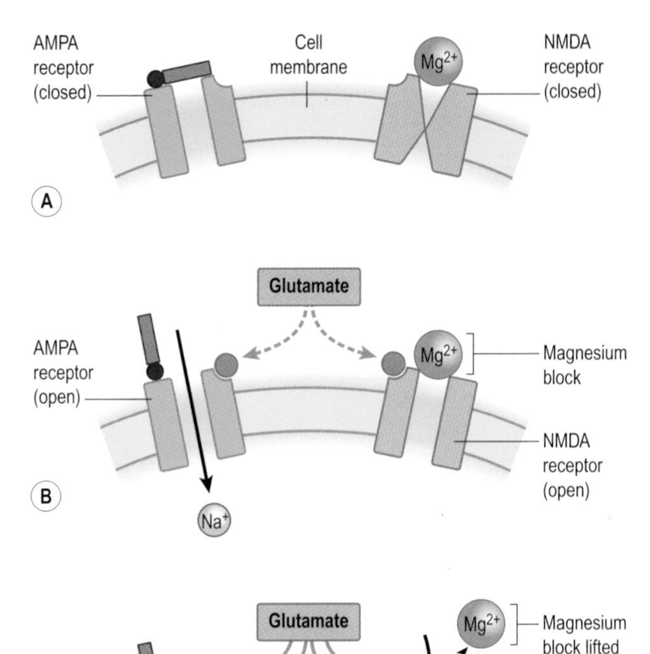

Fig. 7.12 **NMDA glutamate receptors and calcium. (A)** NMDA receptors co-exist with non-NMDA (e.g. AMPA) receptors in the neuronal membrane; **(B)** Stimulation by glutamate opens AMPA receptors which depolarizes the cell by admitting sodium ions. NMDA receptors are also stimulated but the channel pore is occluded by magnesium ions; **(C)** With prolonged stimulation the magnesium block is lifted (as magnesium ions are repelled from the mouth of the channel pore by the increasingly positive interior face of the membrane). Once this has happened, calcium is able to enter the cell via the liberated NMDA channels.

metabotropic receptors, which can be assembled from an array of subunits (Fig. 7.11).

Ionotropic glutamate receptors

Three types of glutamate receptor are linked to ion channels. They are classified by their response to the exogenous ligand **N-methyl-D-aspartate (NMDA)** as NMDA and non-NMDA and each consist of a tetrameric assembly of subunits.

Non-NMDA receptors

The **AMPA** (α-amino-3-hydroxy-5-methyl-4-isoxazole propionic acid) subtype of glutamate receptor is responsible for the majority of fast excitatory transmission in the central nervous system. **The kainate receptor** is similar and the term 'AMPA-kainate' is sometimes used to describe them collectively. AMPA channels are mainly permeable to sodium and gating therefore leads to membrane depolarization. The receptor is an oligomeric assembly of four subunits (selected from GluR1-R4, in various combinations). Most central AMPA receptors incorporate the **GluR2 subunit** which makes them impermeable to calcium. Those lacking the GluR2 subunit permit calcium influx which may trigger long-term changes in biochemistry and gene expression.

NMDA receptors and calcium

At the resting membrane potential the ion channels of NMDA receptors are inactivated by magnesium ions (Mg^{2+}), as shown in Figure 7.12. Once the neuronal membrane has been depolarized and this **magnesium block** is lifted, sodium and calcium ions are able to enter the cell. NMDA receptors therefore have the unique property of being both ligand-gated and voltage-sensitive. Also, because of their high calcium permeability, they are able to effect long-term changes in neuronal biochemistry by initiating downstream, calcium-dependent events.

Metabotropic glutamate receptors

Numerous G-protein-coupled glutamate receptors have been identified, many of which consist of a heterodimeric assembly of subunits (selected from mGLUR1-8; see Fig. 7.11). They fall into three main groups, but the majority are postsynaptic and excitatory. Some are **presynaptic autoreceptors** which help to regulate transmitter release at the synapse.

Memory and learning

The biological basis of memory is not fully understood, but one element appears to be that synaptic strength is able to increase or decrease, depending on usage: **synaptic plasticity** (Greek: plastikos, able to be moulded). A use-dependent increase in the efficacy of central synapses is termed **long-term potentiation (LTP)**. An excitatory synapse that is used frequently is 'potentiated' (made stronger) by increased release of neurotransmitter from the presynaptic cell and increased sensitivity to transmitter in the postsynaptic cell (e.g. by inserting more receptors in the postsynaptic membrane). The presynaptic neuron is therefore more likely to depolarize the postsynaptic cell in future. **Nitric oxide** contributes to this process by acting as a **retrograde messenger**. Glutamate-mediated depolarization of the postsynaptic cell leads to an elevation of cytosolic calcium which trigger nitric oxide release. This then diffuses backwards across the synapse to influence the presynaptic element.

Associative phenomena

When a nerve cell is depolarized to threshold, any synapses that are active at the same time (and have contributed to the successful depolarization of the postsynaptic cell) may also be strengthened. This is referred to as an **associative phenomenon** (sometimes stated as 'neurons that fire together, wire together'). Conversely, an incoming excitatory projection that is consistently active when the target neuron is not depolarized to threshold is progressively weakened ('neurons that fire apart, fall apart'). Long-term weakening of a synapse, perhaps as a result of low or reduced levels of firing leads to **long-term depression (LTD)**. This is important in the cerebellum during motor learning.

The mechanism of long-term potentiation, which depends upon controlled elevation of free cytosolic calcium, explains why glutamate is neurotoxic at high levels. Very strong glutamatergic stimulation leads to **excessive calcium influx** via NMDA receptors and GluR2-negative AMPA receptors, which damages the cell and may trigger programmed cell death. This process is termed **excitotoxicity** and is important in several nervous system disorders (see Ch. 8). Glutamate is therefore described as an **excitotoxin** when present at abnormally high concentrations.

GABA receptors

There are two types of GABA receptor: a fast (ionotropic) **$GABA_A$** receptor that is mainly distributed within the limbic lobe, in areas that are concerned with emotion and memory; and a slow (metabotropic) **$GABA_B$** receptor which is found throughout the cerebral hemispheres.

Ionotropic GABA receptors

The $GABA_A$ receptor is the target of several **anti-anxiety drugs** and its action is also modulated by alcohol (Clinical Box 7.1). It is a pentameric **chloride ion channel** assembled from more than a dozen varieties of alpha, beta, gamma and delta subunits. The reversal potential is around −65 mV, so that activation tends to maintain the hyperpolarized (inhibited) state of the cell.

Metabotropic GABA receptors

The $GABA_B$ receptor is widely distributed throughout the cerebral hemispheres. It is a heterodimeric G-protein-coupled receptor which leads to opening of **potassium channels** that hyperpolarize the cell membrane. Activation of $GABA_B$ receptors inhibits the cell for a longer period of time, but the effect is slower than at $GABA_A$ receptors.

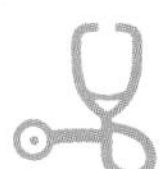

Clinical Box 7.1: Anxiolytic drugs and alcohol

Many anxiolytic, sedative and hypnotic agents (used to treat anxiety or insomnia) act by stimulating $GABA_A$ receptors. These include: (i) **benzodiazepines** such as diazepam, which cause neuronal inhibition by increasing the *frequency* of chloride channel opening; and (ii) **barbiturates** such as phenobarbital, which increase the *duration* of channel opening by acting at a different binding site. One of the many effects of **alcohol** on the central nervous system is potentiation of $GABA_A$ receptors. Antagonism of the $GABA_A$ receptor (with agents such as **picrotoxin**) leads to convulsions, which is used in some animal models of epilepsy (Ch. 11).

Key Points

- Neurotransmitter receptors are of two major types: fast (ionotropic or ion-channel-linked) and slow (metabotropic or G-protein-coupled).
- The majority of fast excitatory neurotransmission in the CNS is mediated by glutamate (or aspartate) acting at ionotropic receptors. These are classified as NMDA and non-NMDA types.
- The non-NMDA receptors include the AMPA and kainate sub-types. NMDA receptors are calcium-permeable and are important for synaptic plasticity, memory and learning.
- An important cellular mechanism in synaptic plasticity is long-term potentiation (LTP), which describes a long-lasting (use-dependent) increase in synaptic efficacy or strength. NMDA glutamate receptors and nitric oxide are important contributors to LTP.
- The main inhibitory transmitter in the CNS is GABA. It acts at ionotropic $GABA_A$ receptors (present mainly in the limbic lobe) and the more widespread metabotropic $GABA_B$ receptors.

Synaptic integration

A typical neuron receives synaptic contacts from around 10,000 other cells. Many different transmitters are released and numerous cell-surface receptors are present to respond to these signals. The small excitatory and inhibitory postsynaptic potentials generated by activity in countless synaptic contacts are continuously integrated and summated. This determines the 'firing rate' of the cell and the frequency of nerve impulse generation from one moment to the next.

Spatial and temporal summation

The impact of a single excitatory postsynaptic potential on a target neuron is small, but if a number of convergent impulses from different nerve cells all reach the postsynaptic neuron together then the combined effect off these disparate influences may be sufficient to depolarize the cell to threshold and generate an action potential (Fig. 7.13). This is referred to as **spatial summation**.

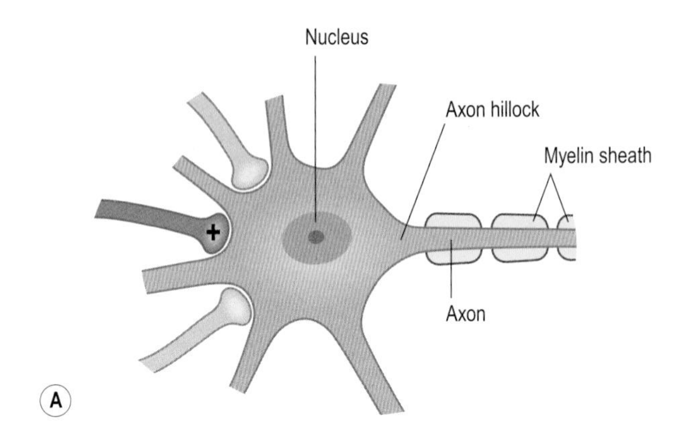

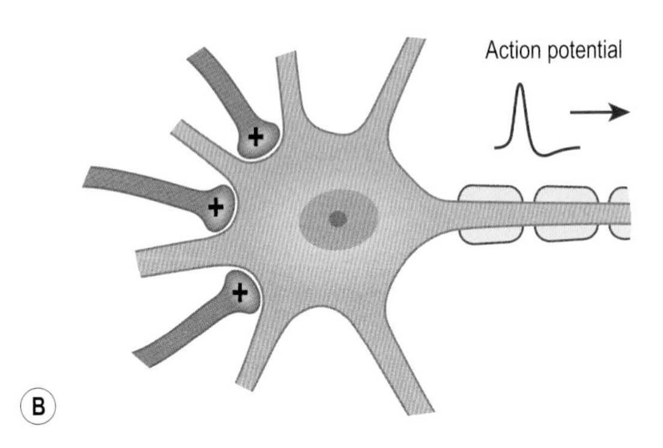

Fig. 7.13 **Spatial summation.** Excitatory projections from one or a small number of afferent fibres may be insufficient to cause depolarization in a target neuron **(A)**, but it may be possible to trigger an action potential if several relatively weak impulses converge on the same target cell **(B)**.

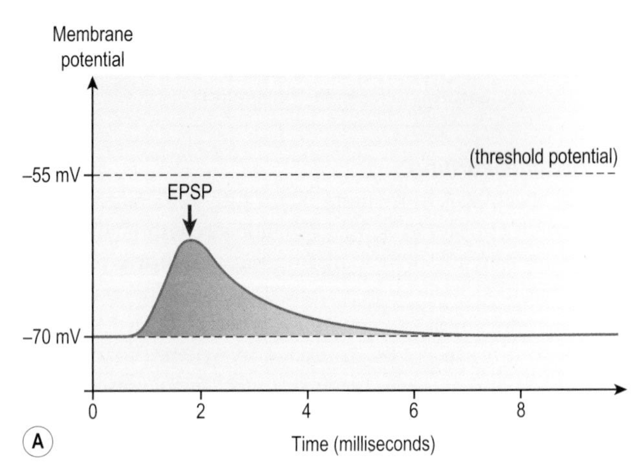

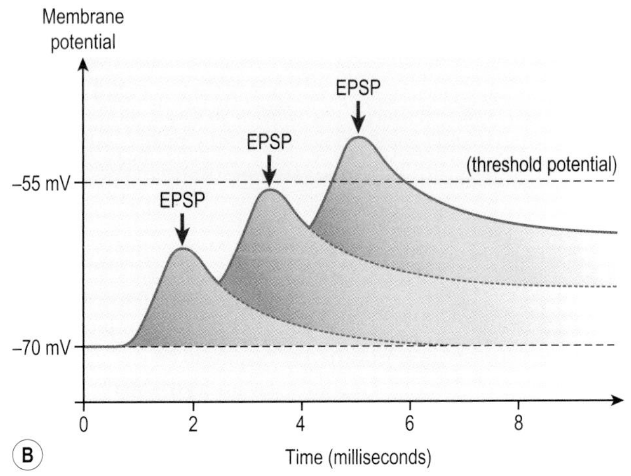

Fig. 7.14 **Temporal summation.** A single, relatively weak excitatory postsynaptic potential (EPSP) may be insufficient to reach the threshold for generation of an action potential **(A)**, but if several excitatory postsynaptic potentials arrive in quick succession (before the previous ones have completely decayed) then they may be additive and take the cell membrane to threshold **(B)**.

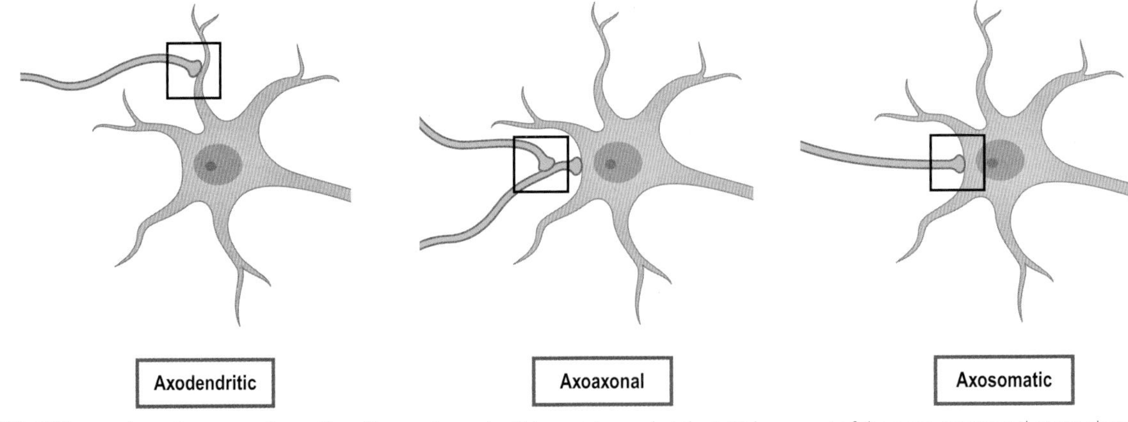

Fig. 7.15 **Different sites of synapse formation.** Since action potentials are triggered at the initial segment of the axon, synapses that are closer to this point (on the proximal dendrites or soma, rather than at the distant reaches of the dendritic tree) have a stronger influence on the target cell.

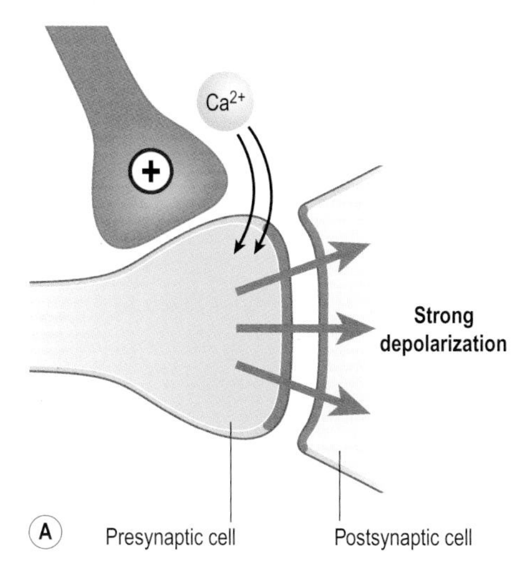

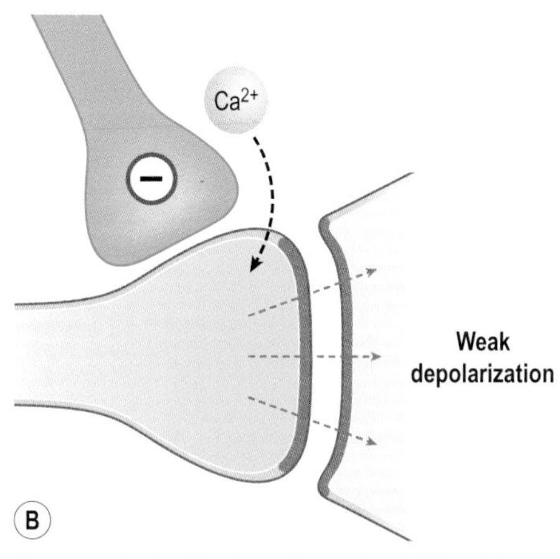

Fig. 7.16 **Presynaptic facilitation (A) and inhibition (B).**

Similarly, although the influence of a single excitatory or inhibitory postsynaptic potential is small, the graded potential takes up to 15 milliseconds to decay – and may be additive if several nerve impulses arrive in rapid succession. This is referred to as **temporal summation** (Fig. 7.14) which operates together with spatial summation.

The trigger zone for action potential generation is the **initial segment** of the axon. Summation of excitatory and inhibitory influences in this region of the membrane is critical for nerve impulse generation, so incoming synapses that are closer to this area stand a better chance of influencing neuronal firing rate than those at the distant reaches of the dendritic tree (Fig. 7.15).

Some neurons exert a more powerful excitatory or inhibitory effect on their targets by making direct synaptic contact with the axon terminal. This is termed **presynaptic facilitation** or **presynaptic inhibition**, illustrated in Figure 7.16.

Key Points

- Excitatory and inhibitory postsynaptic potentials (EPSPs/IPSPs) are constantly integrated by neurons to determine the rate of nerve impulse generation from moment to moment.
- A single neuron may receive as many as 10,000 synapses and the positive and negative influences are integrated at the initial segment of the axon to determine the 'firing rate' of the cell.
- Although the influence of any one postsynaptic potential is small, the target neuron may be brought to its firing threshold as a result of spatial or temporal summation.
- Some neurons exert a more powerful (positive or negative) effect on the target cell by making direct synaptic contact with the axon terminal (presynaptic facilitation or inhibition).

Chapter 8
Cellular mechanisms of neurological disease

CHAPTER CONTENTS

The nervous system is subject to the full range of pathological processes found in other organs, together with a number of unique degenerative and demyelinating diseases. The basic pathological processes underlying these disorders will be discussed in this chapter (including inflammation, gliosis and neuronal cell death) before moving on to specific examples of neurological disorders in the chapters that follow. Demyelination is discussed separately in Chapter 14, in the context of multiple sclerosis.

Neuronal injury and death

Nerve cells have a limited capacity to withstand **pathological stimuli**. Cell death occurs when the neuron reaches a 'point of no return' following irreversible damage to the plasma membrane, nuclear DNA or mitochondria. Since neurons are **post-mitotic** cells (meaning that they are unable to divide) they cannot usually be replaced in most parts of the brain and spinal cord. Exceptions include the hippocampus and olfactory bulb (where neurons can be replenished from a pool of **stem cells**). The two main forms of cell death are illustrated in Figure 8.1 and discussed below.

Necrosis

Tissue death resulting from damage or disease is referred to as **necrosis** (Greek: nekros, corpse). This is the end-point of numerous pathological processes and has features in common with the dissolution of the body that occurs after death

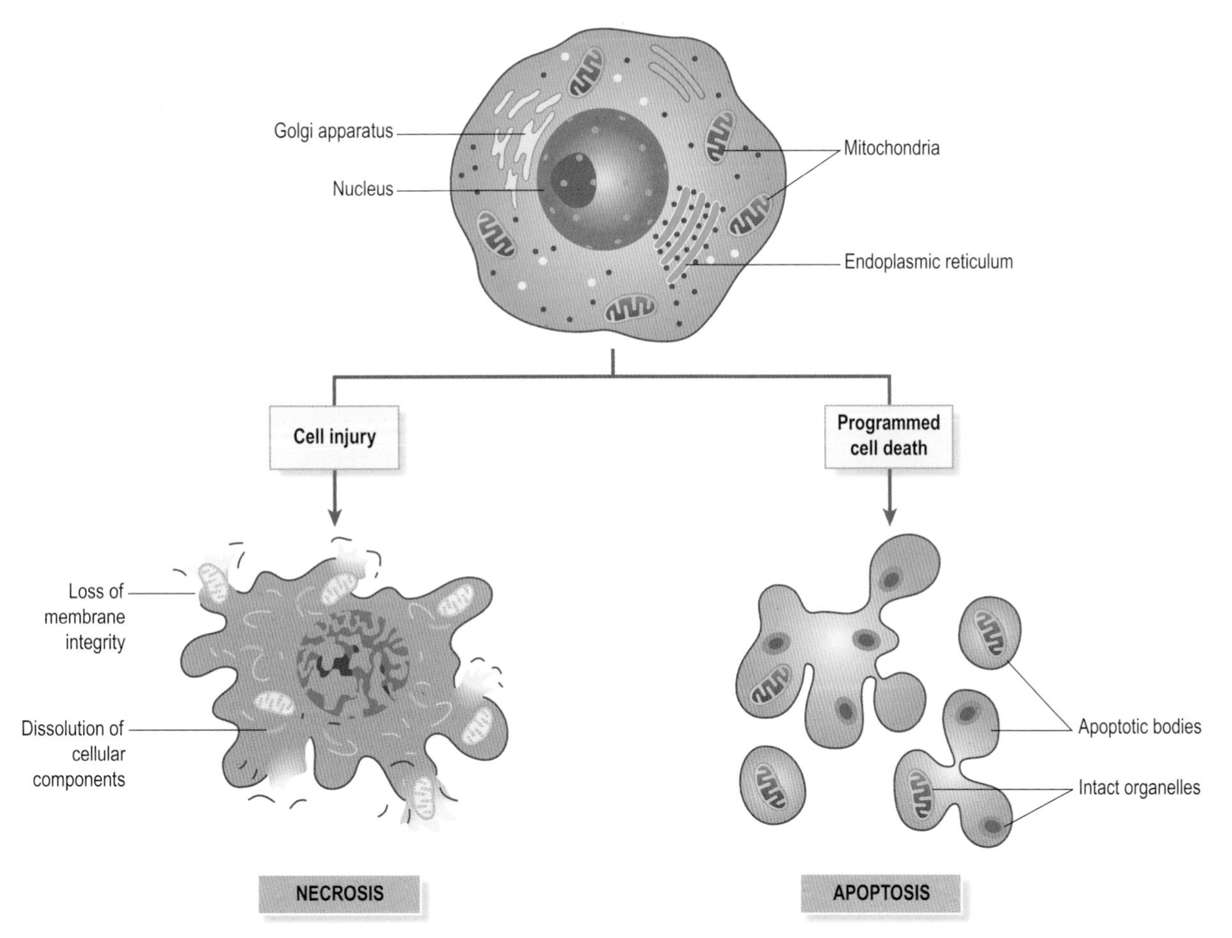

Fig. 8.1 **Types of cell death.**

(**autolysis**). Necrosis is associated with cellular swelling, loss of membrane integrity and influx of sodium and calcium ions, with eventual rupture of the cell. This is followed by digestion of the cellular constituents by **lysosomal enzymes**. As the necrotic cell breaks down, its internal components are discharged into the extracellular space, eliciting an **inflammatory reaction**. Several patterns of necrosis are recognized, but the type usually seen in the brain is called **liquefactive necrosis**. In this process, dead brain tissue is gradually removed by macrophages and liquefied by hydrolytic enzymes. Complete resorption may take several years, ultimately leaving only a fluid-filled cyst.

Apoptosis

Deliberate deletion of unwanted cells is termed **programmed cell death**. This is essential for normal growth and development, but is also responsible for cell loss in a number of CNS pathologies including neurodegeneration, stroke and multiple sclerosis.

The most common and best characterized form of programmed cell death is **apoptosis** (pronounced: apa-TOSIS). The term derives from the Greek and alludes to the deliberate shedding of autumn leaves (Greek: apo, away from; ptosis, falling). Apoptosis has characteristic microscopic features including cell shrinkage, condensation of the nuclear chromatin, cytoplasmic blebbing and formation of membrane-bound **apoptotic bodies** which contain viable organelles.

Most newly formed nerve cells are primed to commit programmed cell death ('cellular suicide') unless rescued by exposure to the appropriate **trophic factors** (Greek: trophē, nourishment). One of the best known examples of this is the dependence of dorsal root ganglion neurons on **nerve growth factor** (**NGF**). During CNS development, up to 50% of neurons are deliberately deleted because they fail to (i) reach their intended targets or (ii) make appropriate connections with other nerve cells.

Apoptosis is also an important mechanism for the destruction of critically injured or abnormal cells and is triggered in diseases where **pathological stress** has compromised key cellular elements beyond repair. Irreparable damage to the nuclear DNA is a potent trigger for apoptosis, contributing to the prevention of tumours. It is also used by activated lymphocytes to sacrifice virus-infected cells and to delete self-reactive T-lymphocytes in the thymus gland (preventing autoimmune disease).

Caspases

Apoptosis is orchestrated by a family of proteolytic enzymes called **caspases** (cysteine-dependent aspartate-specific proteases) which cleave target proteins at aspartate residues. The caspases are synthesized as inactive **procaspases** and once activated are able to cleave parts of the neuronal cytoskeleton and nuclear DNA.

- **Initiator caspases** are activated by intrinsic (cell stress) or extrinsic (cell death) signals. Examples include caspases 2, 8, 9 and 10.
- **Effector caspases** mediate programmed cell death by digesting the nuclear DNA and other key cellular elements. Examples include caspases 3, 6 and 7.

Many components of the caspase cascade converge on the effector (or **executioner**) proteins, such as **caspase-3**, which can be used as a marker of apoptosis. Programmed cell death can be triggered by extrinsic or intrinsic stimuli.

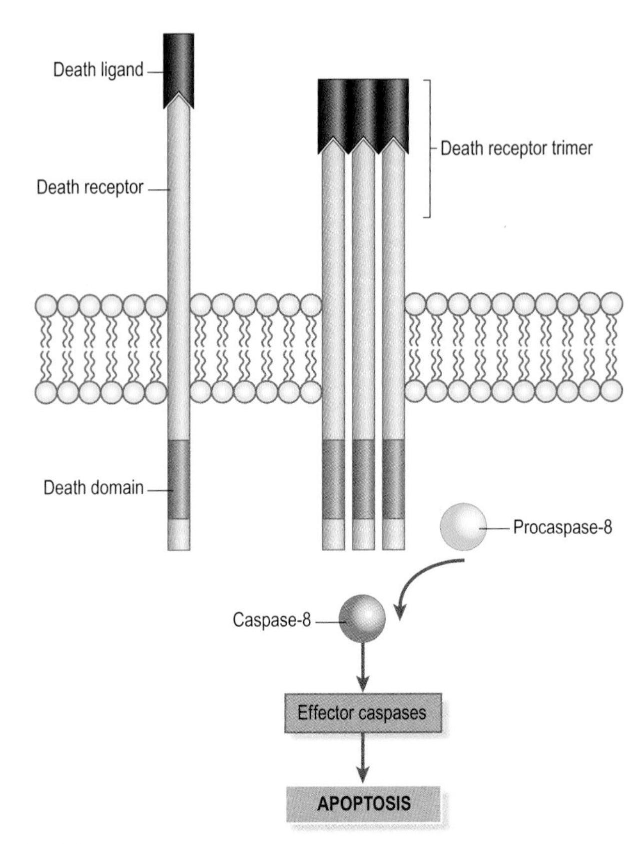

Fig. 8.2 **The extrinsic pathway for apoptosis is triggered by cell death ligands binding to receptors at the cell surface.** This leads to activation of caspase-8 within the cell, which initiates apoptosis.

Extrinsic pathway (Fig. 8.2)

Apoptosis can be triggered by **cell death ligands** in the extracellular fluid. These act on cell-surface receptors belonging to the **tumour necrosis factor** (**TNF**) family. After ligand binding, death receptors cluster within the membrane to form trimers and a conformational change in the cytoplasmic part of the protein exposes an ominously named **death domain**. The intracellular region of the cell death receptor binds apoptotic proteins in the cytoplasm via **adaptor proteins**. The interaction is mediated by **death effector domains** (**DEDs**) that are present in both the adaptor proteins and the procaspases. These interactions lead to formation of a **death-inducing signalling complex** (**DISC**) which activates caspase-8 and thereby initiates programmed cell death.

Intrinsic pathway (Fig. 8.3)

Apoptosis can also be triggered from within the cell if it is exposed to excessive **pathological stress**. Activation of the intrinsic pathway depends upon the balance of pro-apoptotic and anti-apoptotic factors, many of which are members of the **BCL** (**B-cell lymphoma**) family of proteins. Members that tend to oppose programmed cell death include Bcl-2 and Bcl-XL; others, such as Bad and Bax are pro-apoptotic. These molecules act as **stress sensors** in the cytoplasm, responding to pathological stimuli by translocating to mitochondria.

A key event is formation of a **permeability transition pore** (**PTP**) in the mitochondrial membrane, which is a large transmembrane pore (or 'megachannel'). Pore formation allows **cytochrome c oxidase** and **apoptosis inducing**

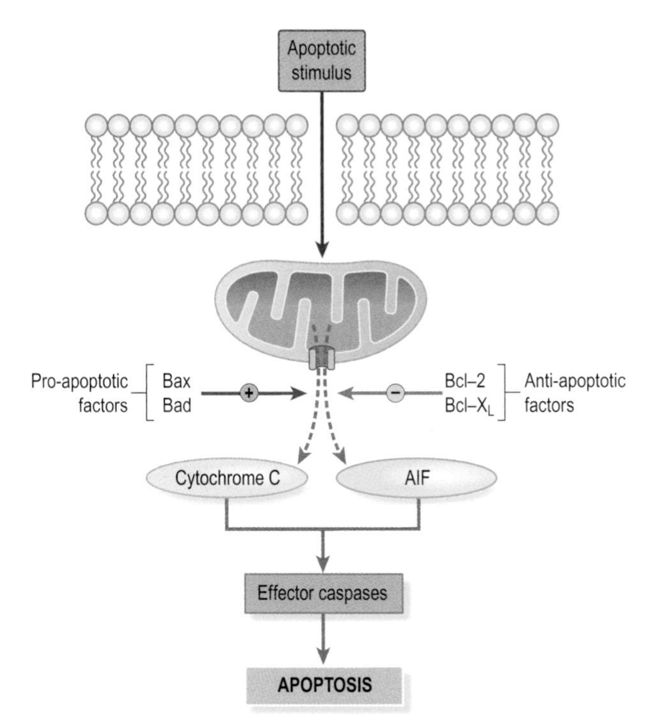

Fig. 8.3 **The intrinsic pathway for apoptosis depends upon the balance of pro-apoptotic and anti-apoptotic members of the Bcl-2 family.** A key event is formation of the permeability transition pore (shown here in orange) in the mitochondrial membrane (coloured purple). This allows apoptosis-inducing factors to be released into the cytoplasm.

factor (**AIF**) to escape from mitochondria and reach the cytoplasm. Cytochrome c then forms a complex with **Apaf-1** (apoptotic protease activating factor 1) which recruits caspase-9 to form a larger multi-protein complex called the **apoptosome**. Following formation of the apoptosome, caspase-9 is activated and apoptosis is triggered, culminating in the upregulation of **cell death genes**.

Disposal of the cell

Once a cell is committed to programmed cell death, its DNA and cytoskeleton are dismantled in an orderly manner. This is an active process that expends energy. A key step is activation of the enzyme **caspase-activated DNAse** (**CAD**) by effector caspases, which breaks down the DNA into nucleosomal units. Organelles are packaged into membrane-bound **apoptotic bodies** (see Fig. 8.1) which contain viable mitochondria. These structures express cell-surface markers that trigger their internalization by neighbouring cells. An example is the membrane constituent **phosphatidylserine**, which translocates from the inner to the outer leaflet of the plasma membrane. Phagocytes recognize and bind these molecules and internalize the apoptotic bodies for degradation. The entire process is carefully orchestrated and, in contrast to necrosis, there is no inflammatory reaction.

Key Points

- The two main types of cell death are necrosis and apoptosis.
- Necrotic cell death is characterized by dissolution of the cell with release of lysosomal enzymes and an inflammatory reaction. Liquefactive necrosis is the most common type in the CNS.
- Apoptosis is the best-understood form of programmed cell death. It is triggered by extrinsic (cell death) and intrinsic (cell stress) pathways and mediated by initiator and executioner caspases.
- Programmed cell death is important in embryogenesis, tumour prevention, deletion of self-reactive (autoaggressive) lymphocytes and destruction of virus-infected cells.
- It also contributes to nerve cell loss in a range of neurological disorders including neurodegenerative diseases, stroke and multiple sclerosis.

Axonal damage

It is possible for axons to undergo selective degeneration without death of the cell body. For instance, following transection of a peripheral nerve, the distal portions of the affected axons degenerate together with their myelin sheaths. This is termed **Wallerian degeneration**, which is accompanied by regenerative changes in the parent cell, called the **axon reaction**. These include swelling of the cell body, dispersal of the Nissl substance (**chromatolysis**) and displacement and enlargement of the nucleus, reflecting increased gene transcription and protein synthesis. If the regenerative attempt fails (which is usually the case in the CNS) then the parent cell will eventually undergo apoptosis.

Transneuronal degeneration (Fig. 8.4)

Following axonal transection, neuronal degeneration may spread to involve other nerve cells, referred to as **transneuronal degeneration**. For instance, following interruption of an anatomical pathway consisting of a linear chain of neurons, there may be subsequent loss of nerve cells 'downstream' (**anterograde**) or 'upstream' (**retrograde**) of the original injury, which may take months or years. This reflects the general principle that nerve cells need to be integrated into a functional network and receive trophic signals from other neurons in order to remain viable.

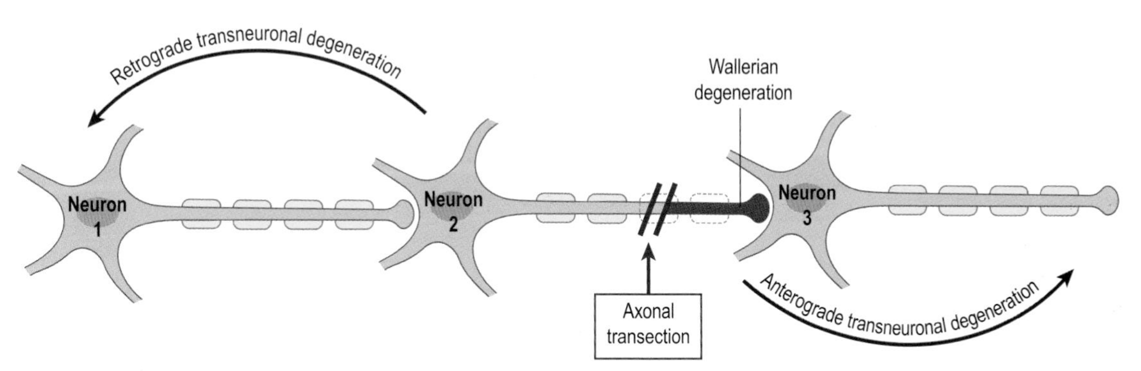

Fig. 8.4 **Degeneration following axonal injury.** Following axonal transection (neuron 2) the distal part of the nerve fibre undergoes Wallerian degeneration. Other neurons may subsequently be lost in an anatomical pathway by transneuronal degeneration (neurons 1 and 3).

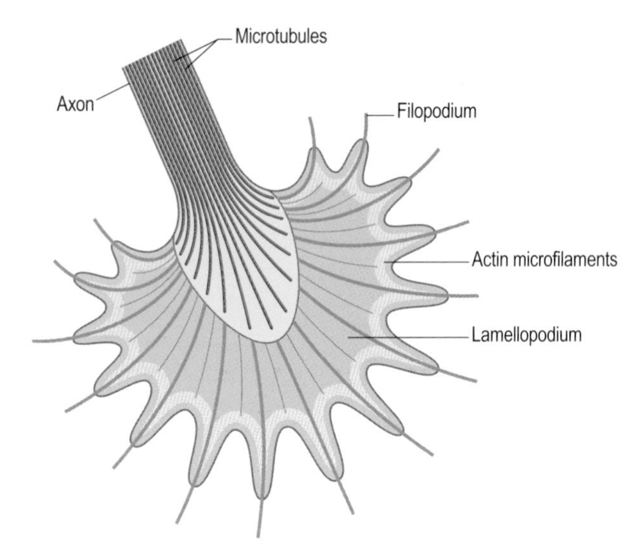

Fig. 8.5 **A growth cone.**

Axonal regrowth

Axons are able to regenerate following peripheral nerve damage and may re-establish connections with muscle fibres or glands. The distal tips of the severed axons form **growth cones** (Fig. 8.5) which 'crawl' along residual Schwann cell basement membranes to reinnervate target structures. This process occurs after peripheral nerve injury (see Clinical Box 8.1) but does not seem to be possible in the brain and spinal cord.

> ### *Clinical Box 8.1: Bell's palsy*
>
> Bell's palsy is a unilateral **facial paralysis** caused by inflammation of the facial nerve. The cause is uncertain, but it may be related to a virus infection. Presentation is abrupt and is sometimes preceded by **otalgia** (earache). Damage to the facial nerve may lead to changes in the sense of taste or sensitivity to loud noises. This is because the facial nerve also supplies taste buds in the anterior two thirds of the tongue and the **stapedius muscle**, which prevents excessive vibration of the ear drum. In most cases symptoms improve spontaneously as the damaged axons slowly grow back. Recovery is often imperfect, with aberrant reinnervation of muscles and glands, leading to symptoms such as eye closure on attempting to smile or **crocodile tears** in place of salivation.

> ### *Key Points*
>
> - Axonal transection leads to degeneration of the distal portion of the axon, together with its myelin sheath (termed Wallerian degeneration).
> - The axon reaction (in the cell body) reflects an attempt by the cell to regrow the axon and establish new connections with the denervated target structures
> - Axonal regrowth is commonly seen following peripheral nerve injury, but does not occur in the brain or spinal cord.
> - Interruption of an anatomical pathway may lead to subsequent degeneration in nerve cells proximal or distal to the original lesion (termed transneuronal degeneration).

Cell death mechanisms

Cells are continuously subjected to physiological and pathological stimuli to which they must adapt in order to survive. **Pathological stimuli** leading to neuronal cell death include excitotoxicity and oxidative stress, with accumulation of excessive intracellular free calcium as a final common event.

Excitotoxicity

Excessive stimulation by excitatory neurotransmitters (such as **glutamate**) can cause neuronal cell death in a process known as **excitotoxicity**. Intense glutamatergic stimulation leads to prolonged neuronal depolarization, lifting the magnesium blockade of **NMDA (N-methyl D-aspartate) receptors**. In this situation, free calcium ions are able to flood the neuronal cytoplasm via liberated NMDA receptors, as well as via calcium-permeable **AMPA (alpha-amino, 3-hydroxy-4-isoxasole-propionic acid) receptors** and **voltage-gated calcium channels** (see Ch. 7). This leads to further depolarization, with additional glutamate release, generating a vicious cycle. In addition to acute excitotoxic injury, there is evidence that low-grade excitotoxicity may cause chronic neuronal damage in some disorders (e.g. **motor neuron disease**; see Ch. 4, Clinical Box 4.9). Accumulation of intracellular free calcium is an important final common event in excitotoxicity neuronal cell death.

The role of calcium

The free calcium ion concentration in the cytoplasm is normally kept very low by several mechanisms including sequestration by **calcium-binding proteins** (e.g. **parvalbumin** and **calbindin**) and export from the cell. The high calcium influxes generated by excitotoxic stimulation overwhelm buffering and extrusion mechanisms, leading to activation of harmful calcium-dependent enzymes, including:

- **Calpains**, which degrade the neuronal cytoskeleton.
- **Proteases**, which digest structural proteins and enzymes.
- **Phospholipases**, which impair the integrity of cell membranes.
- **Endonucleases**, leading to DNA fragmentation.

Several pro-apoptotic genes are also upregulated by calcium-mediated cascades, which promotes degradation of the cytoskeleton and may initiate programmed cell death. Calcium-mediated activation of **xanthine oxidase** and **nitric oxide synthase** may also lead to oxidative stress.

Oxidative stress

Oxidative phosphorylation in normal mitochondria generates potentially harmful **reactive oxygen species (ROS)** or **free radicals**, including **superoxide anion** (O^{2-}) and **hydroxyl radical** (OH^-). These are highly reactive species with unpaired electrons that can damage cell membranes, proteins and DNA. The body has a number of **scavenging mechanisms** and molecules to deal with free radicals, including antioxidant vitamins (especially C and E) and three key enzymes:

- **Superoxide dismutase.**
- **Catalase.**
- **Glutathione peroxidase.**

Mitochondria continuously produce superoxide anion which is catabolized by superoxide dismutase to form **hydrogen peroxide** (H_2O_2). This is also a reactive oxygen species and is

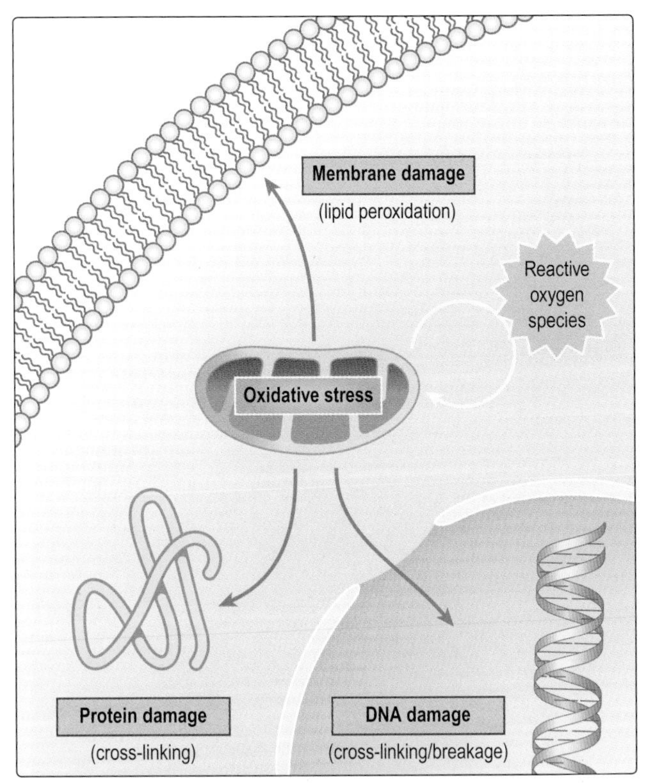

Fig. 8.6 **Oxidative stress.** Reactive oxygen (and nitrogen) species damage key cellular components such a proteins, cell membrane and DNA, leading to cell death.

degraded by catalase. Excessive generation of free radicals or reduced capacity of the normal scavenging mechanisms leads to **oxidative stress**, with abnormal cross-linkages forming between nucleic acids, lipids, carbohydrates and proteins as free radicals react with them indiscriminately (Fig. 8.6). Oxidative stress may be exacerbated by age-related mitochondrial abnormalities due to mutations in **mitochondrial DNA** that accrue during the lifetime of an individual.

Nitric oxide

Nitric oxide gas is synthesized from L-arginine by isoforms of the enzyme **nitric oxide synthase** (**NOS**). It is a free radical species with a number of important physiological roles (e.g. as a vasodilator, transmitter substance and regulator of inflammatory and immune responses). Its synthesis is induced by **glutamate signalling** via the calcium-permeable NMDA receptor and excessive production of nitric oxide is a feature of excitotoxicity.

Nitric oxide reacts with superoxide anion to produce **peroxynitrite** ($ONOO^-$). This is a **reactive nitrogen species** that may damage proteins by interacting with cysteine and tyrosine residues. Although nitric oxide has an anti-apoptotic effect in many cell types, excessive production contributes to cell death in neurodegenerative diseases, multiple sclerosis and stroke.

Inflammation and gliosis

The body responds to pathological insults with an **inflammatory reaction** in which blood vessels become 'leaky' so that protein-rich fluid and inflammatory cells can enter the tissues. **Gliosis** is a unique response to damage that only occurs in the brain and spinal cord.

Key Points

- Glutamate-mediated excitotoxicity is a common cell death mechanism in many neurological diseases, mediated by influx of excessive free calcium via NMDA receptors.
- High intracellular calcium levels trigger enzymes such as calpains, proteases, phospholipases and endonucleases that digest key cellular elements including the cytoskeleton and DNA.
- Reactive oxygen species (ROS) are continuously produced by mitochondria and removed by natural scavenging mechanisms (e.g. superoxide dismutase, catalase, glutathione peroxidase).
- Free radicals (e.g. superoxide anion, O^{2-}; and hydroxyl radical, OH^-) are highly reactive and damage cells by forming abnormal cross-linkages between lipids, carbohydrates and proteins.
- Excessive production of free radicals including nitric oxide contributes to cell death in neurodegenerative diseases, multiple sclerosis and stroke.

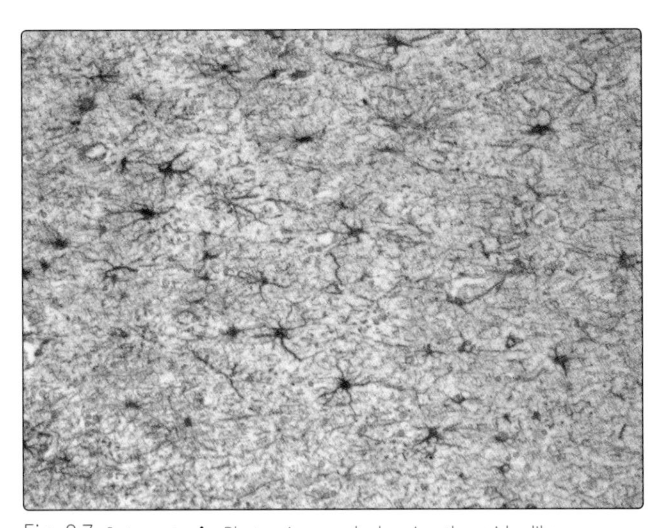

Fig. 8.7 **Astrocytosis.** Photomicrograph showing the spider-like appearance of reactive astrocytes using immunohistochemistry (antibody labelling) for glial fibrillary acidic protein (GFAP).

Reactive gliosis

Gliosis (also known as reactive gliosis) consists of activation and proliferation of glial cells, stimulated by inflammatory cytokines including **interleukin-1** (**IL-1**), **tumour necrosis factor alpha** (**TNF-α**) and **interleukin-6** (**IL-6**). It is a combination of astrocytosis and microgliosis.

Astrocytosis (Fig. 8.7)

Following brain injury, nearby astrocytes enlarge, multiply and increase their expression of **glial fibrillary acid protein** (**GFAP**). Proliferation of astrocytes may be sufficient to fill in a small tissue defect, but larger areas of damage (e.g. following a major stroke, see Ch. 10) are transformed into a fluid-filled cystic cavity lined by a **glial scar**. Astrocytes secrete (i) cytokines that recruit inflammatory cells from the blood and (ii) various **trophic factors**, including:

- Nerve growth factor (NGF).
- Brain-derived neurotrophic factor (BDNF).
- Glial-cell-line-derived neurotrophic factor (GDNF).

These are chemical mediators that promote neuronal survival and axon sprouting. They are released into the extracellular fluid, but can also be delivered directly to the neuronal cytoplasm via intercellular **gap junctions** (see Ch. 7).

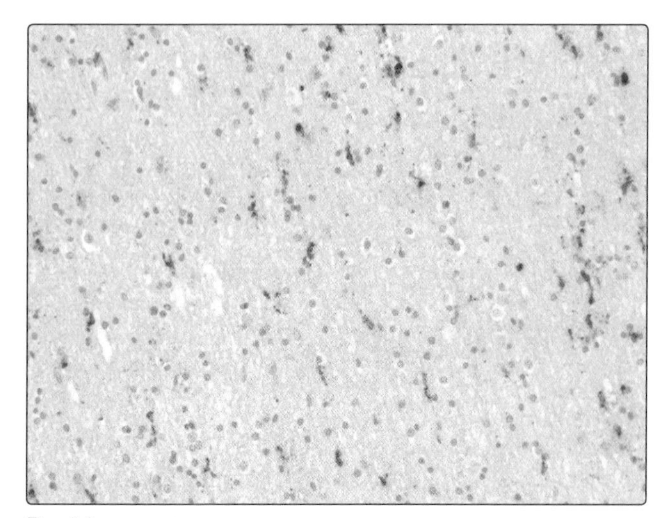

Fig. 8.8 **Microgliosis.** Photomicrograph of reactive microglial cells using immunohistochemistry for the macrophage marker CD68.

Microgliosis (Fig. 8.8)

Microglia are the resident **phagocytes** (scavengers) of the brain. They normally exist in a **ramified**, quiescent state, but following tissue injury they become activated in response to inflammatory cytokines and growth factors. **Activated microglia** migrate towards injured tissues by following chemotactic gradients. They differentiate into **macrophages** and internalize cellular debris and microorganisms. Those that have ingested myelin debris form lipid-laden **foam cells**.

Activated microglia are immunocompetent cells that express MHC class II (major histocompatibility) proteins and are **antigen-presenting cells**. They may therefore contribute to T-cell-mediated immune responses and have been implicated in the inflammatory demyelinating disease **multiple sclerosis** (Ch. 14). Microglial activation is also a component of most neurodegenerative disorders such as **Alzheimer's disease** and **Parkinson's disease** (Chs 12 and 13).

Acute and chronic inflammation

A number of terms are used to describe the site and distribution of acute and chronic inflammation in the nervous system. **Meningitis** is inflammation of the meninges (protective coverings of the brain). The term **pachymeningitis** is used if the dura is predominantly affected or **leptomeningitis** if inflammation is centred on the arachnoid, pia and subarachnoid space (see Ch. 1). The features of **acute bacterial meningitis** are discussed in Clinical Box 8.2.

Inflammation in the CNS

A small focus of inflammation in the brain is referred to as **cerebritis**. More extensive and diffuse brain inflammation is termed **encephalitis**. Encephalitic processes are further subdivided into three main types:

- **Polioencephalitis** (Greek: polios, grey) is grey-matter predominant.
- **Leukoencephalitis** (Greek: leukos, white) is white-matter predominant.
- **Panencephalitis** (Greek: pan-, all) affects both grey and white matter.

The term **myelitis** indicates inflammation of the spinal cord, such as the inflammatory spinal cord disease poliomyelitis

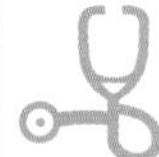

Clinical Box 8.2: Acute bacterial meningitis

The main clinical features of meningitis are fever, headache and drowsiness, together with nausea, vomiting and **photophobia** (sensitivity to light). Clinical examination may show neck stiffness and evidence of raised intracranial pressure including **papilloedema** (swelling of the optic discs; see Ch. 5, Fig. 5.16). Unlike viral meningitis, a self-limiting illness from which most patients make a complete recovery, the mortality in **bacterial meningitis** (Fig. 8.9) is around 10% and a significant proportion of survivors are left with neurological deficits, cranial nerve palsies, hydrocephalus or epilepsy.

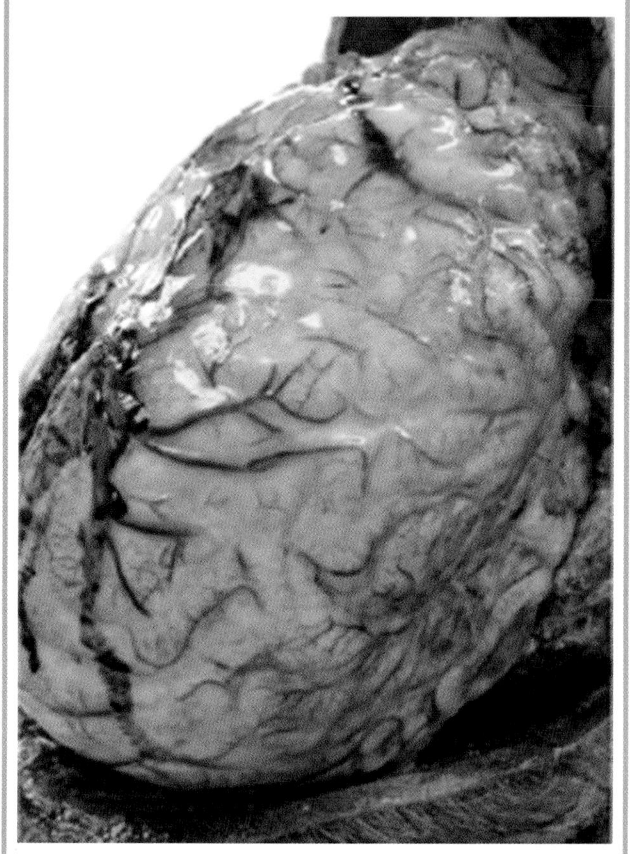

Fig. 8.9 **Acute bacterial meningitis.** Post-mortem photograph showing thick green-yellow purulent exudate filling the subarachnoid space over the surface of the cerebral hemispheres. From Kleinschmidt-DeMasters, BK and Tyler, KL: Practical Surgical Neuropathology: A Diagnostic Approach (Churchill Livingstone 2010) with permission.

Key Points

- Reactive gliosis is the unique CNS response to damage or disease and consists of astrocytosis and microgliosis, coordinated by inflammatory cytokines such as IL-1, TNF-α and IL-6.
- Reactive astrocytes enlarge and proliferate, increasing synthesis of GFAP, to form a glial scar. Astrocytes also release inflammatory mediators and trophic factors.
- Activated microglia differentiate into macrophages and internalize cellular debris and microorganisms. They are also immunocompetent antigen-presenting cells.
- Inflammation of the meninges is referred to as pachymeningitis (if it affects the dura) or leptomeningitis (when it is centred on the pia-arachnoid). Inflammation of the brain is termed cerebritis (if focal) or encephalitis (if diffuse). Myelitis is inflammation of the spinal cord.

(caused by infection with a poliovirus); whereas combined inflammation of the brain and spinal cord is referred to as **encephalomyelitis**. It should be emphasized that these terms are descriptive and do not indicate the underlying cause of the inflammation.

Neurodegeneration

The neurodegenerative diseases are a heterogeneous group of progressive, incurable neurological disorders that are more common in later life. They often present with dementia (e.g. **Alzheimer's disease**; Ch. 12) or as a movement disorder (e.g. **Parkinson's disease**; Ch. 13). Most cases are classified as sporadic or idiopathic, meaning that the cause is not known. Inherited forms often exist, but they are less common and tend to present at an earlier age.

General features

In most neurodegenerative diseases there is a selective loss of certain populations of nerve cells, associated with deposits of an abnormal protein or peptide in neurons and/or glia. These disorders are therefore referred to as **proteinopathies** (Fig. 8.10). In cases where inherited (familial) forms of a disease have been identified, the mutation often affects the protein itself or an enzyme involved in its processing.

Neuronal loss and gliosis

The affected brain regions show **neuronal loss** and **reactive gliosis** in a disease-specific pattern, affecting particular groups of neurons, but sparing others. Importantly, the clinical features in each case are determined by the **anatomical distribution** of the pathological changes rather than the particular protein involved. In most cases it is not clear why specific populations of neurons are susceptible whilst others are resistant (referred to as **selective vulnerability**).

Protein folding and misfolding

An important component of many neurodegenerative diseases is the accumulation of abnormally folded proteins – or failure of the normal cellular mechanisms for their disposal.

Normal protein folding

Nuclear DNA encodes the primary structure of proteins, consisting of the basic amino acid sequence. Attainment of the correct three-dimensional conformation requires **protein folding** (Fig. 8.11). This transforms the linear amino acid sequence into more complex spatial arrangements with **alpha-helices** and **beta-pleated sheets** that make up the secondary structure. Further folding gives rise to a three-dimensional **globular protein** with a particular tertiary structure. Association with other proteins may occur, to form a **multi-protein complex** with its own quaternary structure. Protein folding relies on physical and chemical properties of the constituent amino acid residues (i.e. attraction and repulsion by hydrogen bonds, electrostatic forces and hydrophobic interactions).

Unfolded protein response

The **unfolded protein response** (**UPR**) is triggered by the presence of misfolded proteins in the endoplasmic reticulum or as a result of errors in post-translational modification. It is a type of **cell stress response** characterized by upregulation of **molecular chaperone proteins** that attempt to refold abnormally configured proteins. In the event of an overwhelming pathological stimulus or major dysfunction of the normal mechanisms for protein disposal, large numbers of misfolded proteins may aggregate in the cytoplasm. When this happens they tend to precipitate out of solution as insoluble clusters called **micelles**, since hydrophobic groups that would normally be buried are exposed to the aqueous environment of the cell.

Disposal of abnormal proteins

Abnormal proteins are earmarked for destruction by tagging them with the 8.5 kDa protein **ubiquitin** (Fig. 8.12). This is attached in a series of enzyme-catalysed steps involving activating (E1), conjugating (E2) and ligating (E3) enzymes. These add a **polyubiquitin chain** that is composed of multiple ubiquitin monomers. Once ubiquitinated, the abnormal protein is targeted to the **proteasome**. This is a large multi-subunit protein complex that digests proteins into peptide fragments and amino acids in an active (ATP-dependent) process.

	Main clinical features	Protein	
Parkinson's disease	Parkinsonism	Alpha-synuclein	Synucleinopathies
Dementia with Lewy bodies	Dementia	Alpha-synuclein	Synucleinopathies
Multiple system atrophy	Parkinsonism, cerebellar ataxia	Alpha-synuclein	Synucleinopathies
Alzheimer's disease	Dementia	Tau	Tauopathies
Progressive supranuclear palsy	Parkinsonism	Tau	Tauopathies
Dementia pugilistica (boxers)	Dementia, parkinsonism	Tau	Tauopathies
Motor neuron disease	Progressive paralysis	TDP-43	TDP-43 proteinopathies
Frontotemporal dementia*	Dementia, personality change	TDP-43	TDP-43 proteinopathies
Huntington's disease	Dementia, chorea, personality change	Huntingtin	
Creutzfeldt-Jakob disease	Dementia, ataxia	Prion protein	

Fig. 8.10 **Proteinopathies.** A number of common and/or important neurodegenerative disorders are shown, together with the main protein that accumulates in neurons or glial cells. *[NB: approximately 50% of frontotemporal dementias are TDP43-proteinopathies; in other cases the pathological inclusions are composed of tau (40%) or other proteins (10%)].

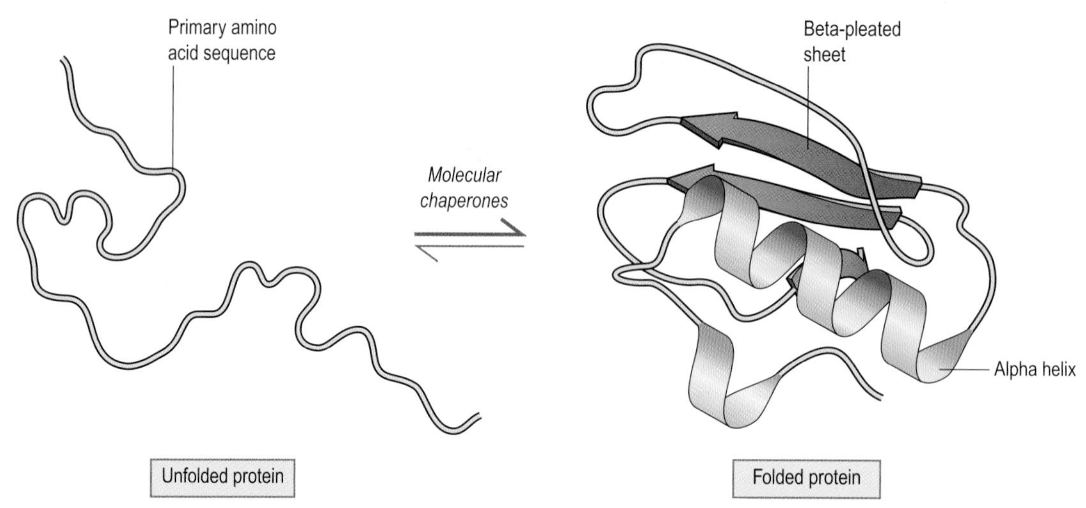

Fig. 8.11 **Protein folding.** The amino acid sequence of an unfolded protein is encoded by the nuclear DNA (primary structure). This leads to spontaneous formation of alpha helices and beta-pleated sheets (secondary structure) and further folding to produce a globular protein (tertiary structure). The process of protein folding is promoted and accelerated by molecular chaperone proteins.

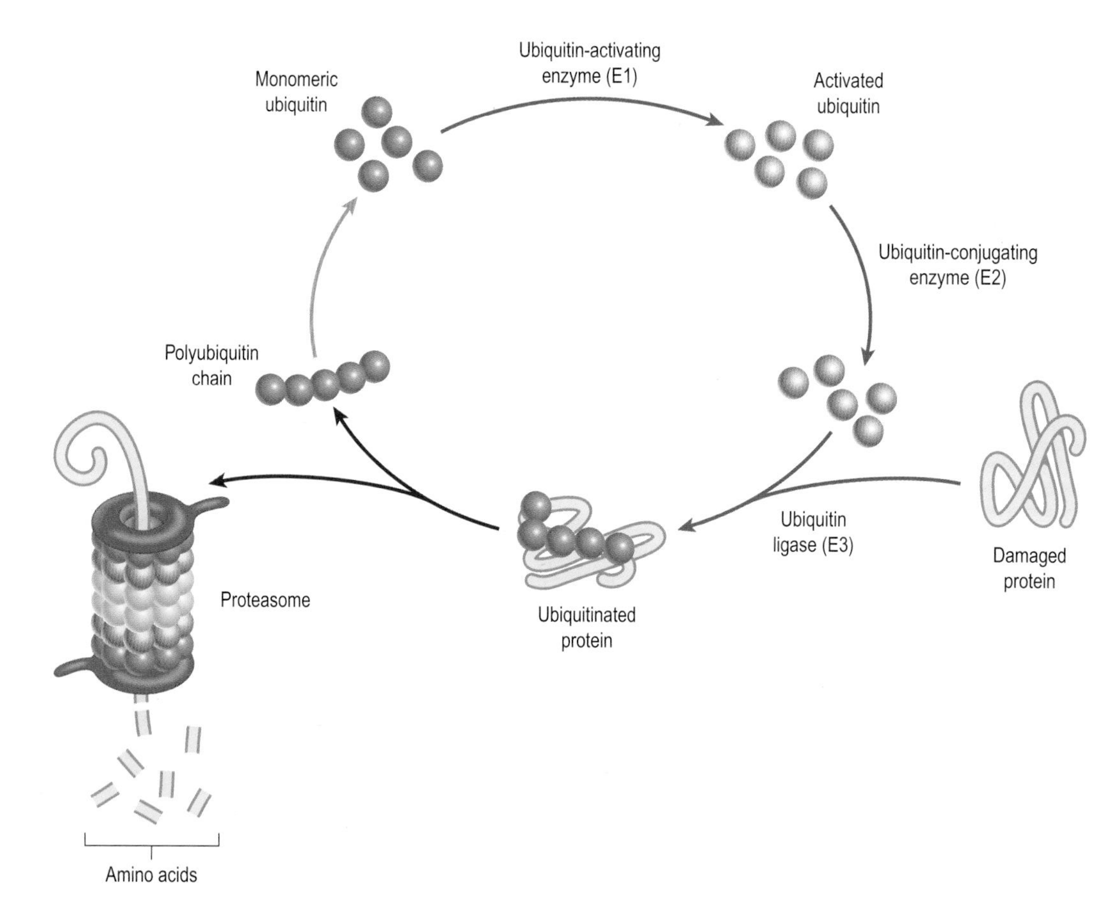

Fig. 8.12 **The ubiquitin-proteasome system.** Damaged or incorrectly folded proteins are tagged with ubiquitin and earmarked for degradation (to amino acids) by the proteasome. Digestion within the proteasome is an ATP-dependent process that consumes cellular energy. Conversion of monomeric ubiquitin to its active form (see upper part of figure) is also an ATP-dependent step.

The proteasome consists of a cylindrical **core region** (the **20S core particle**) composed of four rings stacked around a central pore. This is capped at either end by **regulatory particles** (**19S** or **11S**) which also have a central pore that allows access to a hollow **degradation chamber**. The entire assembly is the **26S proteasome**. Proteins are fed into the proteasome and digested, whilst the polyubiquitin chain is recycled. Accumulation of ubiquitin-tagged proteins is a feature of many neurodegenerative disorders, sometimes due to disturbance or overload of the ubiquitin-proteasome system.

The autophagy-lysosomal pathway

A second disposal mechanism for proteins and other cellular components is **autophagy** (Greek: autos, self; phagein, eat). The abnormal protein is first enveloped in an **autophagic vacuole**. This then fuses with a **primary lysosome** which contains powerful hydrolytic enzymes that digest the contents. Any materials left over from the process, such as undigested cell membrane constituents, remain within membrane-bound **residual bodies**. This mechanism is particularly important for protein aggregates that cannot be cleared by the proteasome. Disruption of the autophagy pathway is important in some

> ### *Key Points*
> - Deposition of abnormal proteins occurs in most neurodegenerative diseases, which can therefore be classified as proteinopathies.
> - This is accompanied by neuronal death and reactive gliosis and the clinical features depend mainly on the extent and distribution of neuronal loss rather than the particular protein involved.
> - In some degenerative diseases there is abnormal protein folding or disturbance of the normal cellular mechanisms that deal with (or dispose of) improperly folded proteins.
> - These include the unfolded protein response, molecular chaperone proteins, the ubiquitin–proteasome system and the autophagy–lysosomal pathway.

forms of familial Parkinson's disease caused by mutation in the ***ATP13A2*** gene (encoding a lysosomal ATPase).

Protein aggregation

Aggregation of abnormal proteins in neurons (or glial cells) gives rise to structures called **inclusion bodies**. These are difficult to identify by routine light microscopy and are better visualized by **silver staining** or **immunohistochemistry** (antibody-labelling of specific proteins). Intracellular inclusions are often cytoplasmic (e.g. in Alzheimer's and Parkinson's diseases; Fig. 8.13) but in some cases are found within the nucleus. Abnormal proteins may also accumulate in the extracellular compartment (between nerve cells).

Amyloid

Many proteins and peptides that form pathological aggregates have a **beta-pleated sheet** structure. This enables monomers to stack together to form elongating **protofibrils** and **fibrils** of around 10 nm in diameter, stabilized by **hydrogen bonds**. Deposits of these insoluble protein fibrils are referred to as **amyloid**. It is important to emphasize that the term 'amyloid' does not refer to one particular protein and that many different peptides with a beta-sheet structure can form 'amyloid deposits'. The name derives from the Greek, meaning starch-like.

All forms of amyloid take up certain tissue stains such as **Congo red** and **thioflavin S**. Due to the regular, crystalline arrangement of the amyloid fibrils, the deposits also have the ability to rotate the plane of polarized light, termed **birefringence**. As a result, amyloid deposits stained with Congo red have a characteristic apple green colour when viewed under polarized light (Fig. 8.14).

Amyloid fibril formation

The process of amyloid formation is illustrated in Figure 8.15. **Fibrillogenesis** is the process by which a peptide forms insoluble aggregates of amyloid. It involves three sequential steps. A peptide with a **beta-pleated sheet** structure must first be produced in sufficient quantities. The second step is **nucleation**, which starts the process of fibril formation. It requires a supportive microenvironment with a sufficiently high protein concentration, together with various permissive factors including appropriate acidity (pH), temperature or the presence of certain metallic ions. Finally, the phase of **fibril growth** involves the sequential addition of monomeric peptide units (each with a beta-sheet structure) to form an extending chain. This leads to the gradual assembly of **oligomeric species** (or **protofibrils**) which associate to form mature **amyloid fibrils**.

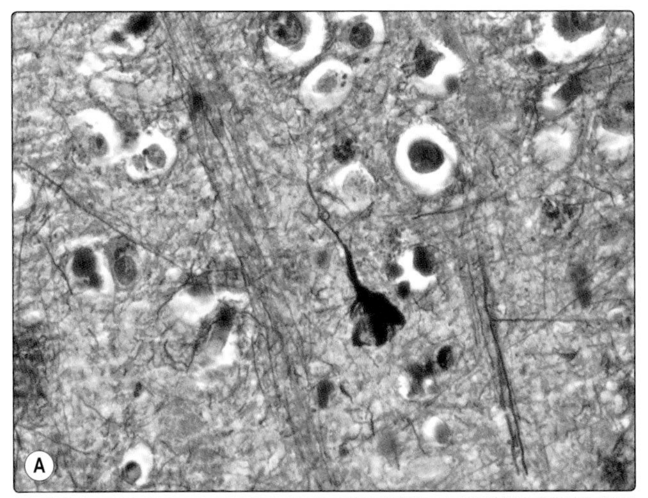

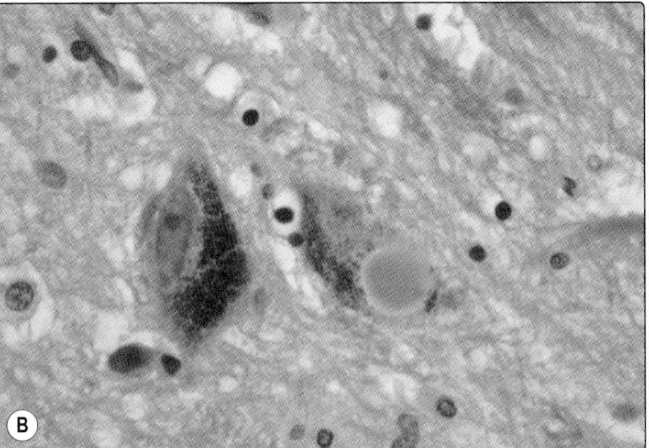

Fig. 8.13 **Neuronal inclusions. (A)** A neurofibrillary tangle (composed of abnormally phosphorylated tau protein) in the cytoplasm of a cortical pyramidal neuron in a patient with Alzheimer's disease [demonstrated using the modified Bielschowsky silver stain]. From Prayson, R: Neuropathology 1e (Churchill Livingstone 2005) with permission; **(B)** Micrograph showing two neurons in the substantia nigra in a patient with Parkinson's disease. The neuron on the left has a large nucleus and prominent nucleolus with abundant brown (neuromelanin) pigment in the cytoplasm. The nucleus of the neuron on the right is not fully seen in this section, but the cytoplasm contains a bright pink Lewy body which is surrounded by a characteristic pale halo [Routine haematoxylin and eosin (H&E)-stained section]. Courtesy of Professor Steve Gentleman.

Amyloid diseases

Deposition of amyloid is responsible for diseases in many different organ systems, but the most common and best understood amyloid disorder is **Alzheimer's disease**. It is characterized by the deposition of **amyloid beta** (Aβ) **peptide** in the extracellular compartment of the brain (between nerve cells) in the form of **amyloid plaques**. Secondary pathological changes occur in the neuronal cytoplasm, with accumulation of an abnormally phosphorylated form of the microtubule-associated protein **tau**. Hyperphosphorylated tau is found within nerve cells as filamentous structures called **neurofibrillary tangles**. Since neuronal injury and tau deposition appear to occur as a consequence of amyloid accumulation, Alzheimer's disease is referred to as a **secondary tauopathy**. This is in contrast to the **primary tauopathies**, in which abnormal tau-positive inclusions are present in the absence of Aβ.

Amyloid toxicity

It is not certain how abnormal protein aggregates cause neuronal damage, but factors that have been implicated include inflammation, gliosis, oxidative stress and production

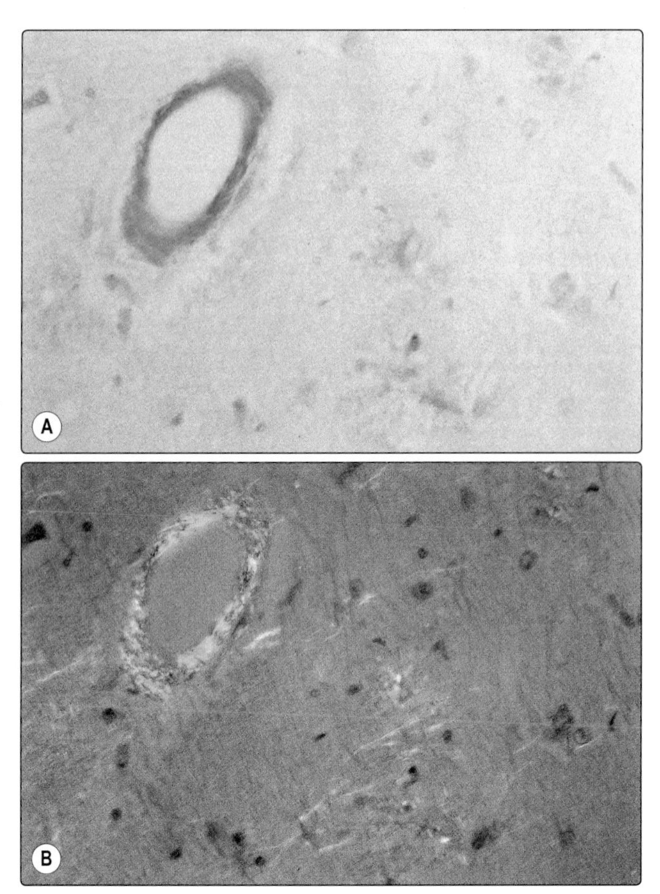

Fig. 8.14 **Amyloid. (A)** Photomicrograph showing deposition of amyloid in a blood vessel in a case of cerebral amyloid angiopathy [stained with Congo red]; **(B)** Fluorescence microscopy showing the characteristic apple-green birefringence of amyloid [Congo red stain]. From Ellison and Love: Neuropathology 2e (Mosby 2003) with permission.

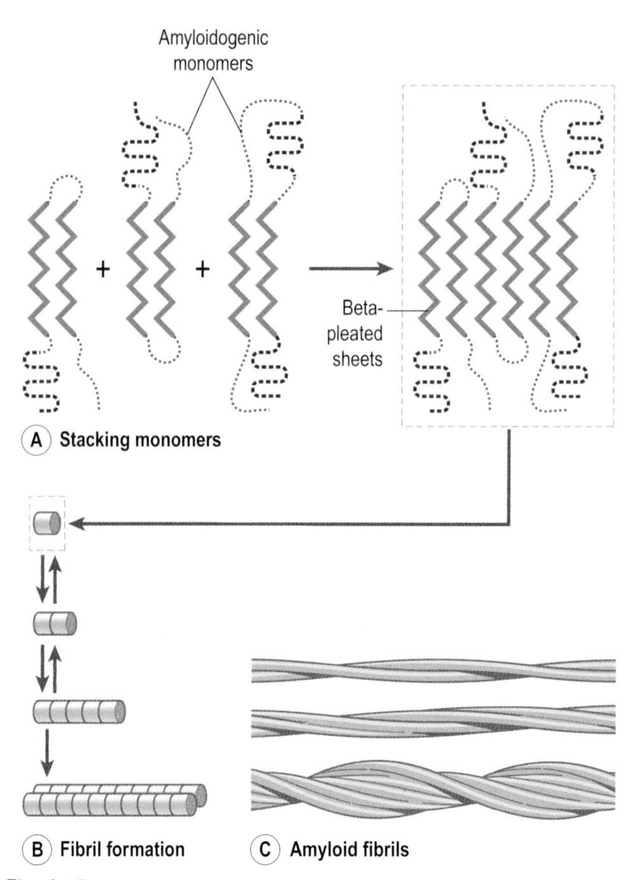

Fig. 8.15 **Amyloid formation.** Amyloidogenic monomers with a beta-pleated sheet structure are able to stack together **(A)** to form elongating chains that are stabilized by hydrogen bonds. These gradually grow to form protofibrils **(B)** and mature amyloid fibrils **(C)**.

of toxic intermediates during fibrillogenesis. There is growing evidence that **oligomeric intermediates** generated during amyloid fibril formation may be primarily responsible for neurotoxicity in a number of neurodegenerative disorders (including Alzheimer's disease and Parkinson's disease).

In particular, it has been shown in cultured cells that oligomeric prefibrillary species of amyloid beta are able to form a **membrane attack complex** that can perforate the neuronal cell membrane. This leads to cellular swelling, loss of transmembrane gradients and influx of free calcium ions – all of which promote neuronal cell death. A similar phenomenon has been described with oligomers of **alpha-synuclein** protein (the main pathological species implicated in Parkinson's disease and related **synucleinopathies**).

Key Points

- Amyloid is a general term used to describe insoluble aggregates of various types of protein, all of which have a beta-pleated sheet structure that enables them to stack together and form fibrils.
- Many different proteins and peptides can form amyloid deposits, all with properties in common (e.g. staining with Congo red and showing apple-green birefringence under polarized light).
- The most common amyloid disorder is Alzheimer's disease, in which Aβ (amyloid beta) peptide forms insoluble aggregates (plaques) in the cerebral cortex.
- Amyloid deposition is neurotoxic, but the mechanism of neuronal injury is not certain and may include oxidative stress, abnormal phosphorylation and calcium influx.
- Oligomeric intermediates created during the process of amyloid formation have been particularly implicated and may form 'pores' in the plasma membrane that compromise the cell.

Prion diseases

The prion diseases are a group of extremely rare neurodegenerative disorders characterized by vacuolar degeneration of the cerebral cortex, which is termed **spongiosis**. They are caused by a unique form of infectious pathogenic agent composed only of protein: the **prion** ('proteinaceous infectious particle').

General characteristics

Prion diseases have been described in a number of animals including sheep (scrapie) and cattle (bovine spongiform encephalopathy or BSE) in which they cause a rapid and devastating neurological decline that quickly ends in death. In humans, the classical form of prion disease is **Creutzfeldt–Jakob disease** or **CJD**, a sporadic disorder of later life characterized by an aggressive and rapidly fatal dementia (Clinical Box 8.3). There are a few very rare genetic forms of prion disease including **fatal familial insomnia** (**FFI**) and **Gerstmann–Sträussler–Scheinker syndrome** (**GSS**) that are all inherited in an autosomal dominant manner. Each of these has distinguishing clinical and pathological features, but all are incurable and ultimately fatal.

Clinical Box 8.3: Sporadic CJD

Creutzfeldt–Jakob disease is a sporadic neurodegenerative disease which affects one in a million people worldwide per year, most of whom are over the age of 65. It is characterized by a very **aggressive dementia** that leads to death in a matter of weeks. This is often accompanied by abnormal movements including electric-shock-like **myoclonic jerks**. The EEG shows characteristic **periodic complexes** in 60–80% of cases, consisting of biphasic or triphasic 'sharp waves' at a frequency of 1–2 Hz. The cerebrospinal fluid may contain increased levels of certain proteins (e.g. **14-3-3** and **S100b**). Examination of the brain after death shows widespread **spongiform degeneration** of the cerebral cortex (Fig. 8.16), accompanied by neuronal loss, gliosis and deposition of abnormal prion protein.

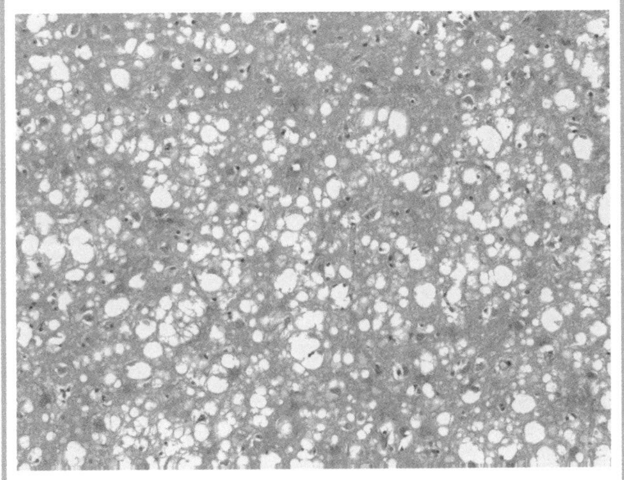

Fig. 8.16 **Spongiform degeneration of the cerebral cortex ('spongiosis') in Creutzfeldt–Jakob disease (CJD).** Routine haematoxylin and eosin (H&E) stain.

Clinical Box 8.4: New variant CJD

The new variant of CJD was first identified by its microscopic appearance. This differs from that of classical CJD and includes characteristic **florid plaques**, named for their resemblance to flowers (Fig. 8.17). The new variant affects younger people (usually below the age of 30) and has a longer duration, typically a year or more. **Psychiatric features** and **cerebellar ataxia** are also common and myoclonic jerks are absent. MRI scanning characteristically shows T2-hyperintensity in the posterior thalamus (the **pulvinar sign**). As with classical CJD, the condition is incurable and fatal, but it is much rarer, with fewer than 180 cases reported in the UK (representing 80% of the worldwide total).

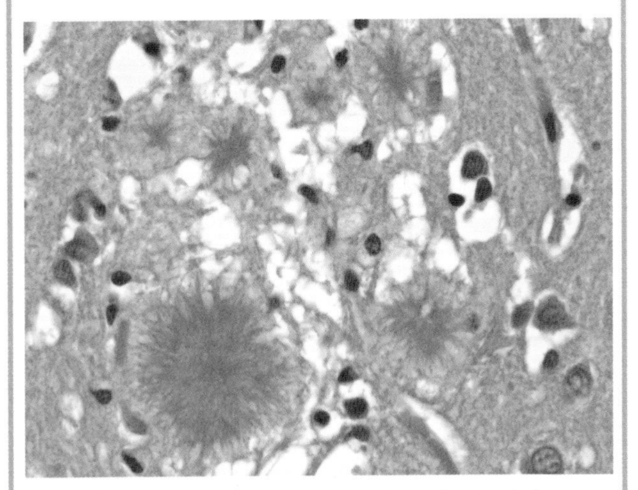

Fig. 8.17 **Florid plaques in new variant Creutzfeldt–Jakob disease (vCJD).** Several plaques are shown, consisting of a central amyloid core, composed of abnormal prion protein, surrounded by coarse vacuoles, which creates a 'florid' or floral appearance [routine haematoxylin and eosin (H&E) stain].

Infectivity

In addition to sporadic and inherited forms, prion diseases have the unique property (among degenerative diseases) of **infectivity**. They are therefore also referred to as **transmissible spongiform encephalopathies (TSEs)**. In the 1990s in the UK and Europe, bovine spongiform encephalopathy entered the human food chain via contaminated beef and led to a **new variant of CJD** (Clinical Box 8.4). Prion diseases have also been transmitted **iatrogenically** (Greek: iatros, doctor) by blood transfusions and growth hormone supplements (obtained from human donors) and various neurosurgical procedures (via contaminated instruments or dural grafts).

Prion protein

The infective agent in prion disease is unique since it is non-cellular, has no DNA or RNA and appears to be composed entirely of protein (the 'protein only hypothesis'). It is an abnormally folded form of cellular prion protein (or **PrP^c^**) which is present in many different tissue types. The pathogenic form has the same primary amino acid structure, but a different secondary structure that is rich in **beta-pleated sheets** rather than alpha-helices and is able to form amyloid deposits. This infective form is designated **PrP^{Sc}** (scrapie variant). The classical model of normal and abnormal prion protein structure is illustrated in Figure 8.18, but the actual three-dimensional structure is not known with certainty.

Key Points

- CJD is a very rare neurodegenerative process, affecting one in a million people each year worldwide, characterized by aggressive dementia, ending in death within a matter of weeks.
- The pathological features include spongiosis (vacuolar degeneration of the cerebral cortex) and deposition of abnormal prion protein, together with neuronal loss and gliosis.
- Most cases of prion disease are sporadic (and some are inherited) but can also be transmitted as an infectious disease and are known as transmissible spongiform encephalopathies.
- In the UK in the 1990s, contaminated beef from BSE-infected cattle entered the human food chain, leading to a new variant of CJD which has distinct clinical and pathological features.

Codon 129

There is a common polymorphism in the general population that affects codon 129 of the prion gene (***PRNP***, located on chromosome 20) which codes either for methionine (M) or valine (V). Since each gene has two alleles, there are three possible genotypes with different population frequencies:

- **MV** (50%)
- **MM** (40%)
- **VV** (10%)

All pathologically confirmed cases of variant CJD have occurred in people who are homozygous for methionine at

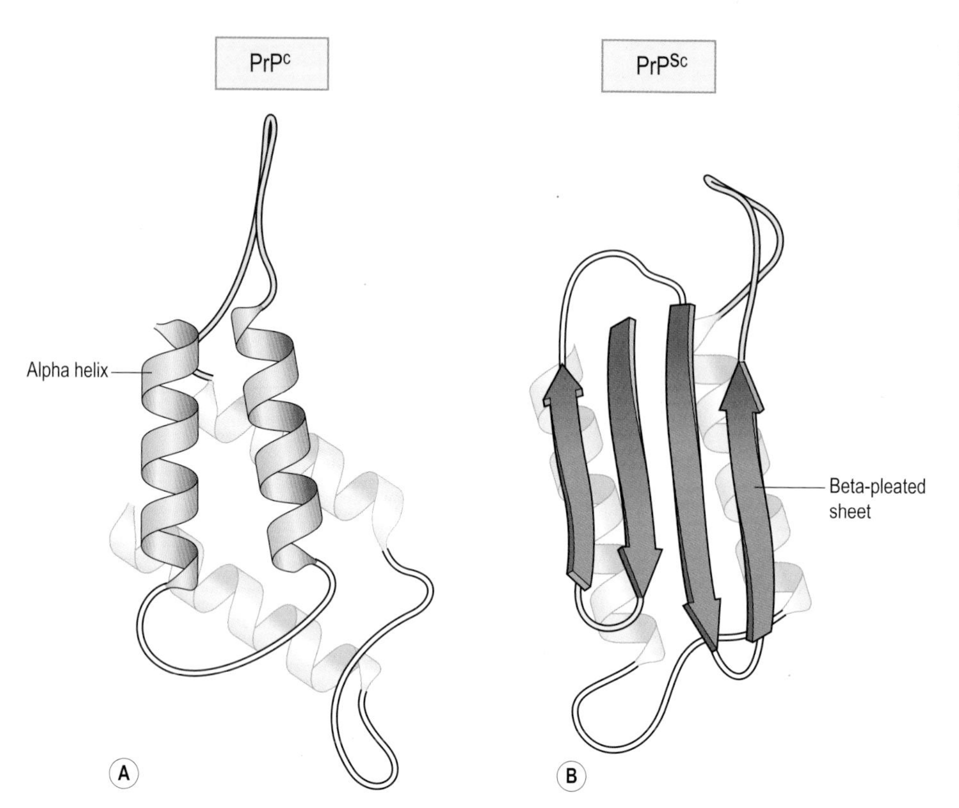

Fig. 8.18 **Structure of prion protein.** **(A)** Normal prion protein, with a secondary structure that is rich in alpha helices; **(B)** Abnormal prion protein has an identical amino acid sequence but is abnormally folded; abnormal prion protein is rich in beta-pleated sheets.

codon 129 (MM). This has therefore been referred to as the **susceptibility genotype**, which implies that the other forms confer resistance to infection. In keeping with this idea, mice that are homozygous for valine (VV) are virtually immune to inoculation with abnormal prion protein whereas heterozygotes (MV) show intermediate susceptibility. However, since the **incubation period** for prion diseases is sometimes measured in decades, the possibility remains that new cases of variant CJD will eventually emerge in people who do not have the susceptibility genotype.

Conversion of PrP^c to PrP^{Sc}

In sporadic disease the abnormal prion protein is assumed to arise by **spontaneous transformation** of native prion protein to the abnormal (scrapie) form. This is thermodynamically unfavourable and is an extremely unlikely spontaneous event, which presumably explains why sporadic disease is so rare.

Animal models have shown that propagation of abnormal prion protein can only take place if the normal cellular protein is present. For instance, **prion-knockout mice** are completely resistant to infection, but infectivity can be restored if native prion protein is reintroduced.

Conversion models

There are two main models that attempt to describe how cellular prion protein may be converted to the abnormal form. The first is the **template-directed refolding (heterodimer) model** (Fig. 8.19). This suggests that

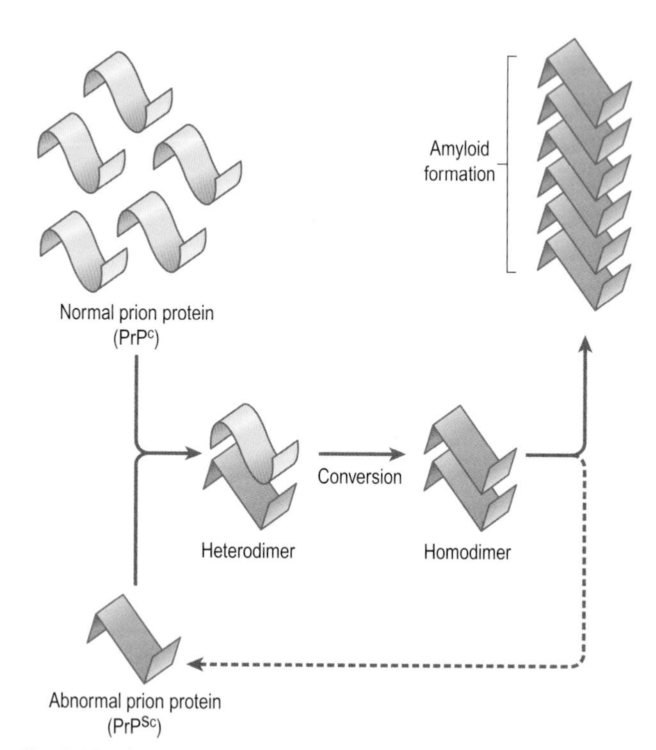

Fig. 8.19 **A model of prion replication.** One possible mechanism of prion formation [illustrated here] is called template-directed refolding. The abnormal prion protein recruits normal (cellular) prion protein and induces a conformation change, converting it to abnormal prion protein. The abnormal protein is rich in beta pleated sheets which can stack to form amyloid.

abnormal prion protein is able to recruit the cellular form and form a heterodimer with it, acting as a template to catalyse its conversion to the scrapie form. The converted prion can then recruit more cellular protein or polymerise to form amyloid fibrils.

Another possibility is described by the **nucleation–polymerization model** which suggests that the critical event is the formation of a nucleus (which consists of an oligomeric aggregate of prion protein). This initial 'seeding' event is highly unlikely since it is thermodynamically unfavourable – but once the nucleus has formed, polymerization and fibril elongation proceed rapidly.

Key Points

- The pathogenic agent in transmissible spongiform encephalopathies such as CJD and variant CJD is the prion (proteinaceous infectious particle). This is a unique pathogen that appears to be composed entirely of protein.
- The pathogenic (scrapie) form of prion has the same primary structure as the native protein, but a different secondary structure that is rich in beta-pleated sheets.
- Animal models show that infection and propagation can only take place if the normal cellular protein is present, since prion-knockout mice are resistant.
- The template-directed refolding and nucleation-polymerization models are attempts to explain how abnormal prion protein might recruit and convert native (cellular) prion protein.

Chapter 9
Head injury

CHAPTER CONTENTS

In the UK, trauma is the leading cause of death in people under the age of 45, with head injury making a substantial contribution in more than 50% of cases. Approximately half of patients admitted to hospital with a serious head injury are under the age of 20, two-thirds are male and alcohol is frequently a contributing factor. Some head injuries are due to assaults, but the vast majority are accidental. Road traffic incidents are an important cause of more serious head injuries, accounting for 60% of fatal traumatic brain injury cases. Survivors are likely to be left with long-term physical and intellectual impairments and may require a prolonged period of neurological rehabilitation.

Clinical aspects

A distinction is made between primary and secondary brain damage. The term **primary brain injury** refers to direct (impact-related) damage which cannot be reversed. The main aim of medical treatment is to prevent or minimize **secondary brain injury** which is often due to hypoxia, ischaemia or infection. These complications develop in the hours or days after the initial injury and are usually associated with brain swelling and raised intracranial pressure.

Assessment and management

The best indicator of head injury severity is impairment of consciousness. This either reflects brain stem dysfunction or diffuse hemispheric damage. Level of consciousness is assessed using the **Glasgow Coma Scale (GCS)** which quantifies responses to verbal and painful stimuli in terms of eye opening, speech and movement (Fig. 9.1). The aggregate score ranges from a maximum of 15 (alert and orientated) to a minimum of 3 (comatose or dead).

A GCS score of 13–15 corresponds to **mild head injury**, accounting for the majority of cases. A total score of 9–12 represents **moderate head injury**, whilst a score of 3–8 signifies **severe head injury**. In addition to providing an initial assessment of severity, any reduction in the GCS score is a sensitive indicator that the clinical state has deteriorated. This may signify development of a **secondary complication** requiring urgent intervention. The role of imaging in the assessment of head injury is discussed in Clinical Box 9.1.

GLASGOW COMA SCALE		Score
Eye opening **E**	Spontaneously	4
	To speech	3
	To pain	2
	None	1
Verbal response **V**	Orientated	5
	Confused	4
	Inappropriate words	3
	Incomprehensible sounds	2
	None	1
Motor response **M**	Obeys commands	6
	Localizes to pain	5
	Withdraws from pain	4
	Abnormal flexion to pain	3
	Abnormal extension to pain	2
	None	1
Maximum score		15

(A)

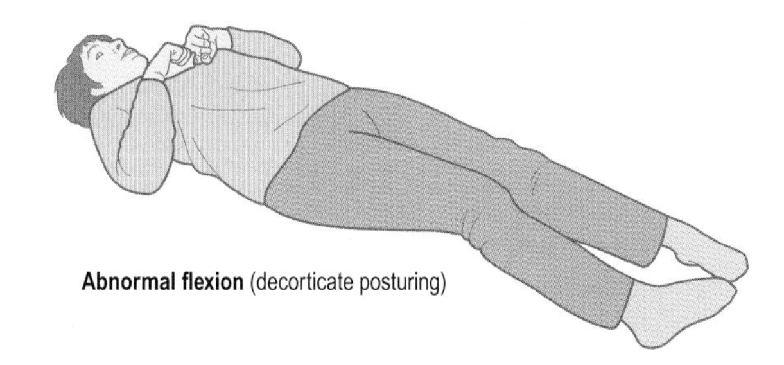

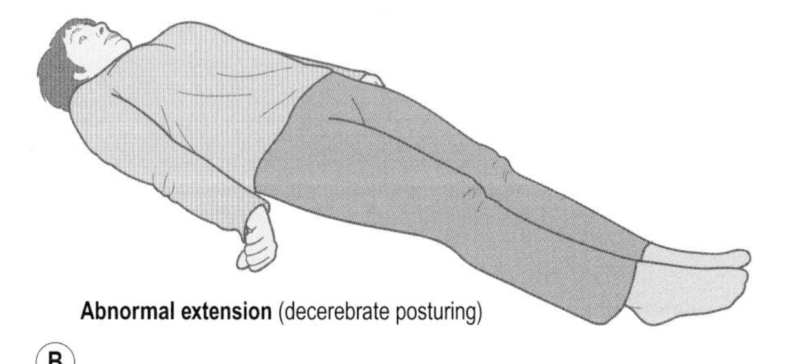

(B)

Fig. 9.1 **The Glasgow Coma Scale. (A)** Response to verbal and painful stimuli is assessed in terms of eye opening, verbal response and motor response. The minimum score is 3 (even in death) and the maximum score is 15 (alert and orientated); **(B)** Abnormal flexion to pain (an 'M' score of 3 out of 5) is also known as decorticate posturing, whereas abnormal extension to pain (an 'M' score of 2 out of 5) is called decerebrate posturing. From Teasdale, G and Jennett, B: LANCET (ii) 81-83: (1974) with permission.

The initial management of head injury is the same as for any other major trauma and begins with the 'ABC' of **basic life support** (airway, breathing, circulation). Attention is then directed to any potentially life-threatening pathologies in the chest, abdomen or pelvis. Once the patient has been stabilized they can be assessed for head and spinal injuries and any appropriate medical or surgical treatments initiated.

Outcome following head injury

The long-term outcome after moderate or severe head injury depends on the extent and severity of the damage, including any **co-existing injuries**. It also varies with the age and general health of the patient. Although the mortality rate is declining, around a third of patients with severe head trauma will ultimately die as a result of their injuries. Another third will eventually recover sufficiently to return to work, whilst the remainder will be left with at least moderate mental or physical disability.

A small proportion of people (less than 3%) enter a **persistent vegetative state**, in which there is partial arousal or apparent wakefulness without full conscious awareness; this is considered permanent if it lasts more than 12 months.

Factors that predict a less favourable outcome include increasing age (>60 years), an initial GCS score below 5, a fixed and dilated pupil, a prolonged period of hypotension/hypoxia or a haemorrhage requiring surgical decompression. Late complications may include **hydrocephalus** due to obstruction of CSF drainage pathways (see Ch. 2, Clinical Box 2.2) or **seizures** (Clinical Box 9.2).

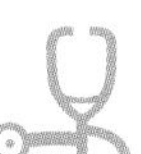

Clinical Box 9.1: Neuroimaging in head injury

Brain imaging is important in the assessment of moderate and severe head injury. The investigation of choice is **computed tomography** (**CT**), which is able to demonstrate lesions of the scalp, skull and brain. This can be supplemented by plain radiographs of the spine in cases with possible vertebral trauma. In severe head injury (GCS <9), significant focal lesions such as cerebral haemorrhages and contusions are identified in more than 50% of cases. The remainder often show small haemorrhages scattered throughout the white matter and at grey-white matter junctions. This is suggestive of **diffuse axonal injury** and is associated with increased morbidity and mortality.

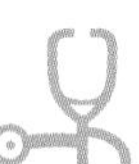

Clinical Box 9.2: Post-traumatic epilepsy

Seizures occur in approximately 2–3% of patients with traumatic head injury (10–15% of those with severe injuries). **Post-traumatic epilepsy** is described as 'early' if it occurs within the first week or 'late' when the onset is beyond this point. Seizure risk is higher with penetrating trauma, depressed skull fractures and in the presence of an intracerebral haemorrhage. The focus may be an area of **gliosis** (glial 'scarring' ; see Ch. 8) resulting from a focal brain lesion. Individuals experiencing early post-traumatic seizures are at most risk of longer-term recurrent seizures.

Key Points

- In the UK, trauma is the leading cause of death in people under the age of 45 and head injury makes a substantial contribution in more than 50% of cases.
- A distinction is made between primary (irreversible, impact-related) damage and secondary brain injury (preventable, by avoiding complications such as hypoxia, ischaemia or infection).
- GCS score indicates severity after head injury: 13–15 (mild); 9–12 (moderate); 3–8 (severe). Any subsequent reduction in GCS score is a sensitive indicator of deterioration in the clinical state.

Pathology of head injury

Most traumatic brain damage is caused by **blunt-force** trauma. This usually results in a **closed head injury**. **Penetrating** (or **missile**) trauma such as stab wounds and gunshot injuries are less common and carry the additional risk of infection (e.g. meningitis or brain abscess).

Contact (or **impact-related**) damage occurs when the head collides with a hard surface or object. The energy from the impact is rapidly dissipated, causing direct mechanical injury such as **cerebral contusion** (bruising) and **laceration** (tearing; from the Latin lacerāre, to tear).

In addition, **acceleration–deceleration** (**inertial**) injury occurs when the head is suddenly set in motion – or is moving at high velocity and comes to an abrupt halt. The brain slides forwards or backwards within the cranial cavity and strikes the inside of the skull, which is most likely to damage the frontal, temporal or occipital poles. Complex **rotational** ('**swirling**') **movements** are also generated within the brain, which has a very soft, gelatinous consistency. This leads to widespread compressive, tensile and **shearing forces**, causing diffuse damage to axons and blood vessels.

Three main patterns of traumatic brain damage are found at **post-mortem examination** in people who died as a result of serious head injuries (due to a mixture of contact-related and acceleration–deceleration injury): cerebral contusions, intracranial haemorrhages and diffuse axonal injury.

Cerebral contusions

Cerebral contusions (bruising) and lacerations (tears) are common in traumatic brain injury, occurring in more than 90% of fatal cases. Contusions are most pronounced at the crests of gyri in the frontal and temporal lobes, particularly in places where the brain comes into contact with the irregular contours of the skull base (Fig. 9.2). Cerebral contusions may be associated with haemorrhage into the overlying subarachnoid or subdural spaces and if blood continues to accumulate it will begin to act as an intracranial mass lesion. The combination of a cerebral contusion with an overlying subdural haemorrhage is called a **burst lobe**. This most often occurs at the frontal and temporal poles.

Coup and contrecoup lesions (Fig. 9.3)

Contusions that occur at the point of impact are referred to as **coup lesions** (from the French, meaning shock or blow). These result from direct mechanical trauma, often from small, hard objects. Contusions may also be present on the opposite side of the brain, well away from the point of impact. These are **contrecoup lesions** which may be more severe and extensive than those at the impact site. This phenomenon is particularly common at the frontal and temporal poles in association with a blow to the back of the head. The mechanism is not fully understood. It is sometimes said that the contrecoup lesion is due to 'rebound' of the brain against the opposite side of the skull, but this does not explain why it is often more severe (as the kinetic energy of the second impact would be less). Experiments suggest that it may be due to a pocket of negative pressure (a 'vacuum') caused by rapid separation of the brain from the overlying skull.

Intracranial haemorrhage

Bleeding may occur at the moment of impact or as a secondary complication, leading to formation of a **haematoma** (blood clot) which acts as a mass lesion. If the haematoma becomes sufficiently large it may compress the underlying brain or cause a life-threatening rise in intracranial pressure. The three main types of intracranial haemorrhage are: extradural, subdural and intracerebral.

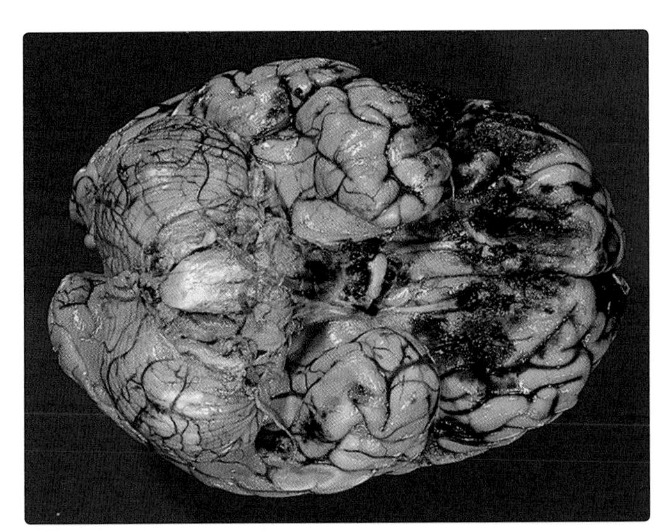

Fig. 9.2 **Post-mortem photograph in a case of severe head injury showing widespread cerebral contusions.** They are particularly marked in the orbital cortex and frontal/temporal polar regions. From Prayson, R: Neuropathology 1e (Churchill Livingstone 2005) with permission.

Key Points

- Most traumatic brain damage is caused by blunt-force trauma, often in association with a closed head injury. Penetrating (missile) injuries are less common and carry an additional infection risk.
- Contact (impact-related) brain damage includes cerebral contusions, intracranial haemorrhages and lacerations (tears). The indirect (contrecoup) lesion may be more severe than the direct (coup) lesion.
- Widespread shearing of axons and small blood vessels is caused by acceleration–deceleration (inertial) forces and complex rotational (swirling) movements in the gelatinous brain tissue.

Extradural haemorrhage

This typically occurs when the **middle meningeal artery** is torn by a skull fracture in the region of the pterion, where the bone is thin and is closely related to the underlying vessel (Fig. 9.4). Arterial blood escapes into the extradural space (between dura and bone) and strips the tightly adherent dura from the inner table of the cranial vault (Fig. 9.5).

An **extradural haematoma** occurs in around 10% of severe head injuries and this is associated with a skull fracture in four out of five cases. Classically, a brief loss of consciousness at the time of impact is followed by a **lucid interval** which may last minutes or hours. Later, there is a sudden deterioration in consciousness which may rapidly lead to death without urgent surgical intervention (the patient is said to 'talk and die'). Extradural haematoma is therefore a surgical emergency.

Subdural haemorrhage

Subdural haemorrhage is caused by tearing of **bridging veins** that pass between the cerebral cortex and dural venous sinuses (see Ch. 1). These vessels pass through a potential plane between the dura and arachnoid membranes. A **subdural haematoma** results from the accumulation of venous blood in this potential space, which is easily expanded by blood under venous pressure because the dura and arachnoid are only loosely attached to each other (Fig. 9.6).

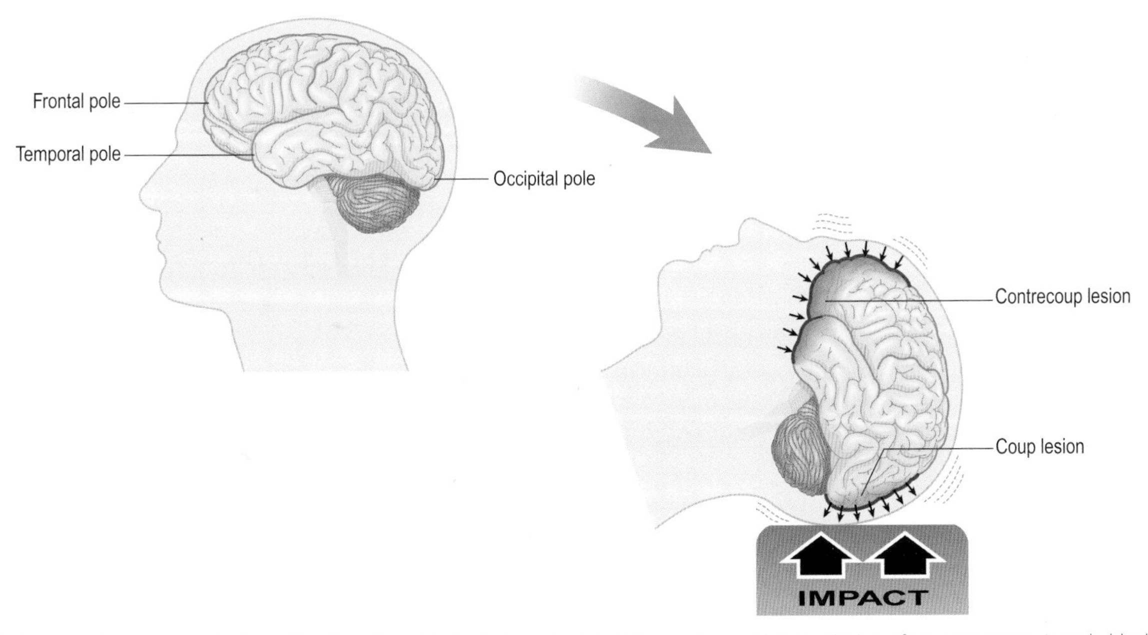

Fig. 9.3 **Coup and contrecoup lesions.** The direct (coup) lesion is impact-related. The contrecoup lesion, which is often more severe, is probably due to extreme pressure changes which may damage thin-walled blood vessels as the brain is violently wrenched away from the overlying skull.

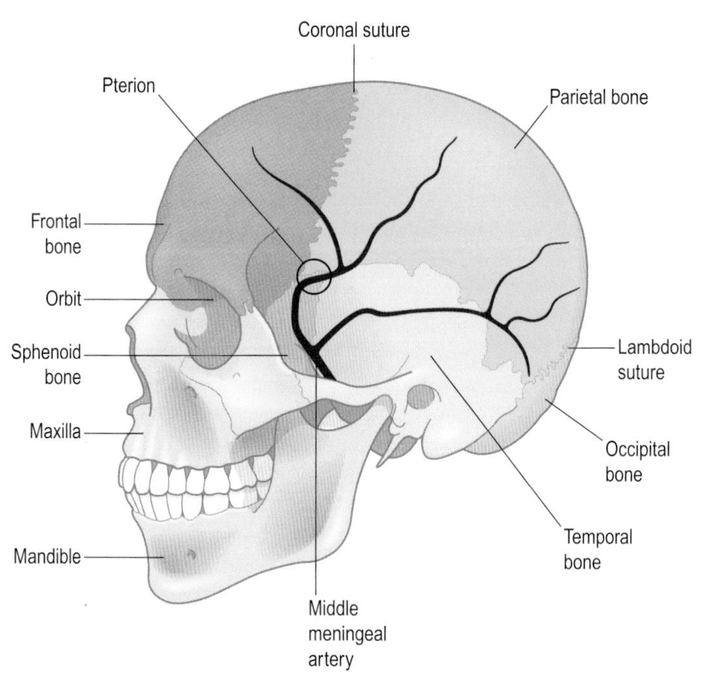

Fig. 9.4 **The middle meningeal artery is closely related to the pterion, which is the thinnest part of the cranial vault.** The underlying vessel is therefore vulnerable to damage in association with a skull fracture.

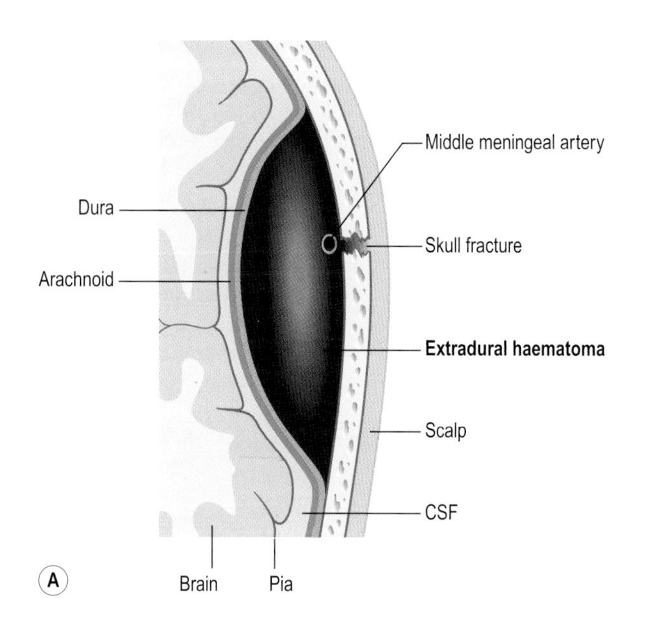

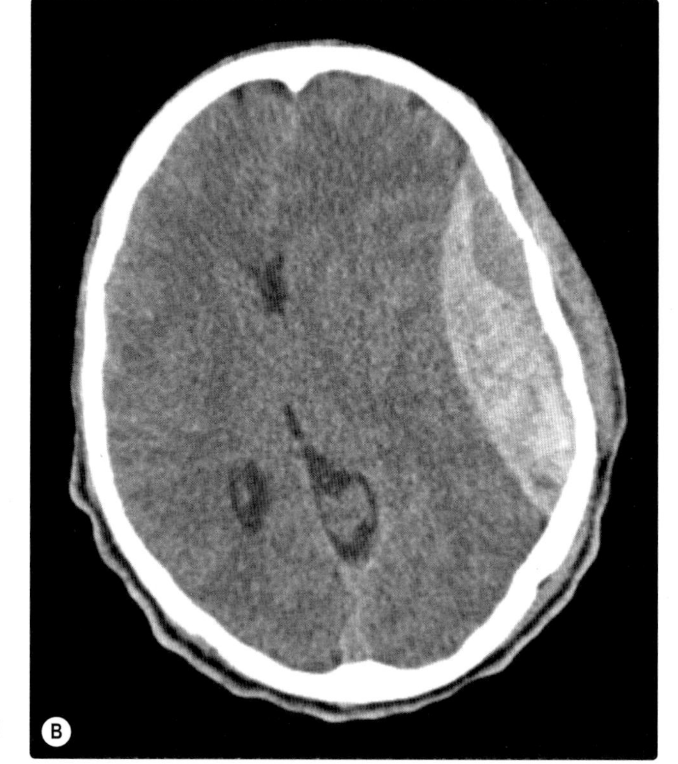

Fig. 9.5 **Extradural haematoma shown diagrammatically (A) and on CT scanning (B).** On brain imaging, the typical biconvex shape is due to the fact that the dura is firmly anchored to the overlying skull and the accumulating blood is not able to cross suture lines (between adjacent cranial bones). Note the considerable 'midline shift' caused by the expanding mass lesion. Courtesy of Dr Andrew MacKinnon.

Acute subdural haematoma usually follows an obvious head injury, is more common in younger people and is likely to require surgical evacuation. In contrast, **chronic subdural haematoma** is often seen in the elderly, particularly in those with some degree of brain atrophy and in many cases there is no recollection of a head injury.

Intracerebral haemorrhage

Traumatic **intracerebral haemorrhage** may occur at the time of impact or as a secondary complication. It is more likely in people with pre-existing vascular disease or high blood pressure. In some cases a spontaneous (non-traumatic) intracerebral haemorrhage leads to an accidental fall or road traffic accident, but it is not always easy to tell which came first.

Intraventricular haemorrhage is seen in a proportion of cases, mainly in association with severe head injury. It may be a primary event, due to rupture of vessels in the **choroid plexus** (within the ventricles) or it might be due to dissection of blood into the ventricular system from an intracerebral or subarachnoid haemorrhage.

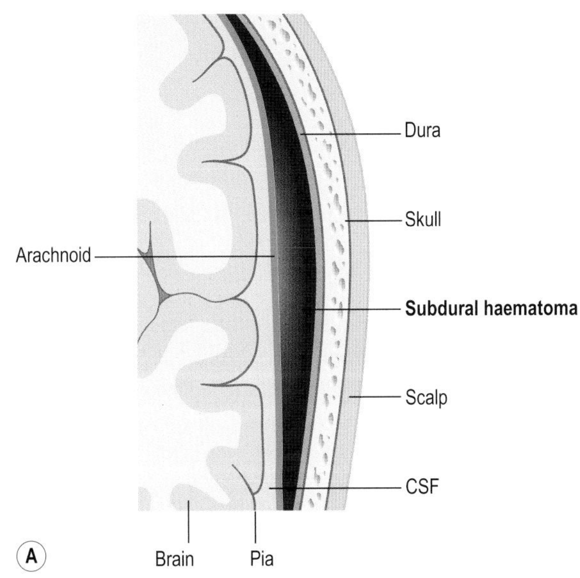

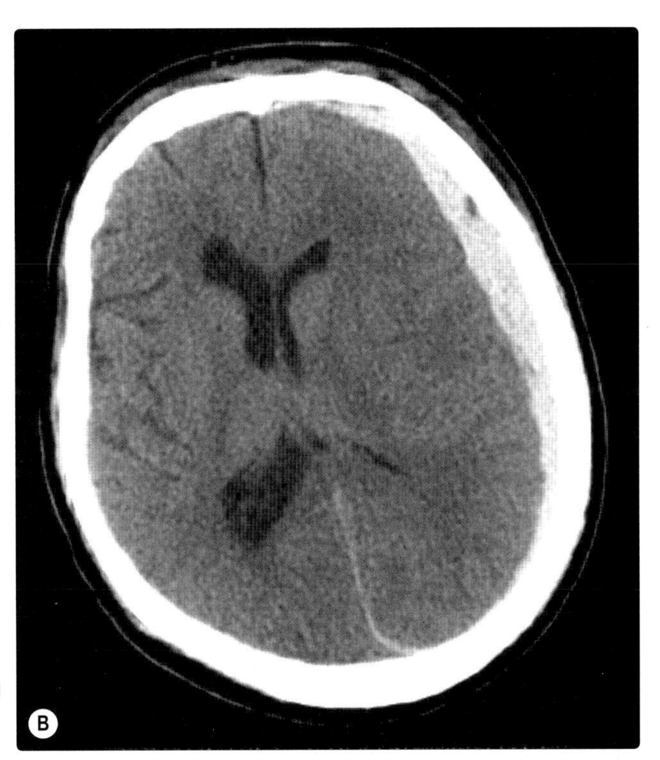

Fig. 9.6 **Subdural haematoma shown diagrammatically (A) and on CT scanning (B).** On brain imaging, subdural haematomas spread further over the surface of the brain and cause less mass effect. This is because the blood is able to track freely between the arachnoid and dura (within the subdural space). Courtesy of Dr Andrew MacKinnon.

Key Points

- The three main types of intracranial haemorrhage are extradural, subdural and intracerebral.
- Extradural haematoma is most often caused by rupture of the middle meningeal artery following a fracture in the region of the pterion. It is a surgical emergency with significant risk of death.
- Subdural haematoma may be acute (e.g. as a result of head trauma) or chronic (more often encountered in older people, often with no recollection of a head injury).

Diffuse axonal injury

Perhaps the most significant pathological change in severe head injury is widespread damage to axons in the cerebral hemispheres and brain stem, termed **diffuse traumatic axonal injury** (TAI). Some axons are transected at the moment of impact (**primary axotomy**) whilst others degenerate later (**secondary axotomy**).

Diffuse axonal injury appears to be a major determinant of impaired consciousness in head injury across the full spectrum of severity and it is thought to be an important factor in determining **long-term disability**. Brain imaging in patients with diffuse axonal injury is sometimes normal or may show only non-specific changes such as generalized **brain swelling**, but neuropathological examination of the brain shows characteristic findings.

Microscopic appearances

Diffuse axonal injury can only be detected reliably by microscopic examination of the brain after death. This shows **axonal swellings** throughout the cerebral hemispheres and brain stem (Fig. 9.7). Large white matter bundles such as the corpus callosum and internal capsule are particularly vulnerable, together with the dorsolateral sector of the upper brain stem.

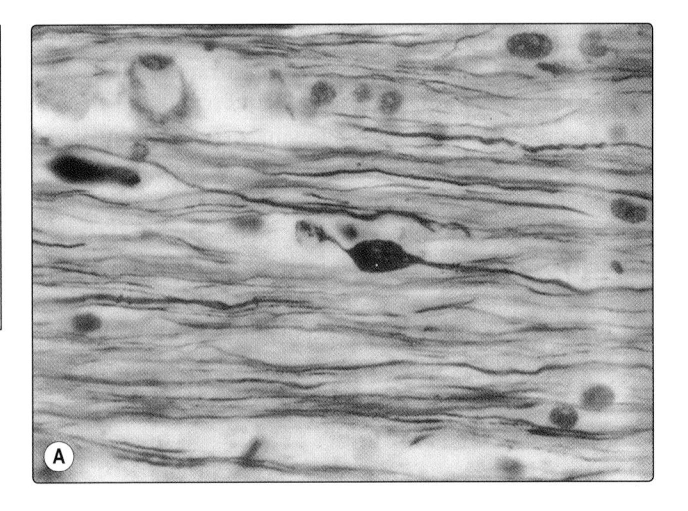

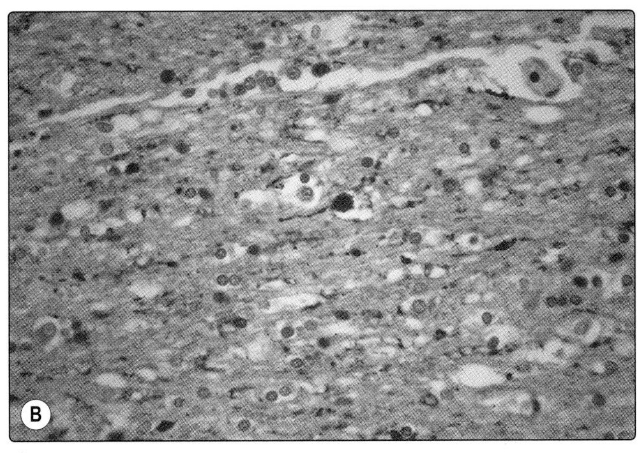

Fig. 9.7 **Microscopic appearances of diffuse axonal injury. (A)** Axon swellings, demonstrated using silver staining. From Stevens and Lowe: Pathology 2e (Mosby 2000) with permission; **(B)** Antibody-labelling (immunohistochemistry) for beta-APP. From Prayson, R: Neuropathology 1e (Churchill Livingstone 2005) with permission.

Axonal swellings can be highlighted by **silver stain** preparations (Fig. 9.7A). They can also be demonstrated by immunohistochemistry (antibody-labelling) of proteins that are normally transported along axons, including **beta amyloid precursor protein (β-APP)**. Positive labelling for β-APP can be seen within two hours of head injury (Fig. 9.7B).

In the most severe cases, axonal transection is accompanied by tears in small blood vessels, leading to **microhaemorrhages**. These form small haematomas at the junction between grey and white matter (Fig. 9.8).

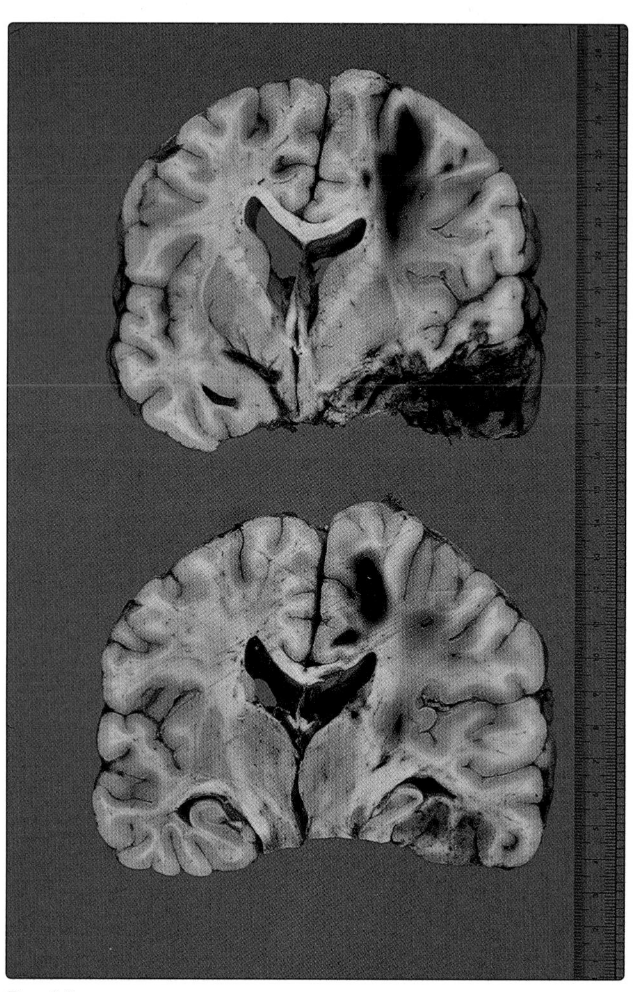

Fig. 9.8 **Gliding contusions.** Post-mortem photograph in a case of traumatic head injury. The upper and lower images show large gliding contusions in the parasagittal white matter, close to the overlying cortex. There is also severe contusion of the temporal lobe. From Ellison and Love: Neuropathology 2e (Mosby 2003) with permission.

Confusingly, these small haemorrhages are known as **gliding contusions**.

Skull fracture

Head injury is often associated with damage to the scalp, skull and dura. The presence of a skull fracture does not necessarily imply damage to the underlying brain, but does give some indication of impact force. Conversely, there may be significant brain injury in the absence of a skull fracture.

Most are simple **linear fractures** of the skull vault, usually occurring at the site of impact (Fig. 9.9A). The term **depressed fracture** is used when a piece of bone becomes detached and is displaced towards the brain (Fig. 9.9B).

A **compound** (or **open**) fracture is a depressed fracture that is associated with an overlying scalp tear; this poses an infection risk and requires antibiotic prophylaxis. **Skull base fractures** require much greater force and are considerably less common. They may be associated with cranial nerve damage or ascending infection from the ear or nose.

Key Points

- One of the most significant pathological changes associated with impairment of consciousness and long-term neurological disability in severe head injury is widespread damage to axons.
- This is called diffuse traumatic axonal injury (TAI) which is characterized by axonal swellings, accumulation of beta-APP and microhaemorrhages ('gliding contusions').
- Skull fracture gives some indication of impact force but is not necessarily associated with brain injury. Conversely, there may be significant brain injury in the absence of a skull fracture.

Brain swelling and intracranial pressure

An important consequence of head injury is **brain swelling**. This includes generalized increase in brain water content (**cerebral oedema**) and focal swelling in association with haematomas or other lesions. Brain swelling is dangerous because it leads to **raised intracranial pressure**, which may in turn compromise cerebral blood flow or result in potentially fatal brain herniation (discussed below).

Raised intracranial pressure

The cranium is a rigid structure with non-compressible contents (Fig. 9.10A). Any increase in the total volume of the cranial contents will therefore lead to a steep rise in intracranial pressure, but this is initially prevented by

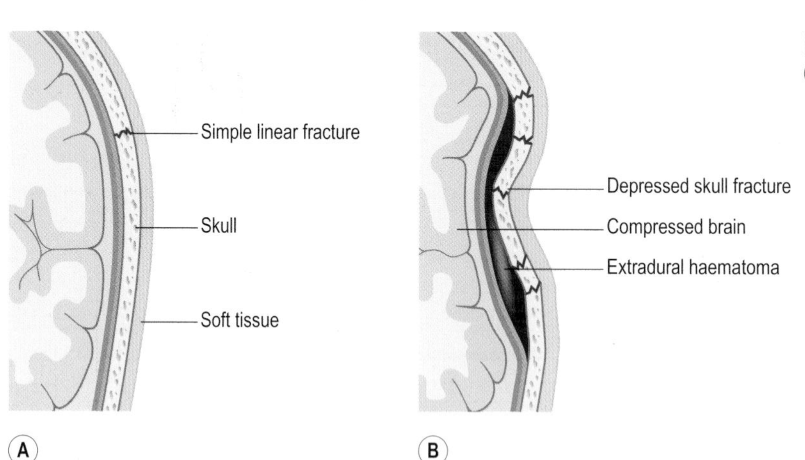

Fig. 9.9 **Skull fracture. (A)** Simple linear fracture; **(B)** Depressed fracture.

compensatory mechanisms which modify the volume–pressure curve (Fig. 9.10B). These include redistribution of CSF from the ventricles to the lumbar subarachnoid space and compression of the dural venous sinuses (thereby reducing the total intracranial blood volume).

Once the compensatory mechanisms have been exhausted (the point of **decompensation**) the volume–pressure relationship becomes linear and the intracranial pressure rises steeply. This may lead to brain shift and herniation.

In general, the impact of a **space-occupying lesion** is less if the rate of expansion is slow, since this allows more time for compensation. Individuals with some degree of brain atrophy (e.g. the elderly) are also more tolerant of an expanding intracranial mass, since there is more free space inside the skull.

Brain shift and herniation

The cranial cavity is incompletely divided into **compartments** by two dural partitions: the falx cerebri (in the midline) and the tentorium cerebelli (forming a roof over the posterior fossa) (see Ch. 1). A **pressure gradient** may be created by an expanding mass lesion, displacing part of the brain from one intracranial compartment to another. This is termed **brain shift** (or **internal herniation**).

Types of herniation (Fig. 9.11)

Displacement of the cingulate gyrus under the free edge of the falx cerebri is termed **subfalcine herniation** and usually results from a focal lesion in one cerebral hemisphere (see Figs 9.11a and 9.12a).

Downward displacement of the medial temporal lobe (the parahippocampal gyrus and uncus) through the tentorial hiatus is referred to as **transtentorial** (or **uncal**) **herniation** (Fig. 9.11A). This may cause pupil changes due to compression of the oculomotor nerve (Clinical Box 9.3).

Diffuse swelling of both cerebral hemispheres is likely to produce downward displacement of the entire diencephalon (thalamic region). This is called **diencephalic**

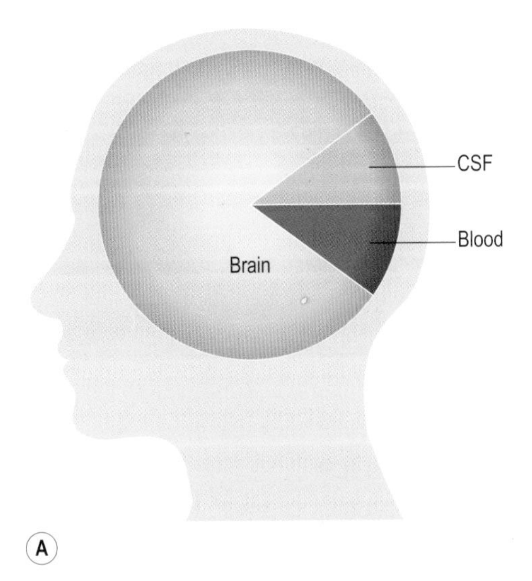

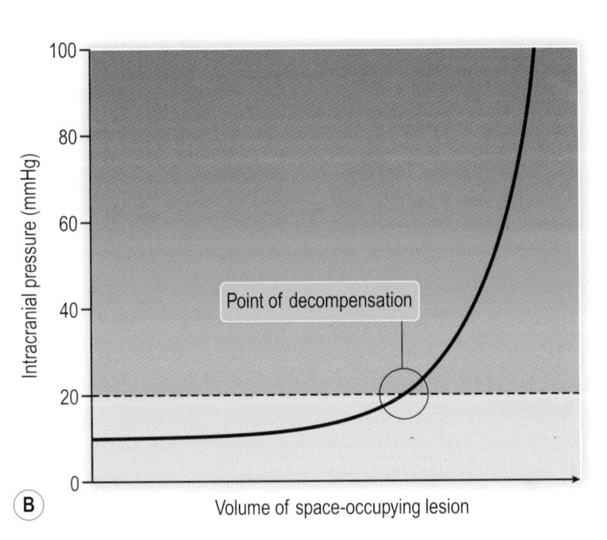

Fig. 9.10 **Pressure–volume relationship with an intracranial mass lesion. (A)** The cranium can be regarded as a rigid box with non-compressible contents; **(B)** This figure illustrates the pressure–volume relationship with an expanding intracranial mass lesion.

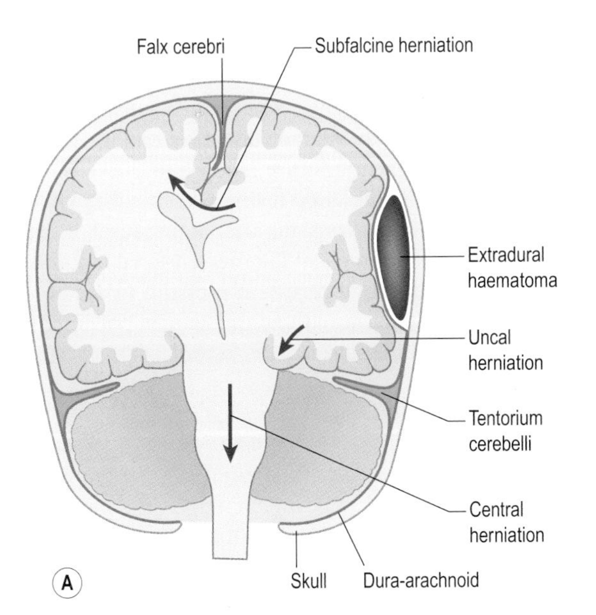

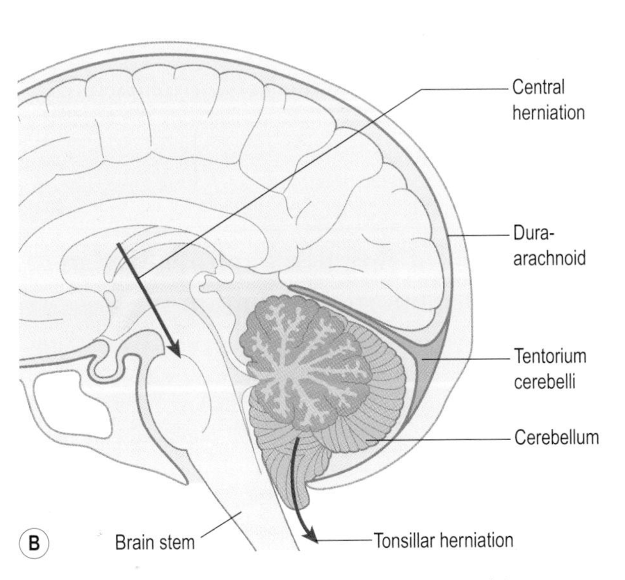

Fig. 9.11 **Brain shift and internal herniation. (A)** Coronal section illustrating the main types of internal herniation; **(B)** Sagittal section of the posterior fossa showing tonsillar and central (diencephalic) herniation.

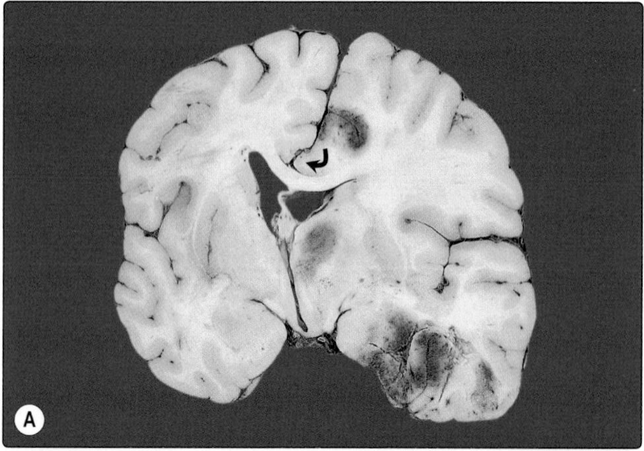

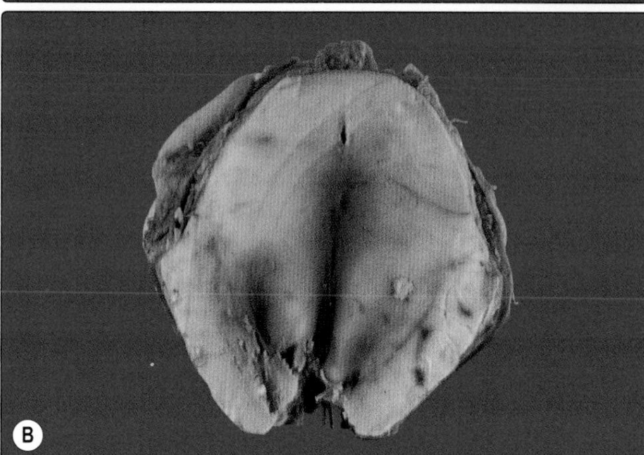

Fig. 9.12 **Internal herniation after traumatic head injury. (A)** Coronal section showing subfalcine herniation of the right cingulate gyrus (arrow) with marked midline shift. There is also haemorrhage in the medial temporal region due to transtentorial herniation; **(B)** Displacement of the brain stem may lead to a fatal midline haemorrhages (Duret or 'flame' haemorrhages), shown here in the midbrain. From Ellison and Love: Neuropathology 2e (Mosby 2003) with permission.

(or **central**) **herniation** and may be associated with tearing of brain stem blood vessels, causing fatal haemorrhage (Fig. 9.12B).

Herniation of the cerebellar tonsils through the foramen magnum in the base of the skull is called **tonsillar herniation** (or **coning**). This can be rapidly fatal due to compression of the medulla oblongata, leading to respiratory arrest.

A sign of critical brain stem compression (compromising the cardiorespiratory centres of the medulla) is the **Cushing response**, consisting of (i) raised intracranial pressure, leading to (ii) arterial hypertension and (iii) bradycardia.

Secondary infarction

In addition to the direct effect of cerebral herniation, which damages the compressed brain tissue, obstruction of cerebral blood vessels may lead to **secondary infarction** (tissue death due to impaired blood flow; see Ch. 10). For instance, subfalcine herniation may be associated with compression of the anterior cerebral artery with consequent infarction of the medial frontal lobe, whereas transtentorial herniation may obstruct the posterior cerebral artery, with infarction of the occipital and inferior temporal lobes.

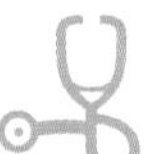

Clinical Box 9.3: Pupil reflexes in transtentorial herniation

Transtentorial herniation is often associated with compression of the **oculomotor (III) nerve** which runs alongside the free edge of the tentorium cerebelli. This results in a dilated pupil due to involvement of parasympathetic **pupilloconstrictor fibres** (see Ch. 3) which travel in the peripheral part of the nerve and are therefore vulnerable to compression. Reduction in GCS and sluggish pupillary light reaction on one side is therefore an early sign of a transtentorial herniation. At a later stage, the pupil will become fixed (unresponsive to light) and dilated.

Key Points

- Brain swelling (cerebral oedema) is an important consequence of primary and secondary brain injury. It may lead to raised intracranial pressure and brain shift or herniation.
- An expanding intracranial mass can be tolerated for a short period of time due to compensatory mechanisms including CSF redistribution and reduced volume of the dural venous sinuses.
- Beyond the point of decompensation the volume–pressure curve becomes linear and the intracranial pressure rises rapidly.
- This may cause brain shift or internal herniation within the cranium. The main types of internal herniation are subfalcine, transtentorial, diencephalic and tonsillar.
- Coning (medullary compression due to tonsillar herniation through the foramen magnum) is an important cause of respiratory arrest and death in patients with raised ICP.

Brain blood flow and ICP

The main factors determining **cerebral blood flow** (**CBF**) are illustrated in Figure 9.13. Blood flow to the brain is proportional to the **cerebral perfusion pressure** (**CPP**) and inversely proportional to the **cerebral vascular resistance** (**CVR**). The cerebral perfusion pressure can be thought of as the 'driving force' for cerebral blood flow.

Under normal circumstances perfusion pressure is mainly determined by the **mean arterial blood pressure** (**MABP**) which is essentially unopposed when the intracranial pressure is normal (0–10 mmHg). If the ICP rises significantly, the mean arterial blood pressure is gradually offset and it becomes increasingly difficult to drive blood into the cranium. In other words, the net cerebral perfusion pressure drops as the ICP increases (assuming constant arterial pressure). If the intracranial pressure were to equal the mean arterial blood pressure, then the net cerebral perfusion pressure would be zero (and brain blood flow would cease). Raised intracranial pressure thus compromises cerebral perfusion.

Regulation of brain blood flow

The cerebral blood flow is normally maintained at a constant level in a process termed **autoregulation**. With normal intracranial pressure, flow depends mainly upon the mean arterial blood pressure, which is approximately equal to the **diastolic blood pressure** plus one third of the **pulse pressure** (the 'pulse pressure' is the difference between systolic and diastolic pressures). The brain compensates for fluctuations in the arterial perfusion pressure by altering the

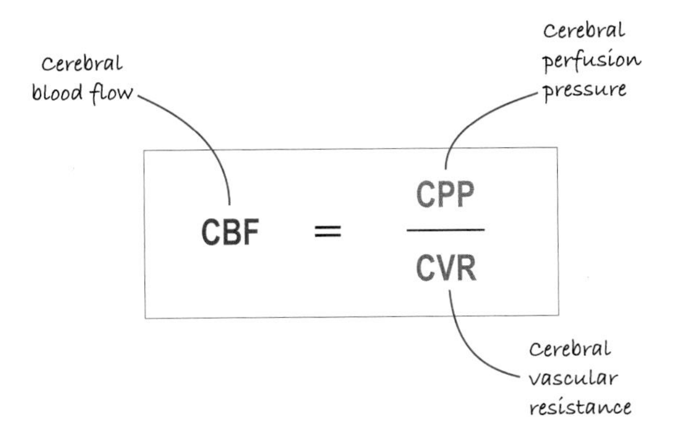

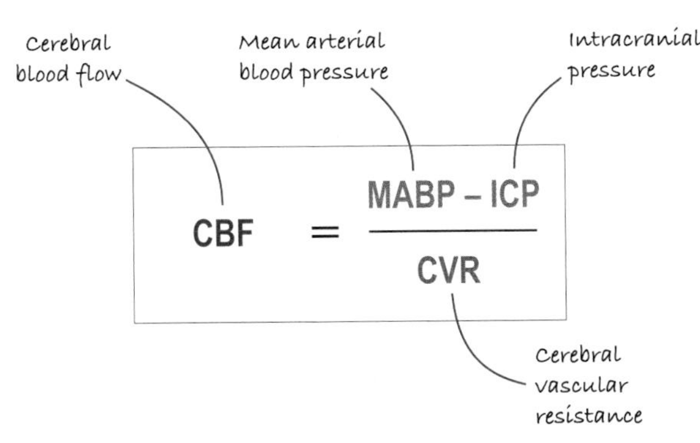

Fig. 9.13 **The relationship between cerebral blood flow and intracranial pressure.** NB: The upper and lower expressions are the same, but the lower part of the figure shows the main determinants of the cerebral perfusion pressure (coloured purple).

vascular resistance of the brain, achieved by contraction and relaxation of smooth muscle in cerebral arterioles. Autoregulation is effective over a very wide range of mean arterial blood pressures (see Fig. 9.14). Following head injury the normal autoregulatory mechanisms may not be effective, so that relatively small falls in perfusion pressure (caused by low blood pressure or high intracranial pressure) may be associated with precipitous drops in cerebral blood flow. Management of raised ICP is discussed in Clinical Box 9.4.

Clinical Box 9.4: Management of raised ICP

It is important to keep intracranial pressure under control after head injury and some patients may be fitted with an **implantable pressure transducer** to monitor it. Raised intracranial pressure can be treated acutely with an intravenous bolus of **mannitol**. This is an **osmotic diuretic** which does not cross the **blood–brain barrier** and reduces cerebral oedema by drawing water away from the brain (into the bloodstream) but the effect is short-lived. Another option that may 'buy time' prior to decompressive surgery is **forced hyperventilation**. Over-breathing reduces the arterial concentration of carbon dioxide (a vasodilator) resulting in cerebral vasoconstriction and reduced intracranial blood volume. In cases with extreme brain swelling it may be necessary to remove part of the skull vault temporarily to relieve the pressure (**hemicraniectomy**). Steroids such as **dexamethasone** are not effective in reducing brain swelling after head injury.

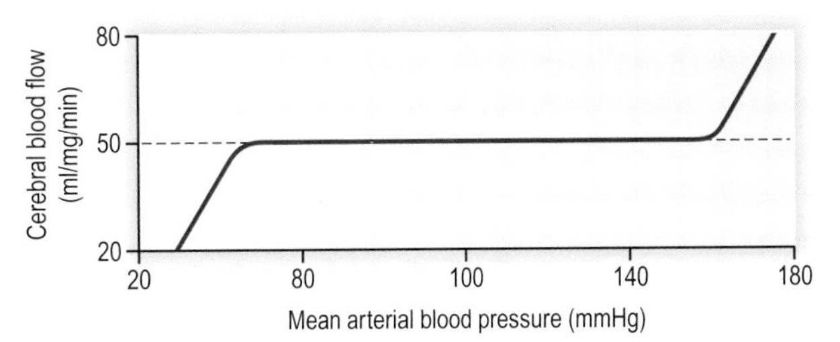

Fig. 9.14 **Cerebral autoregulation.** Cerebral blood flow normally remains constant over a very wide range of mean arterial blood pressures.

Key Points

- Cerebral blood flow is proportional to the cerebral perfusion pressure (which is mainly determined by the mean arterial blood pressure) and inversely proportional to the cerebral vascular resistance.
- In addition to the risk of brain shift and internal herniation, raised intracranial pressure reduces cerebral blood flow (by offsetting the mean arterial blood pressure).
- Raised ICP may be reduced in the short term using the osmotic diuretic mannitol or by forced hyperventilation (which causes cerebral vasoconstriction by reducing arterial CO_2 levels).

Minor head injury

Minor head injury that is severe enough to cause loss of consciousness is referred to as **concussion** (Latin: concutere, to shake violently). There is usually complete recovery with no long-term consequences, but repeated episodes may lead to cumulative brain damage.

Concussion

Concussion is characterized by a brief period of unconsciousness with confusion and **post-traumatic amnesia** (disruption of new memory formation for a short period after the event). There may also be headache, nausea or vomiting. Memory for events prior to the head injury are sometimes affected (**retrograde amnesia**) but this tends to diminish over time and is a less useful marker of severity.

Concussion is thought to be caused by **acceleration–deceleration injury** leading to shearing forces and **diffuse axonal dysfunction**. Pathological studies show that concussion may be associated with lasting changes in the brain and these may be responsible for the long-term alterations in mood, memory and concentration that occur in some people (Clinical Box 9.5).

Repeated minor head injury

There is increased risk of cumulative **mild traumatic brain injury** in certain sporting activities. It is well known in boxing as the '**punch drunk**' **syndrome**, but may also occur in other sports such as football or horse racing. Examination of the brain in such cases often reveals signs of old contusions (especially in the frontal and temporal lobes) together with generalized cerebral atrophy, enlargement of the ventricles and tearing of the septum pellucidum. Microscopic examination may show neuronal loss in the cerebral cortex and substantia nigra of the midbrain. Surviving neurons often contain **neurofibrillary tangles** similar to those found in Alzheimer's disease (Ch. 12); and selective loss of neurons in the substantia nigra may lead to features mimicking Parkinson's disease (Ch. 13).

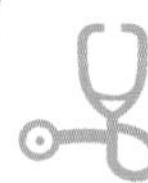

Clinical Box 9.5: Post-concussion syndrome

Some patients experience on-going symptoms after relatively trivial head injury. Typical features include headaches, dizziness and **emotional changes** (irritability, fatigue, depression) together with **impaired memory** and **concentration**. This may lead to problems coping at work or at home. The emotional and cognitive changes might represent mild diffuse axonal injury in the frontal and temporal lobes.

Key Points

- Concussion is a form of minor head injury in which there is a brief loss of consciousness followed by a variable period of post-traumatic amnesia and confusion.
- Some patients have on-going problems with memory, mood and concentration (post-concussion syndrome) that may interfere with work or social activities.
- Repeated minor head injury can lead to lasting changes in the brain (e.g. 'punch drunk' syndrome) including neurofibrillary tangles, similar to those found in Alzheimer's disease.

Chapter 10
Stroke

CHAPTER CONTENTS

Stroke follows heart disease and cancer as the third leading cause of death in developed countries, accounting for 10% of overall mortality in the UK. It is defined clinically as an acute neurological deficit of vascular origin that lasts more than 24 hours or causes death.

Types of stroke

Stroke is caused by inadequate tissue perfusion or **ischaemia** (Greek: isch-, restriction; haema, blood). The brain is particularly sensitive to ischaemia because neurons have a high metabolic rate and can only survive a few minutes without oxygen and glucose. Tissue death as a result of inadequate blood flow (e.g. due to an occluded blood vessel) is called **infarction** (Latin: infarctus, stuffed). The area of dead tissue is referred to as 'an infarct'. There are two main types of stroke (Figs 10.1 and 10.2):

- **Ischaemic stroke** (85% of cases) is caused by reduced blood flow to a particular part of the brain, usually following occlusion of a cerebral artery.
- **Haemorrhagic stroke** (15% of cases) is due to a ruptured blood vessel. This is commonly associated with high blood pressure and diseases that weaken the arterial wall.

In both types of stroke the brain tissue normally supplied by the vessel is suddenly deprived of blood and its function is lost. This causes focal neurological deficits that develop very rapidly (e.g. sudden weakness or loss of speech) and **abrupt onset** is the clinical hallmark of stroke. In haemorrhagic stroke, there may also be mechanical damage, such as tearing and compression of brain tissue, caused by blood escaping under arterial pressure.

Key Points

- Stroke follows heart disease and cancer as the third leading cause of death in developed countries, accounting for 10% of overall mortality in the UK.
- It is defined as an acute neurological deficit of vascular origin that lasts more than 24 hours or causes death. Abrupt onset is the clinical hallmark of stroke.
- The two main types of stroke are ischaemic (85%) and haemorrhagic (15%); in most cases, inadequate tissue perfusion (ischaemia) leads to death of brain tissue (infarction).

Ischaemic stroke

Ischaemic stroke can be divided into five groups based on cause: (i) large-artery atherosclerosis; (ii) cardioembolism; (iii) small vessel occlusion; (iv) other defined cause; and (v) unknown cause (cryptogenic stroke). This classification is derived from a multicentre **trial of acute stroke treatment** ('TOAST') in the 1990s and continues to be widely used in UK stroke trials. The 'other defined cause' category incorporates many uncommon and rare causes of stroke

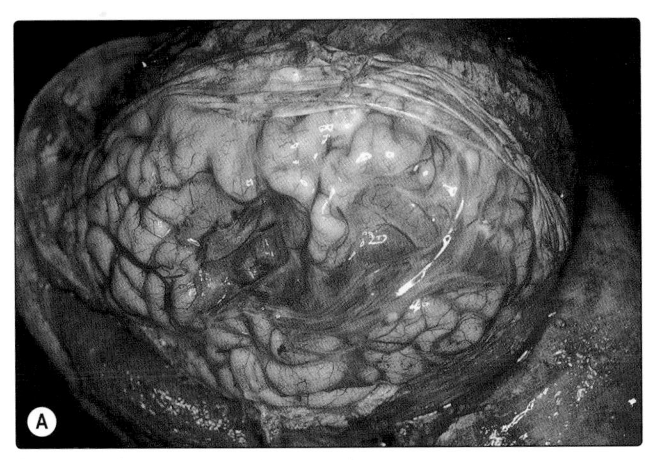

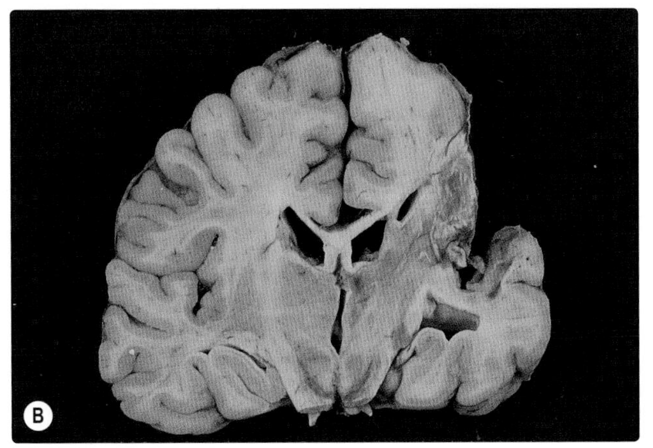

Fig. 10.1 **Ischaemic stroke. (A)** Photograph taken during a post-mortem examination in a patient with an old ('healed') left hemisphere ischaemic infarct in the territory of the middle cerebral artery. Extensive resorption of brain tissue (leaving only a fluid-filled cyst cavity) indicates a prolonged period of survival after the stroke; **(B)** Coronal section of a fixed (preserved) brain slice in a different patient showing an old ischaemic stroke, also in the territory of the middle cerebral artery. From Ellison and Love: Neuropathology 2e (Mosby 2003) with permission.

including abnormalities of blood coagulation, infectious diseases, arterial damage and inflammatory disorders.

Large vessel and cardioembolic stroke

Cerebral blood vessels may be occluded by an **embolus** (Greek: embolos, wedge or plug). This is a small piece of coagulated blood (or occasionally some other material such as fat) that travels in the circulation and lodges in the vascular tree of the brain. Emboli often originate from the heart (**cardioembolic stroke**) in association with valve disease or an abnormal heart rhythm (Clinical Box 10.1). Disease in the neck vessels or aortic arch may also give rise to emboli.

Some ischaemic strokes are caused by coagulation of blood within a cerebral vessel, termed **in situ thrombosis** (Greek: thrombos, blood clot) or **large artery intracranial occlusive disease**. This is more common in people of Asian and African origin, but is increasingly recognized in Caucasians.

Small vessel disease

Small vessel disease is particularly common in patients with **arterial hypertension** together with other vascular risk factors (e.g. diabetes, cigarette smoking, elevated cholesterol). High blood pressure damages the arterial wall and its smooth muscle is gradually replaced by collagen, termed **hyaline arteriosclerosis**. In some cases there is vessel wall necrosis with accumulation of lipid-laden foam cells, which is referred to as **lipohyalinosis**.

Both types of pathology cause **arteriosclerosis** or 'hardening' of the arteries (Greek: sklerōs, hard). Sclerotic vessels are unable to dilate in response to reduced flow, leading to **lacunar infarcts** (see Ch. 12, Figs 12.18 and 12.19). These are small areas of ischaemic tissue damage (often in the basal ganglia or internal capsule) measuring less than 1 cm in diameter (Latin: lacūna, hole or gap). Small vessel disease is also an important cause of **vascular cognitive impairment** and **dementia** (Ch. 12).

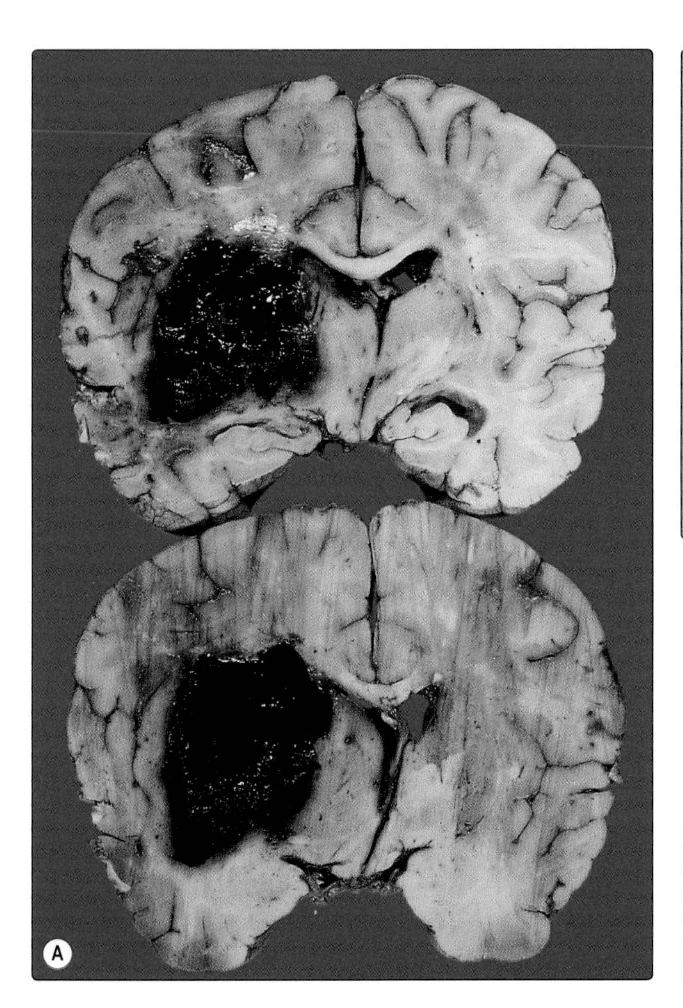

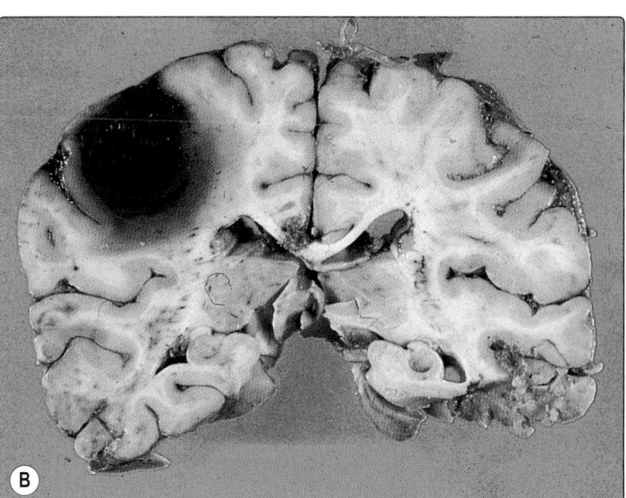

Fig. 10.2 **Haemorrhagic stroke. (A)** Coronal sections showing a typical hypertension-associated haemorrhagic stroke replacing the basal ganglia; **(B)** Coronal section showing an atypical ('lobar') haemorrhage due to cerebral amyloid angiopathy affecting the cortical and meningeal arteries. Note the superficial (cortical) position of the atypical haemorrhage. From Ellison and Love: Neuropathology 2e (Mosby 2003) with permission.

Clinical Box 10.1: Atrial fibrillation

This is the most common type of **abnormal heart rhythm**, affecting 1% of people over the age 65 and 10% of those over 80. It is characterized by disorganized atrial contraction (**fibrillation**) with an **irregular heartbeat**. There may be palpitations, fainting episodes or chest pain, but it is often asymptomatic. Blood tends to pool and coagulate in the poorly contracting atria, increasing the risk of **cardioembolic stroke** (from the left atrium to the brain) up to ten-fold. Predisposing factors for atrial fibrillation include hypertension, heart disease, hyperthyroidism and excessive alcohol consumption. It can be treated with **anticoagulants** (e.g. warfarin or newer agents such as the direct thrombin inhibitor dabigatran). Alternatively, drugs may be given to control the heart rate if it is fast (which can compromise cardiac output) or a defibrillator can be used to restore a normal heart rhythm (called **cardioversion**).

Transient ischaemic attacks

A brief period of cerebral ischaemia may cause a reversible neurological deficit that resolves when the blood flow is restored. This is a **transient ischaemic attack** (TIA). Involvement of the retinal blood supply causes temporary blindness in one eye, termed **amaurosis fugax** (Greek: amaurosis, dark; Latin: fugax, fleeting). Symptoms usually resolve within minutes (and never last more than 24 hours, by definition) but neuroimaging evidence suggests that permanent damage occurs in 10–20% of cases. TIAs are associated with increased risk of both stroke and heart attack.

Haemorrhagic stroke

Spontaneous intracerebral haemorrhage is more common in people with **high blood pressure** and frequently occurs in the basal ganglia, cerebellum or pons (Fig. 10.2A). However, the incidence of hypertensive intracerebral haemorrhage is declining in the UK and USA and an increasingly important cause is **cerebral amyloid angiopathy**, particularly in the elderly (see Ch. 12, Clinical Box 12.5). This is caused by deposition of **amyloid beta peptide** in the walls of cortical and meningeal arteries, leading to **atypical** (or **lobar**) **haemorrhages** that are close to the cortical surface (Fig. 10.2B).

Up to a third of spontaneous intracranial haemorrhages are caused by rupture of an **aneurysm** (a dilatation in the wall of an artery). Since the cerebral blood vessels travel and branch within the subarachnoid space, this results in **subarachnoid haemorrhage** (Clinical Box 10.2). Aneurysms that rupture in the substance of the brain may cause devastating brain damage or sudden death.

> ### *Clinical Box 10.2: Subarachnoid haemorrhage*
>
> Bleeding into the subarachnoid space accounts for a third of intracranial haemorrhages. Although this does not necessarily cause a focal neurological deficit, **subarachnoid haemorrhage** is normally regarded as a type of stroke, accounting for 5% of cases overall. It classically presents with a severe headache ('the worst headache I have ever had'). The most common cause is a ruptured **berry aneurysm**, a medical emergency with a high mortality rate (Fig. 10.3). Berry aneurysms are small vascular swellings which develop at congenital weak spots in the arterial wall. They are usually found at points where blood vessels branch, especially in the **circle of Willis** at the base of the brain. Ischaemic stroke may occur as a late complication. This is due to blood in the subarachnoid space acting as an irritant and triggering **vasospasm**. Unruptured berry aneurysms are found incidentally in up to 2% of post-mortem examinations.
>
> 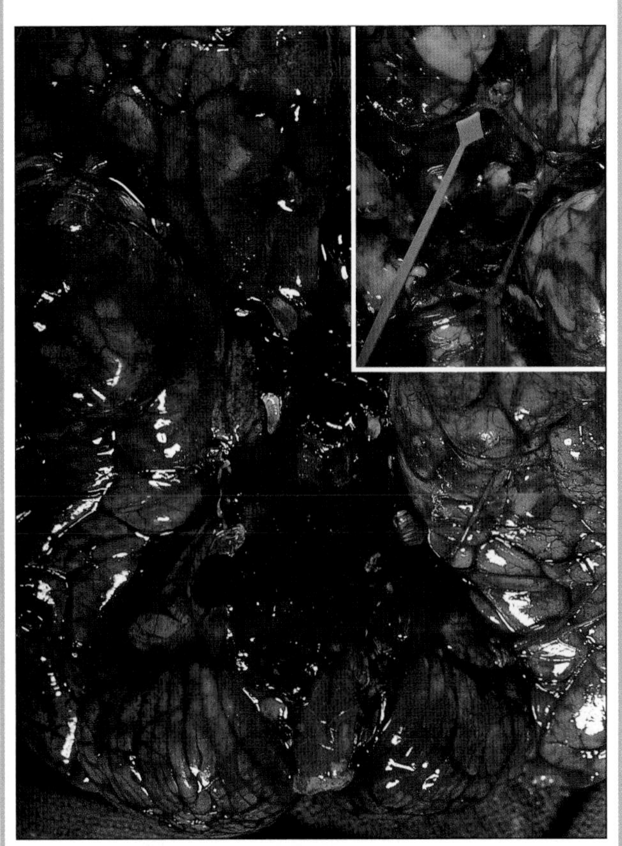
>
> Fig. 10.3 **Subarachnoid haemorrhage.** Post-mortem photograph of the brain (ventral aspect) in a patient who collapsed and died after a sudden, severe headache. The subarachnoid space at the base of the brain is filled with fresh blood, obscuring the circle of Willis. *Inset*: after removal of the blood a ruptured berry aneurysm was found in the region of the anterior communicating artery, indicated by the pointer. From Ellison and Love: Neuropathology 2e (Mosby 2003) with permission.

Blood supply to the brain

The brain is supplied by two pairs of arteries that arise from branches of the aortic arch (Fig. 10.4):

- The **internal carotid arteries** ascend in the anterior part of the neck, arising from the bifurcation of the common carotid arteries.
- The **vertebral arteries** arise from the subclavian arteries and ascend in the lateral cervical region, passing through foramina in the transverse processes of the upper six cervical vertebrae.

The arteries at the base of the brain are linked by **communicating vessels** to form the **circle of Willis**. This gives rise to **anterior**, **middle** and **posterior cerebral arteries** on each side, which supply most of the cerebral hemisphere. The cerebral blood supply can be divided into anterior and posterior circulations (Fig. 10.5A).

Anterior circulation

The internal carotid artery divides at the base of the brain, giving rise to the **middle cerebral artery** (**MCA**) and the **anterior cerebral artery** (**ACA**). The MCA is the larger of the two and receives 80% of the internal carotid blood flow. For this reason, **cardiogenic emboli** are much more likely to enter the MCA than the ACA. The middle cerebral artery continues laterally between the frontal and temporal lobes and emerges from the lateral sulcus to supply most of the hemispheric convexity (Figs 10.6A and 10.7).

The anterior cerebral artery passes forward and medially to meet its partner between the cerebral hemispheres. It winds around the corpus callosum and supplies the medial aspect of the hemisphere as far back as the **parieto-occipital sulcus** (Figs 10.6 and 10.8). Posterior to this point the posterior cerebral artery takes over to supply the occipital lobe. Perforating branches of the anterior circulation supply the **optic radiations**, so that anterior circulation strokes may cause a contralateral visual field defect.

Posterior circulation

The posterior circulation supplies the remainder of the cerebral hemisphere and the **posterior fossa contents**

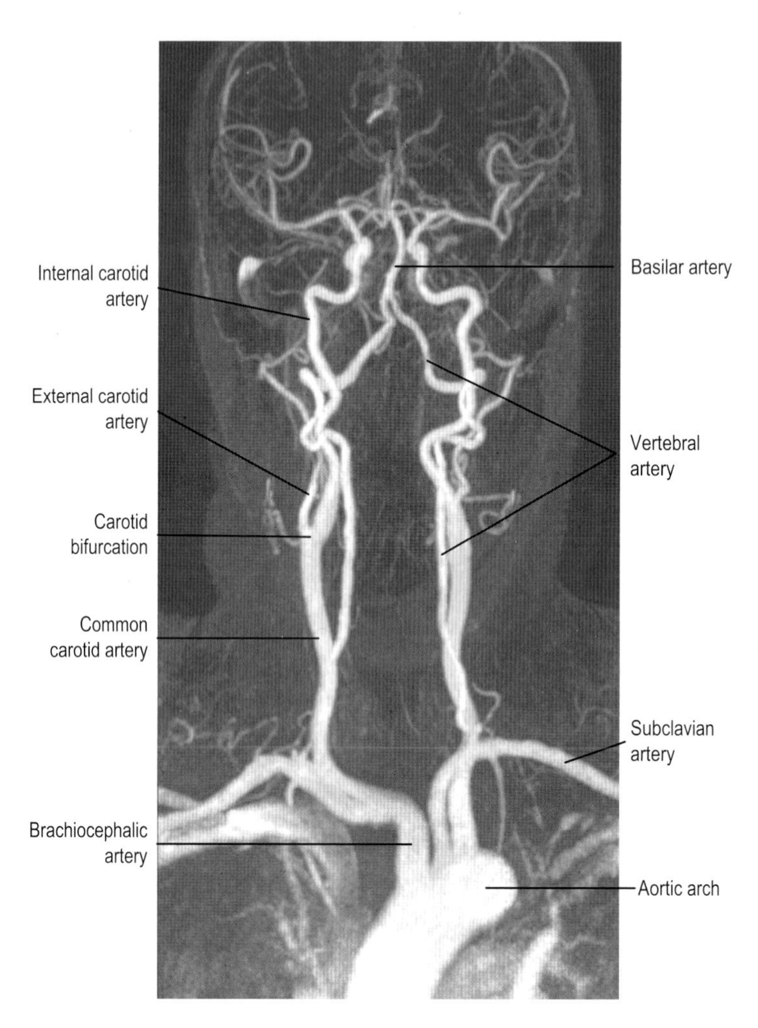

Fig. 10.4 **MRI-angiogram showing the aorta and neck vessels.** Note that the right common carotid and right subclavian arteries [seen here on the left side of the image, following radiological convention] both arise from a single brachiochephalic artery. In contrast, the left common carotid and left subclavian arteries each arise separately as direct branches of the aortic arch. Courtesy of Dr Andrew MacKinnon.

Key Points

- Cerebral blood vessels are most commonly occluded by emboli. These are often cardiogenic (e.g. due to atrial fibrillation or valve disease) but may also arise from the aortic arch or neck vessels.
- Small vessel disease is associated with hypertension and other cardiovascular risk factors. In addition to stroke, it is an important cause of vascular cognitive impairment and dementia.
- Large artery intracranial occlusive disease (in situ thrombosis) is often associated with vessel wall disease, leading to a regional infarct. It is more common in people of African and Asian origin.
- Brief periods of cerebral ischaemia cause transient ischaemic attacks which usually resolve within a few minutes and never last more than 24 hours (by definition).
- Spontaneous intracerebral haemorrhage is more common in people with arterial hypertension and frequently occurs in the basal ganglia, cerebellum or pons. Cerebral amyloid angiopathy is an increasingly recognized cause, leading to 'atypical' (superficial/lobar) haemorrhages.
- Subarachnoid haemorrhage usually presents with a sudden, severe headache and is most often due to a ruptured berry aneurysm. It is a medical emergency with a high mortality rate.

(brain stem and cerebellum). The two vertebral arteries unite in front of the brain stem, at the junction between pons and medulla, to become the **basilar artery**. For this reason, the posterior circulation is also known as the **vertebrobasilar circulation**. The basilar artery ascends along the basal pons to reach the midbrain where it splits into the two **posterior cerebral arteries** (**PCA**). These vessels wind around the midbrain and pass posteriorly, above the tentorium cerebelli, to supply the occipital lobe and the inferior surface of the temporal lobe (Figs 10.6B, 10.7 and 10.8).

Circle of Willis

The circle of Willis is a polygonal arrangement of blood vessels surrounding the optic chiasm and pituitary stalk. It connects the anterior and posterior circulations via the single **anterior communicating artery** and the paired **posterior communicating arteries** (Figs 10.5B and 10.9). The circle of Willis shows considerable anatomical variation and is incomplete in 50% of people. It is an example of a **collateral circulation**, an arrangement of interconnected vascular channels permitting blood flow via an alternative route in the event of an obstruction. Interconnections between vessels exist elsewhere (e.g. between the distal territories of the three main cerebral blood vessels) but are not always effective, particularly in the elderly. Some structures do not have a collateral blood supply (e.g. the internal capsule and basal ganglia) and are therefore more vulnerable to stroke.

Perforating vessels

The circle of Willis gives rise to a number of **central perforating vessels** which supply the internal substance of the brain. Perforating vessels from the anterior circulation enter the brain just lateral to the optic chiasm on each side, via the **anterior perforated area**. A second group arises from the posterior circulation and enters the brain at the

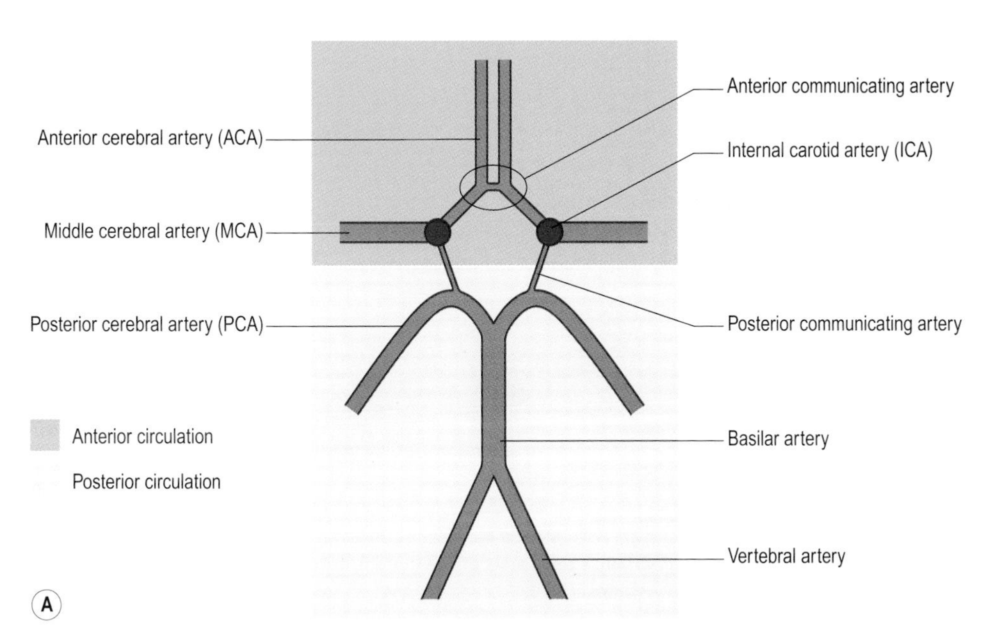

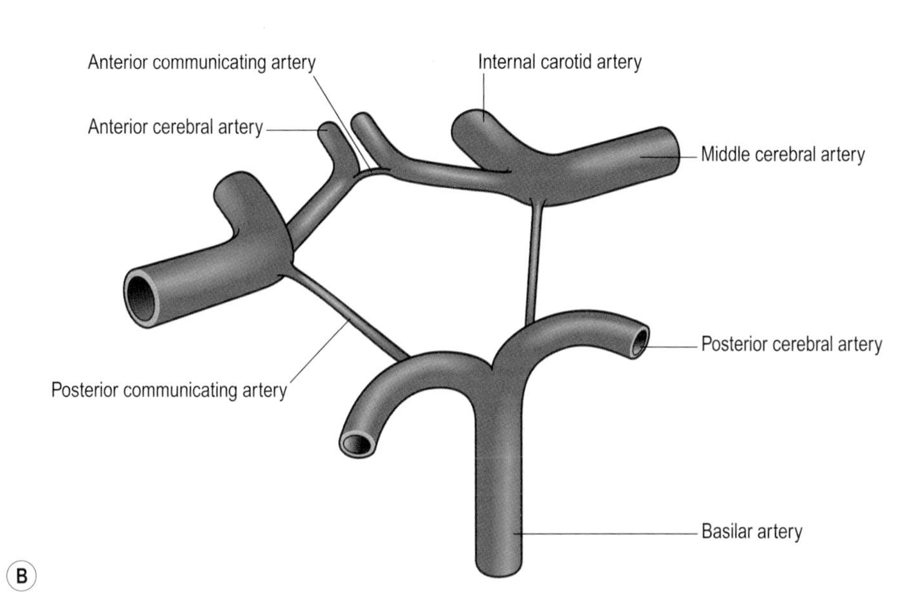

Fig. 10.5 **The anterior and posterior circulations and their origins from the circle of Willis. (A)** Schematic, two-dimensional, representation of the circle of Willis, showing the anterior (internal carotid) and posterior (vertebrobasilar) circulations; **(B)** Illustration of the three-dimensional arrangement of the circle of Willis.

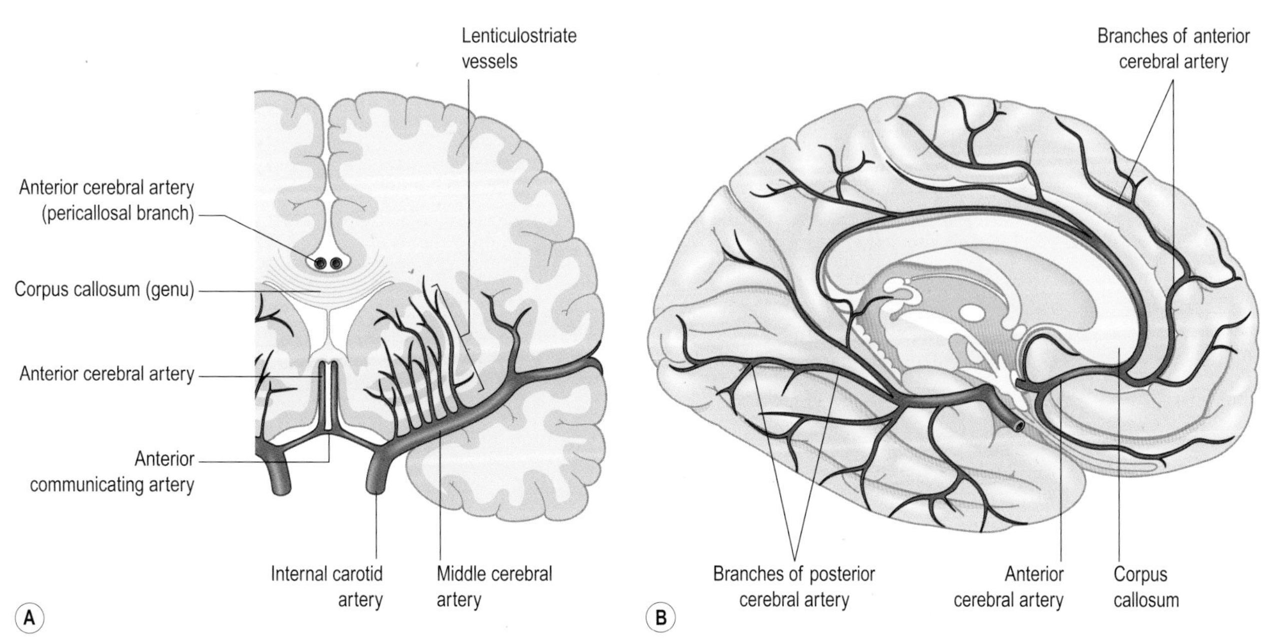

Fig. 10.6 **The anterior, middle, posterior and lenticulostriate arteries. (A)** Coronal view of the cerebral hemisphere showing the anterior and middle cerebral arteries. The lenticulostriate (deep perforating) vessels can be seen arising at right-angles from the middle cerebral artery; **(B)** Midsagittal view of the cerebral hemisphere showing the anterior and posterior cerebral arteries.

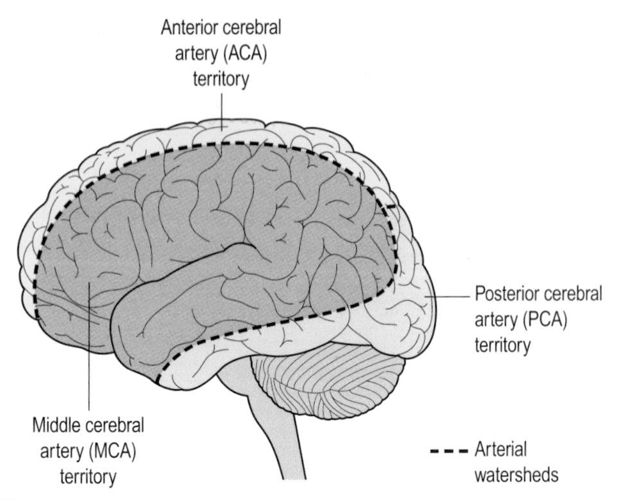

Fig. 10.7 **Lateral view of the cerebral hemisphere showing the vascular territories of the middle, anterior and posterior cerebral arteries.** The dashed line indicates the arterial watershed zone between the main vascular territories.

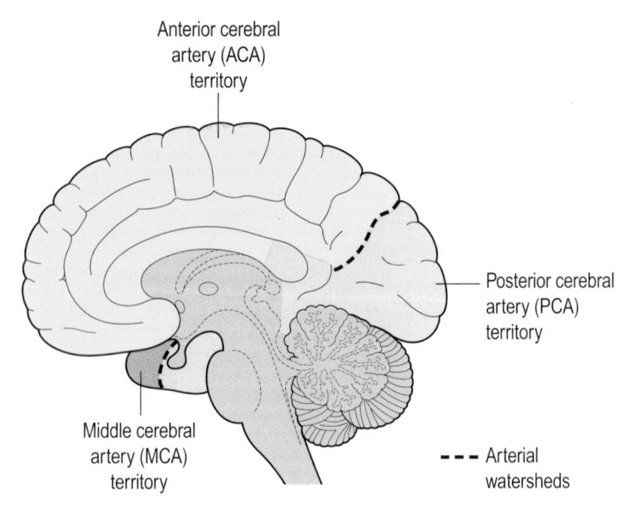

Fig. 10.8 **Medial view of the cerebral hemisphere showing the vascular territories of the middle, anterior and posterior cerebral arteries.** The dashed line indicates the arterial watershed zone between the main vascular territories.

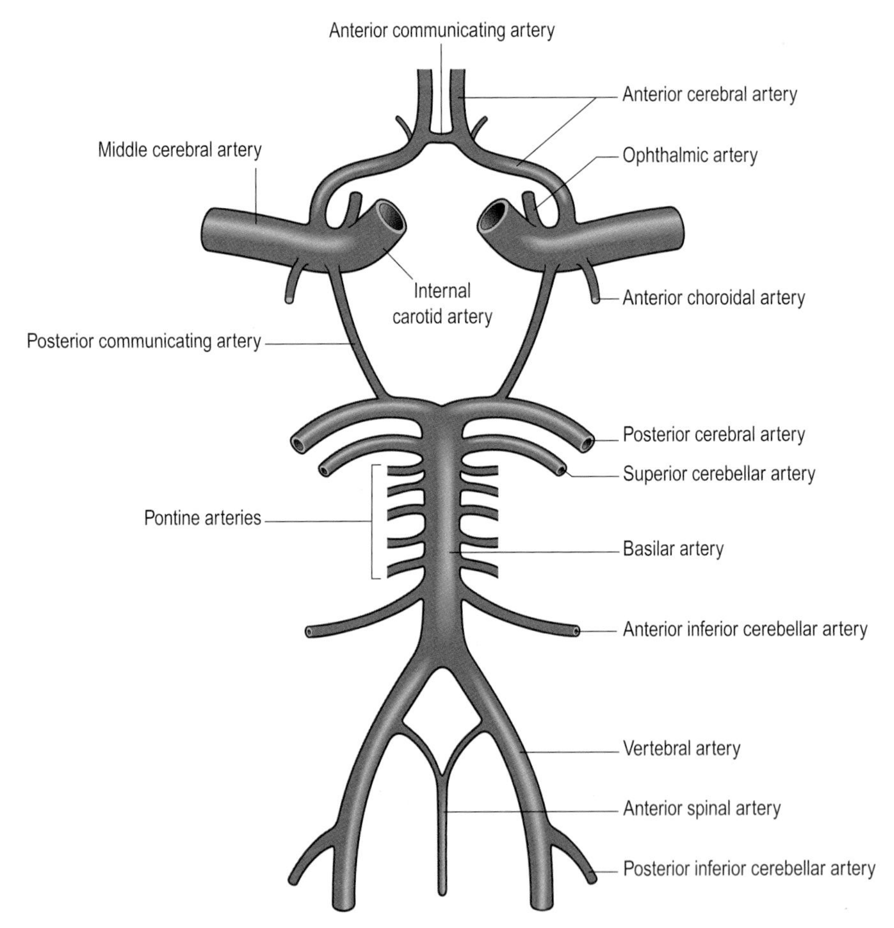

Fig. 10.9 **More detailed representation of the circle of Willis, including the main branches to the brain stem and cerebellum.** The ophthalmic artery is the first branch of the intracranial portion of the internal carotid artery and supplies the orbital contents. The anterior choroidal artery is the final branch of the internal carotid artery (or an early branch of the MCA); despite being a small vessel, it supplies portions of the central visual pathways, medial temporal lobe (e.g. hippocampus, amygdala) and part of the basal ganglia and internal capsule. The anterior spinal artery supplies the basal portion of the medulla and the anterior two thirds of the spinal cord.

interpeduncular fossa of the midbrain, via the **posterior perforated area**. The anterior group includes the **lenticulostriate vessels** (or 'arteries of stroke') which supply the basal ganglia and internal capsule (Fig. 10.6A). They are an important site of spontaneous intracerebral haemorrhage and lacunar infarcts (both caused by small-vessel disease).

The arterial territories of the three main cerebral vessels and deep perforating vessels are illustrated in coronal section in Figure 10.10. The regions between territories are the **watershed zones** and are particularly vulnerable to a sudden reduction in arterial blood pressure. This may lead to a characteristic pattern of **watershed infarction** at the arterial border zones following profound **arterial**

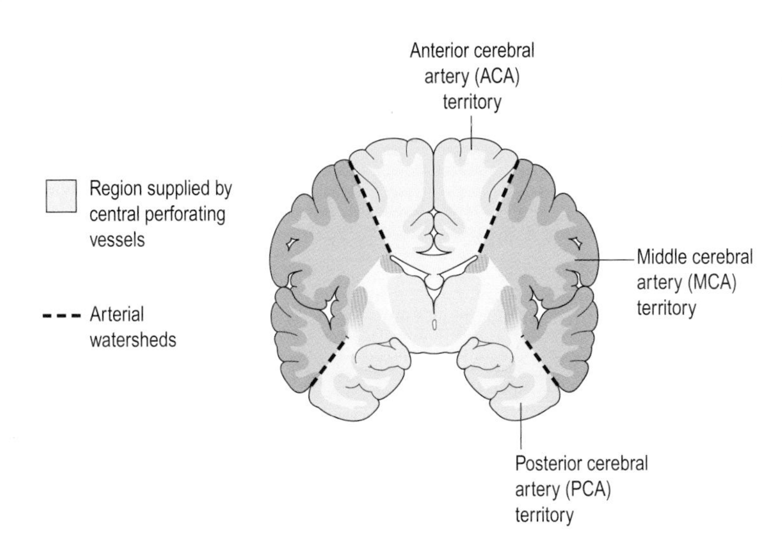

Fig. 10.10 **Coronal section of the cerebral hemispheres showing the vascular territories of the middle, anterior and posterior cerebral arteries and the watershed zones between them.** The grey zone is supplied by deep (perforating) branches of the circle of Willis.

Key Points

- The anterior (internal carotid) and posterior (vertebrobasilar) circulations are united at the base of the brain to form the circle of Willis. This is an example of a collateral circulation.
- The circle of Willis is formed by a single (short) anterior communicating vessel and two (long and thin) posterior communicating vessels.
- The internal carotid artery divides at the base of the brain to become the middle cerebral artery (which passes laterally) and anterior cerebral artery (passing anteriorly and medially).
- The MCA receives 80% of the carotid blood flow and the ACA receives 20%. Cardiogenic emboli are therefore more likely to enter the MCA than the ACA territory.
- The MCA supplies the lateral surface of the cerebral hemisphere, whereas the ACA supplies the medial surface as far back as the parieto-occipital sulcus.
- The posterior cerebral artery is the terminal branch of the basilar artery. The territory of the PCA includes the occipital lobe and the inferior surface of the temporal lobe.

hypotension (e.g. after cardiorespiratory arrest, anaphylactic shock or major blood loss).

Blood supply to the brain stem

The midbrain, pons and medulla are supplied from the posterior circulation by small **perforating vessels**, most of which are not named. They are arranged in three groups: (i) paramedian; (ii) short circumferential; and (iii) long circumferential. The **paramedian vessels** pass directly backwards through the full thickness of the brain stem (to the ventricular floor) to supply a portion of the pons and medulla on either side of the midline. The **short** and **long circumferential vessels** encircle the brain stem to supply more lateral and posterior portions.

Blood supply to the cerebellum

The cerebellum is supplied by three long circumferential vessels that arise from different parts of the posterior circulation (Figs 10.9 and 10.11):

- **The superior cerebellar artery** (**SCA**) arises from the upper part of the basilar artery, immediately below the origin of the posterior cerebral artery.

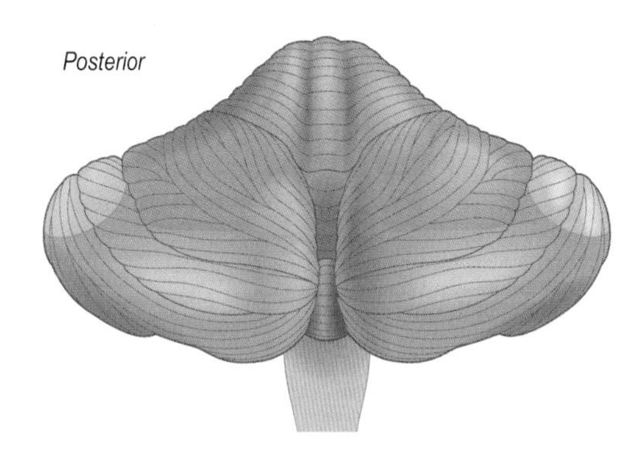

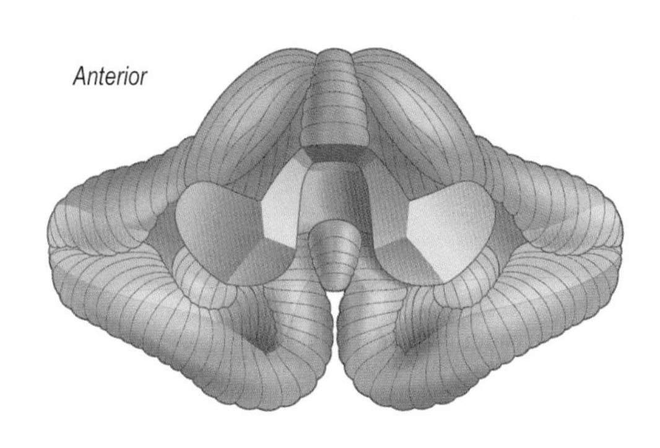

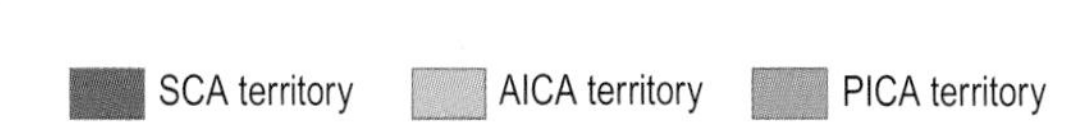

Fig. 10.11 **Blood supply to the cerebellum.** The vascular territories of the three main blood vessels supplying the cerebellum are illustrated. The superior cerebellar artery (SCA) and anterior inferior cerebellar artery (AICA) both arise from the basilar artery; the posterior inferior cerebellar artery (PICA) usually arises from the vertebral artery.

- **The anterior inferior cerebellar artery** (**AICA**) is a caudal (inferior) branch of the basilar artery.
- **The posterior inferior cerebellar artery** (**PICA**) usually arises from the vertebral artery.

The posterior inferior cerebellar artery also supplies the lateral medulla. Occlusion of this vessel is associated with the **lateral medullary syndrome** (Clinical Box 10.3).

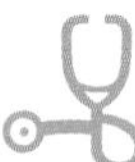

Clinical Box 10.3: Lateral medullary syndrome

Occlusion of the posterior inferior cerebellar artery (PICA), supplying the lateral part of the medulla, causes: (i) **ipsilateral** loss of pain and temperature sensation in the face; and (ii) **contralateral** loss of pain and temperature sensationin in the trunk and limbs. This results from damage to the **trigeminal sensory nucleus** and **spinothalamic tract** respectively (see Ch. 4). Sympathetic fibres passing from the hypothalamus to the spinal cord may also be affected, leading to loss of sympathetic innervation to the ipsilateral face. This is one cause of **Horner's syndrome**, characterized by **ptosis** (drooping eyelid), **miosis** (small, constricted pupil) and facial **anhidrosis** (loss of sweating). Other features of the lateral medullary syndrome reflect damage to local brain stem structures and connections with the cerebellum: difficulty swallowing, double vision, poor coordination, vertigo and nausea.

Stroke syndromes

For practical purposes, ischaemic strokes can be classified into one of four major clinical categories based on the maximum deficit following a single stroke, illustrated in Figure 10.12:

- Total anterior circulation syndrome (TACS).
- Partial anterior circulation syndrome (PACS).
- Posterior circulation syndrome (POCS).
- Lacunar syndrome (LACS).

This system is easy to use and provides useful prognostic information. For example, the proportion of patients dying within the first year in each type is approximately 60% (TACS), 20% (PACS or POCS) and 10% (LACS). In the first week after a stroke, the most common cause of death is raised intracranial pressure due to brain swelling (**cerebral oedema**); this causes herniation of the cerebellar tonsils through the skull base, compressing the brain stem (which is referred to as '**coning**', see Ch. 9).

TACS
- New higher cortical dysfunction (e.g. aphasia)
- AND homonymous visual field defect
- AND sensorimotor deficit (affecting 2 out of 3 of: face, arm, leg)

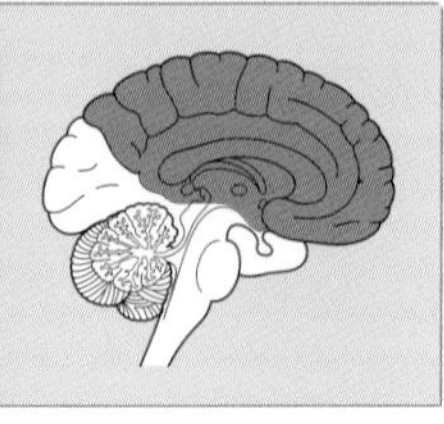

PACS
- Two out of three elements of TACS
- OR higher cortical dysfunction alone
- OR limited sensorimotor deficit (affecting fewer than 2 of: face, arm, leg)

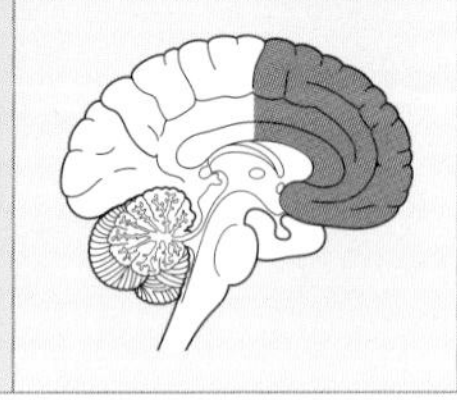

POCS
- Cranial nerve + crossed sensorimotor deficit
- OR bilateral sensory/motor deficit
- OR disorder of conjugate eye movement
- OR isolated cerebellar dysfunction/field defect

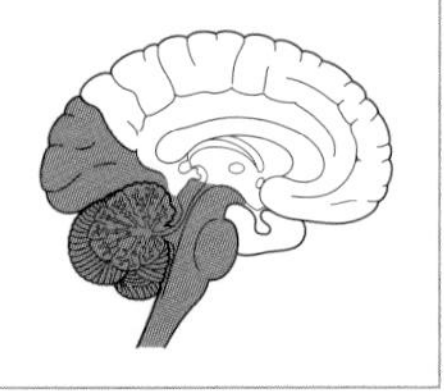

LACS
- Pure motor deficit
- OR pure sensory deficit
- OR sensorimotor deficit
- OR ataxic hemiparesis

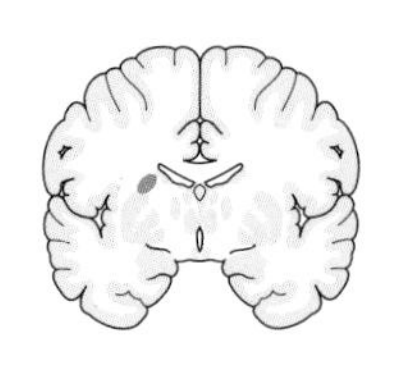

Fig. 10.12 **Clinical classification of stroke syndromes.** Ischaemic strokes can be classified as a total anterior circulation syndrome (TACS), partial anterior circulation syndrome (PACS), posterior circulation syndrome (POCS) or lacunar syndrome (LACS). The classification is based on the maximum observed deficit following a single stroke. For the lacunar syndrome, the sensorimotor deficit must affect at least two out of three areas (i.e. leg, arm and face).

Key Points

- The watershed areas between the territories of the main named cerebral arteries are vulnerable in the event of very low blood pressure, leading to a 'watershed infarction'.
- Perforating branches of the anterior, middle and posterior cerebral arteries (and circle of Willis) supply the basal ganglia, thalamus and internal capsule.
- The lenticulostriate vessels ('arteries of stroke') are prone to hypertension-associated small vessel disease and are a common site of spontaneous intracerebral haemorrhage.
- The brain stem is supplied from the posterior (vertebrobasilar) circulation, via three groups of artery: paramedian, short circumferential and long circumferential.
- The cerebellum is supplied by three long circumferential vessels, the: superior cerebellar artery (SCA), anterior inferior cerebellar artery (AICA) and posterior inferior cerebellar artery (PICA).

Atherosclerosis

The underlying pathology in a significant proportion of cerebrovascular (and cardiovascular) disease is **atherosclerosis**. This is a degenerative process affecting medium and large arteries throughout the body (Greek: sklērōsis, hardening). It is almost universal in the developed world, chiefly as a result of lifestyle factors including poor diet, cigarette smoking and lack of exercise.

Atheromatous plaques

The characteristic lesion in atherosclerosis is called an **atheroma** (from the Latin word for porridge). This is a deposit of lipid-rich material in the vessel wall that develops over many years. The process begins in the innermost (intimal) layer of large arteries and slowly expands. Atheromatous deposits therefore cause progressive **stenosis** (narrowing) of the vessel (Fig. 10.13). This gradually impinges on the lumen, but may remain asymptomatic for many years. The precursor lesions in atherosclerosis are known as **fatty streaks**. These are pale areas beneath the arterial endothelium that can be identified in the arteries of children and consist of lipid-laden macrophages.

The distribution of **atheromatous plaques** is not random. Areas exposed to rapid, turbulent blood flow are particularly susceptible, especially arterial branch-points. These include the aortic arch and large arteries of the neck, both of which may be a source of **emboli** to the brain (Clinical Box 10.4). Atherosclerosis is also common in the intracranial portion of the internal carotid artery and at the origin and major branch-points of the middle cerebral artery.

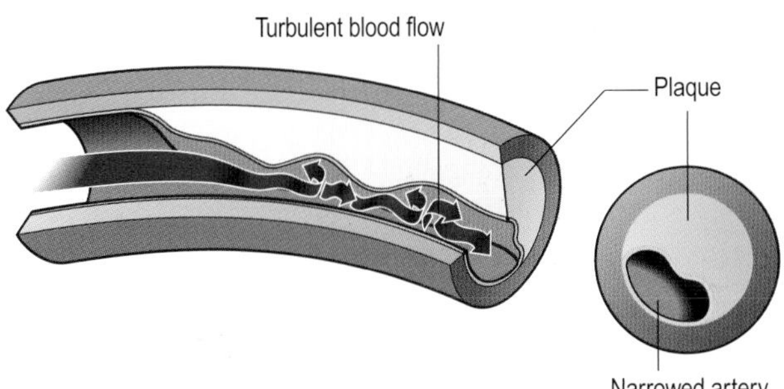

Fig. 10.13 **Effect of atheroma on arterial blood flow.** In a normal artery, the blood flow is smooth and laminar, but development of atheromatous plaques causes progressive stenosis (narrowing) of the arterial lumen and leads to abnormal, turbulent blood flow.

Clinical Box 10.4: Carotid endarterectomy

Atherosclerosis in the neck vessels causes progressive stenosis and increases the risk of TIA and stroke. Patients with moderate to severe stenosis (>50% occlusion) may benefit from **carotid endarterectomy**, a procedure to remove the diseased vessel lining. This can be achieved by open neck surgery or as an **endovascular procedure** (using a catheter introduced via the femoral artery in the groin). Although the risk of stroke is significantly reduced, the surgery itself may precipitate a cerebral infarct (or even death in a small minority of patients) and trial data suggest that it is necessary to treat 80 asymptomatic patients in order to prevent a single adverse event. Current best practice guidelines therefore do not recommend the procedure for asymptomatic individuals, in whom the stroke risk is less than 1% with medical treatment alone.

Plaque formation

A key factor in plaque formation is dysfunction of the endothelium, which normally releases factors such as **nitric oxide** that prevent platelet and leukocyte adhesion. **Endothelial dysfunction** can be caused by toxic agents including **aromatic hydrocarbons** and **free radicals** that are present in cigarette smoke. Damage is also caused by physical shearing forces due to high blood pressure and turbulent flow. Platelets adhere to dysfunctional endothelial cells and become activated, releasing **cytokines** (inflammatory mediators) and **platelet derived growth factor** (**PDGF**). This initiates a chronic inflammatory response in the vessel wall.

Plaque progression

Inflammatory mediators released by activated platelets recruit **monocytes** from the bloodstream. These migrate into the vessel wall and differentiate into **macrophages** where they take up cholesterol and lipids to become **foam cells**. Growth factors and cytokines released by foam cells initiate a cascade of pathological events in which there is further accumulation of cholesterol and proliferation of **intimal smooth muscle**. This process is accelerated if the serum cholesterol is high (Clinical Box 10.5). Smooth muscle cells secrete extracellular matrix proteins including **collagen**, which generates a tough **fibrous cap** over the soft plaque core, creating a relatively stable **fibrous plaque** (Fig. 10.14A). If the fibrous cap ruptures or the overlying endothelial layer becomes ulcerated, the plaque is referred to as **complicated** (Fig. 10.14B). This may trigger **thrombosis**, leading to vessel occlusion and stroke.

Clinical Box 10.5: Good and bad cholesterol

Cholesterol is not water-soluble and is transported through the bloodstream by **lipoproteins**, a family of spherical particles composed of phospholipid and protein. **Low-density-lipoprotein** (**LDL**) particles deliver lipids to peripheral tissues and contribute to the development of atheromatous plaques. Raised LDL levels are therefore harmful and are said to represent 'bad cholesterol'. Excess cholesterol is transported to the liver for disposal in **high-density-lipoprotein** (**HDL**) particles, which are sometimes referred to as 'good cholesterol'. The ratio of HDH:LDL cholesterol may therefore be more important than the total serum cholesterol.

Key Points

- Atherosclerosis is an almost ubiquitous degenerative process of medium and large arteries (e.g. neck vessels, aorta, coronary arteries) and is a major cause of stroke and heart attack.
- Plaque formation is triggered by endothelial dysfunction (e.g. as a result of high blood pressure and toxins in cigarette smoke). This allows platelets to adhere to the blood vessel lining, releasing cytokines and PDGF, triggering an inflammatory response in the vessel wall.
- Monocytes, which have been recruited from the bloodstream, enter the vessel wall and differentiate into macrophages, before taking up lipid and cholesterol to become foam cells.
- Much of the cholesterol is derived from circulating low-density-lipoprotein (LDL) particles and is a key component of the plaque core, which is covered by a collagen-rich fibrous cap.
- If a fibrous plaque ruptures it becomes a 'complicated' plaque, which predisposes to thrombosis and embolism. These events may occlude the vessel, resulting in a stroke (or heart attack).

Stroke management

Several large clinical trials have shown that the best outcomes in stroke care are achieved by dedicated **stroke units** (or by specialist multidisciplinary stroke teams). Key elements include:

- **Good nutrition and hydration**, with early nasogastric or parenteral feeding, if necessary.
- **Speech and language therapy** assessment and treatment in the first few days.
- **Early mobilization and physiotherapy**, avoiding harmful consequences of immobility.
- **Prompt treatment of complications**, such as infection.

The collective impact of these simple measures is a substantial reduction in long-term neurological impairment, with a 25% increase in the number of people returning to work. A small proportion of patients with ischaemic stroke may be suitable for **thrombolysis** (Clinical Box 10.6).

Stroke prevention

Acute stroke treatment is currently limited, which increases the importance of preventative measures including the avoidance of known risk factors. **Primary prevention** aims to avoid a first stroke in someone who is at risk, whereas **secondary prevention** reduces the likelihood of recurrence.

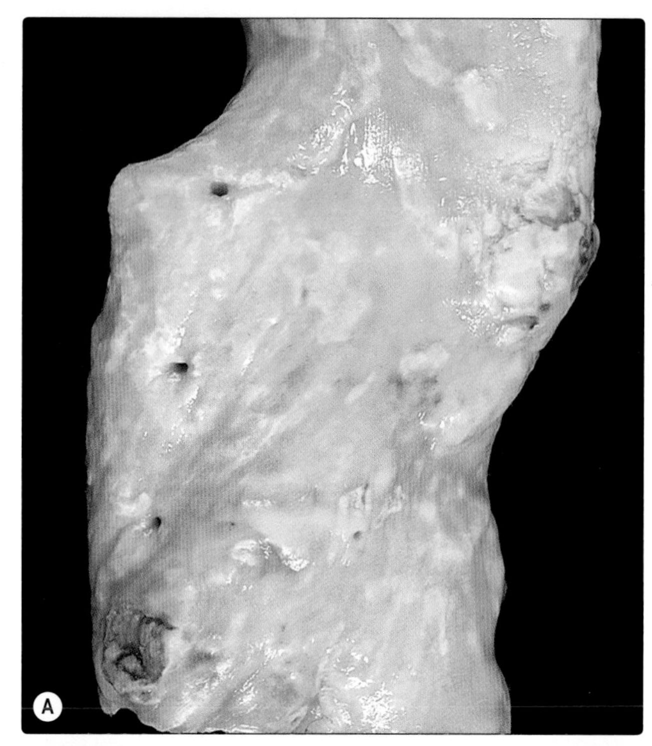

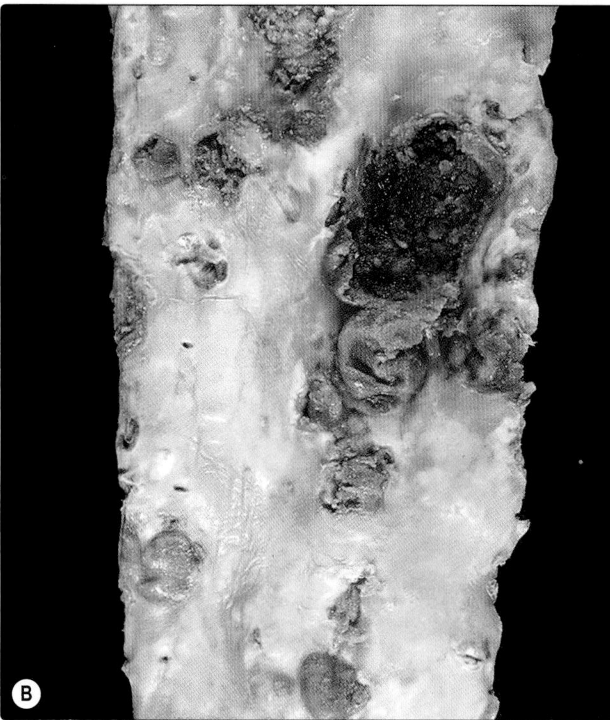

Fig. 10.14 **Post-mortem photographs showing examples of atherosclerotic plaques in the abdominal aorta (the arteries have been opened to expose the endothelial lining). (A)** This image shows numerous yellow-white fibrous plaques in the wall of the aorta. These lesions have a cholesterol-rich core covered by a collagenous cap and they often remain stable (without causing symptoms) for many years; **(B)** This example (in a different patient) shows complicated atheromatous plaques, in which there has been rupture/haemorrhage of the collagenous cap or ulceration of the overlying endothelium – in this case adherent thrombus is clearly visible on some of the plaques. From Kumar et al: Robbins Basic Pathology 8e (Saunders 2007) with permission.

Clinical Box 10.6: Thrombolysis

Thrombus can be dissolved by intravenous administration of **tissue plasminogen activator (tPA)**, an enzyme of the **fibrinolytic (anti-coagulation) cascade**. This must be done within four and a half hours of stroke onset to minimize the risk of a potentially fatal brain haemorrhage. It is therefore extremely important to determine the **exact time of onset** (and to perform a CT scan to rule out a haemorrhage) prior to thyrombolysis. Outcome data from clinical trials show that 10% of patients receiving thrombolysis will have 'minimal or no disability' at three months and another third will have some measurable degree of benefit. The incidence of haemorrhage is approximately 1 in 18, but overall mortality is not increased. It is important to note that most people do not qualify for thrombolysis, but all patients are likely to benefit from specialist care in a stroke unit.

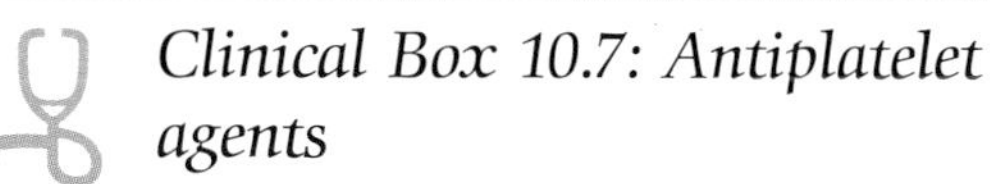

Clinical Box 10.7: Antiplatelet agents

Low-dose aspirin (75 mg/day) reduces the tendency of platelets to adhere to dysfunctional endothelial cells and cuts recurrent stroke risk by up to 25%. Alternative antiplatelet drugs such as **dipyridamole** and **clopidogrel** were previously used only in patients who are unable to tolerate aspirin but are now given in combination with aspirin or as first-line agents. Antiplatelet agents are not recommended for people who have never had a stroke as the increased risk of haemorrhage probably outweighs any potential benefits.

Risk factors for stroke

Arterial hypertension is the most important factor and clinical trials show that a 5 mmHg reduction in diastolic blood pressure cuts stroke risk by around a third, even in patients with normal blood pressure. Decreasing **serum cholesterol** is also highly beneficial, and even people with normal levels may benefit from cholesterol-lowering agents such as **statins** (inhibitors of the cholesterol-synthesizing liver enzyme hydroxy-methyl-glutaryl-CoA reductase). Reduced consumption of **saturated animal fats** is also helpful, together with increased intake of polyunsaturated vegetable fats and fish oils (containing **omega-3 fatty acids**). In patients with **diabetes**, who are particularly predisposed to arterial disease, good control of blood sugar is essential. Daily low-dose aspirin and other **antiplatelet agents** may also of value (Clinical Box 10.7).

Other factors

Oral contraceptives with a **high oestrogen content** increase relative stroke risk by enhancing the tendency of blood to coagulate, but since the background risk is tiny in young females, the **absolute risk** remains extremely low. Elevation of the amino acid homocysteine in the serum, as a result of folate or vitamin B deficiency or in the rare genetic condition **homocysteineuria**, is also associated with premature vascular disease, but it is not clear if reducing homocysteine levels is beneficial in preventing stroke. **Modest alcohol intake** may reduce stroke risk (perhaps in part by increasing plasma HDL concentration) but consuming more than two units per day (i) begins to reverse the benefits, (ii) has other negative effects on health and (iii) is an important cause of haemorrhagic stroke in younger people (Fig. 10.15).

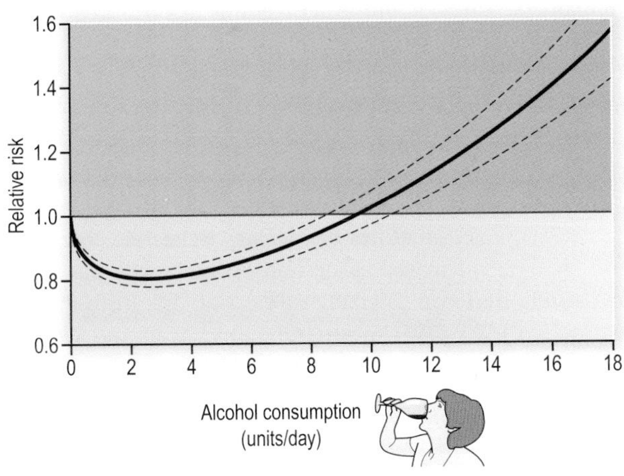

Fig. 10.15 **Moderate alcohol consumption may have a beneficial effect on cardiovascular disease.** With increasing levels of consumption, the negative effects quickly outweigh the benefits. This is described as a J-shaped relationship.

Key Points

- The best outcomes in stroke are achieved by dedicated stroke units, with a significant reduction in long-term neurological impairment and a 25% increase in the number of people returning to work.
- Key elements include: (i) good nutrition and hydration; (ii) early speech and language therapy; (iii) prompt mobilization and physiotherapy; and (iv) aggressive treatment of any complications.
- Thrombolysis is suitable in a minority of cases and must be administered within 4.5 hours of stroke onset, after a CT scan has been performed to exclude haemorrhage.
- The principal modifiable risk factors for primary and secondary stroke prevention are high blood pressure, smoking, elevated cholesterol, diabetes and atrial fibrillation.
- Antiplatelet agents (aspirin, dipyridamole, clopidogrel) reduce the incidence of stroke, but the risk of haemorrhage probably outweighs the benefit in people who have never had a stroke.

Pathophysiology of stroke

The average rate of cerebral blood flow is 50 mL per 100 g of tissue per minute. This high rate of blood flow is required to deliver enough oxygen and glucose to support the intense metabolic demands of neural tissue. If the blood supply fails, neurons begin to die within a few minutes.

The ischaemic cascade (Fig. 10.16)

In acute cerebral ischaemia, **perfusion failure** leads to **energy failure**, due to cessation of oxidative phosphorylation within mitochondria. Without fresh blood flowing through the tissue, toxins such as **lactic acid** and **carbon dioxide** build up and **acidosis** develops. Neurons can tolerate ischaemia in the short term by reducing electrochemical activity and minimizing energy consumption, but prolonged or intense ischaemia inevitably leads to **cell death**.

Failure of ATP production

In the early stages of ischaemia, tissue buffers such as **phosphocreatine** donate high-energy phosphate bonds to replenish **adenosine triphosphate** (ATP). This provides enough energy to drive cellular processes and can maintain ATP levels at about 95% of normal for a short period of time. A small amount of glucose is released from astrocytic glycogen stores, but within five minutes the phosphate buffers and glycogen have been spent and ATP levels are less than 10% of normal.

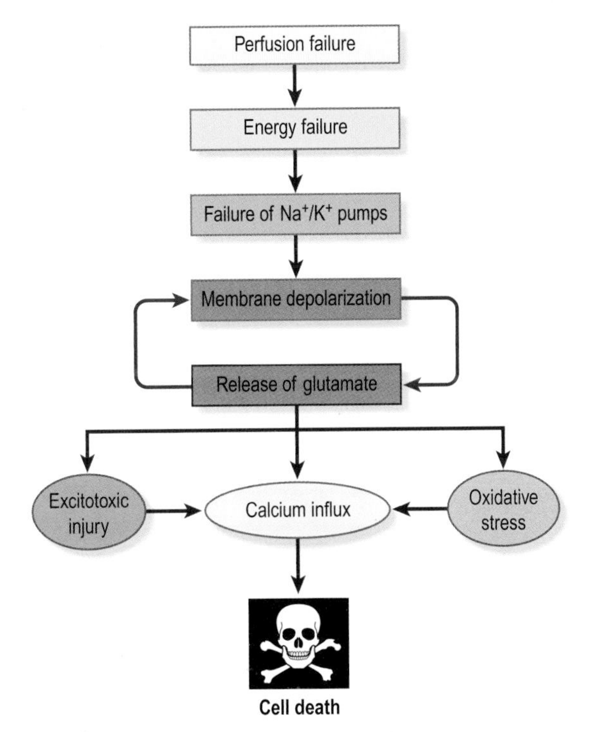

Fig. 10.16 **The ischaemic cascade.**

Anaerobic respiration

In the absence of oxygen, cellular metabolism switches from aerobic respiration to anaerobic glycolysis. This extracts much less energy from the limited glucose available and generates **lactate** as a by-product, exacerbating the developing acidosis. The mitochondrial Na^+/H^+ pump, which expels hydrogen ions from the cell, is retarded as the pH falls below 6.0. This compromises cellular respiration further and a vicious cycle develops. Under these conditions harmful **reactive oxygen species** such as **superoxide anion** (O^{2-}) and **hydroxyl radical** (OH^-) are liberated in large quantities, creating **oxidative stress** and further tissue damage (see Ch. 8).

Failure of the sodium pump

The **sodium pump** (Na^+/K^+**-ATPase**) is responsible for two thirds of the basal energy expenditure of the brain. It works constantly in the background to maintain the intracellular and extracellular sodium and potassium ion concentrations and is therefore essential for electrical activity in nerve cells (see Ch. 6). As the ATP supply falls to critical levels, the sodium pump fails. As a result, the sodium and potassium gradients dissipate and neuronal membranes depolarize. A critical point is reached when cerebral blood flow falls to less than 20% of normal (below 10 mL per 100 g per minute). Depolarized neurons reach their 'firing thresholds' and there is large-scale release of neurotransmitters, including the excitatory amino acid **glutamate** which is toxic at high concentrations.

Calcium and excitotoxicity

As a result of these events the extracellular glutamate concentration is increased to ten times its normal value. At these levels glutamate behaves as an **excitotoxin** by allowing excessive calcium influx through **NMDA channels** (which have been liberated from their normal magnesium block) together with contributions from **voltage-gated calcium channels** and **calcium-permeable AMPA receptors** (see Chs 7 and 8). Elevation of intracellular calcium is a critical event in neuronal cell death since calcium activates a host of harmful enzymes, including calpains, proteases, phospholipases, endonucleases and nitric oxide synthase (see Ch. 8). The final 'point of no return' occurs as plasma membrane integrity is lost and water enters the cell. This is called **cytotoxic oedema** which causes cell rupture and death, followed by an inflammatory response.

Key Points

- In acute cerebral ischaemia, perfusion failure leads to energy failure, combined with a build-up of toxic waste products such as lactic acid.
- The modest energy reserves of the brain and tissue phosphate buffers are spent within five minutes and ATP levels fall to less than 10% of normal.
- Cellular metabolism therefore switches from oxidative phosphorylation to anaerobic glycolysis, with lactate accumulation, acidosis and free radical formation.
- Ionic gradients dissipate as membrane pumps fail, so that neurons depolarize and release glutamate into the extracellular space. At this level, glutamate behaves as an excitotoxin by over-stimulation of NMDA receptors, leading to neuronal calcium overload.
- Excessive intracellular calcium activates calpains, proteases, phospholipases, endonucleases and nitric oxide synthase, with degradation of key structural and functional proteins.
- Loss of membrane integrity ultimately results in cytotoxic oedema and cell death, followed by an acute inflammatory reaction.

The ischaemic penumbra

Within an hour of stroke onset a necrotic **core lesion** is established in which the blood flow is below 20% of normal. This is surrounded by a poorly perfused border zone known as the **ischaemic penumbra** in which blood flow is between 20–40% of normal (Fig. 10.17). Penumbral neurons may remain viable for up to 24 hours and can potentially be salvaged, but if perfusion is not restored the core lesion will gradually expand.

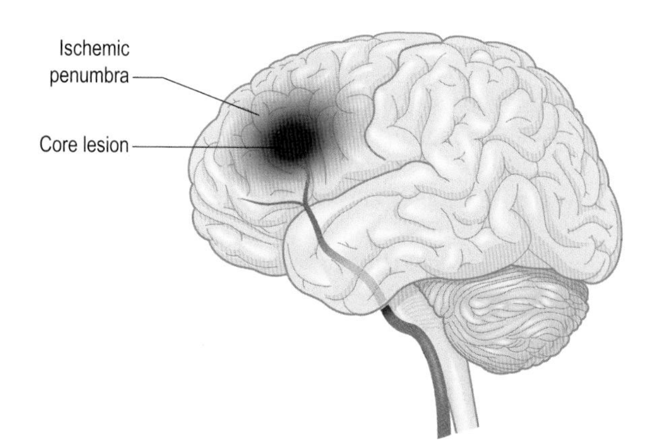

Fig. 10.17 **The ischaemic penumbra.** Following an ischaemic stroke there is often a core lesion of irreversible cell death, surrounded by a poorly perfused penumbral region in which neurons are functionally compromised but may still be salvaged.

The ischaemic penumbra can be visualized using a combination of **perfusion-weighted** and **diffusion-weighted** magnetic resonance imaging (**PWI** and **DWI**). A perfusion-weighted MRI scan provides a semi-quantitative measure of cerebral blood flow whereas the diffusion-weighted sequence identifies the densely ischaemic core lesion, by using increased tissue water content as a marker of **cytotoxic oedema**. Digitally subtracting one from the other gives a **PWI–DWI mismatch**, which corresponds approximately to the ischaemic penumbra and can usually be identified within six hours of stroke onset.

Key Points

- The ischaemic penumbra is a poorly perfused zone of tissue that surrounds the densely ischaemic core lesion. Blood flow in the penumbra is approximately 20–40% of normal.
- Penumbral neurons are functionally compromised but viable for up to 24 hours and are therefore good targets for neuroprotective interventions.
- Radiological techniques such as PWI–DWI mismatch provide a way to visualize the approximate extent of the ischaemic penumbra in life.

Neuroprotection

A major aim of basic stroke research is the development of compounds that are able to protect poorly perfused tissue by interfering with the **ischaemic cascade** or **brain inflammatory response**. Most of this work is first carried out in animal models, before moving on to clinical trials.

Animal models of stroke

Animal models of cerebral ischaemia most often use laboratory rats, mice or gerbils. Rabbits, dogs and cats have also been used, but there are relatively few trials in non-human primates such as chimpanzees because of the major ethical considerations and considerable expense.

Dissociated neuronal cultures

These are the simplest, easiest to use and least expensive systems available. It is difficult to see how **dissociated embryonic cells** can model the multi-cellular anatomical complexity of the human brain, but this method can provide important insights if the data are handled with caution.

Whole animal studies

These include **middle cerebral artery occlusion** (**MCAo**) and the **four-vessel model of transient forebrain ischaemia** (bilateral occlusion of both carotid and vertebral arteries) in the rat. Such models can be used to generate a **reversible ischaemia** of fixed duration (usually 5–30 minutes). Although 'realistic', they are complex, costly and technically demanding. There is also interference from **systemic variables** that are difficult to control such as blood pressure, heart rate, body temperature, circulating hormones – and the effects of the host immune system.

Organotypic cultures

This method employs intact **brain slices** (e.g. rodent hippocampus) that are maintained in an incubated culture

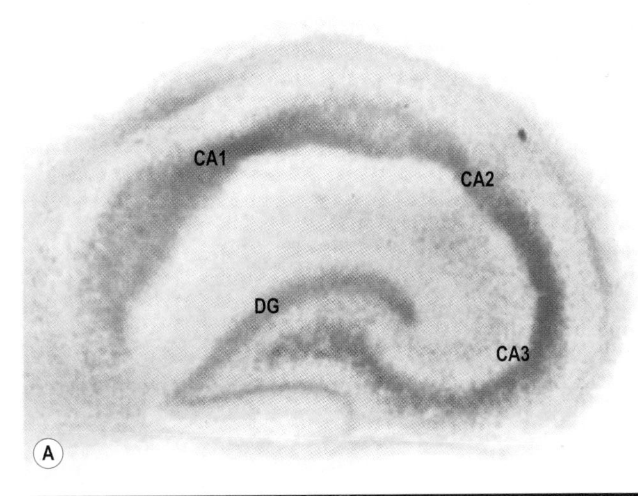

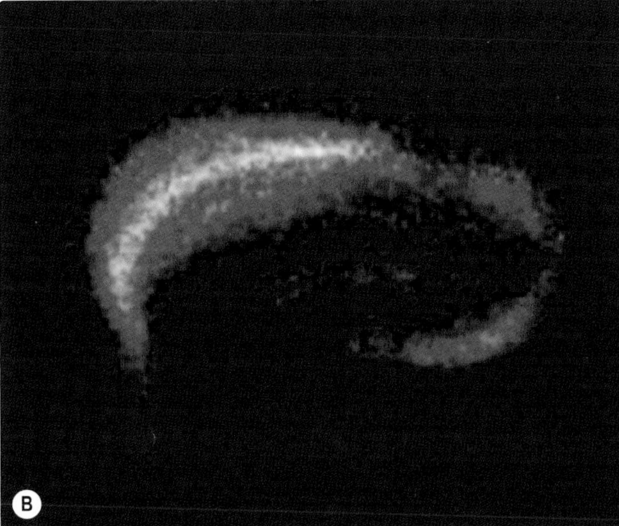

Fig. 10.18 **Organotypic hippocampal slice cultures (OHSC) can be used to model stroke. (A)** A slice culture preparation of rodent hippocampus after two weeks in culture showing normal hippocampal anatomy. The tissue slice has been stained with thionine to demonstrate neuronal cell bodies [DG= dentate gyrus, CA1-3 = subfields of Ammon's horn/cornu Ammonis]; **(B)** Rodent hippocampal slice 24 hours after a 60-minute period of combined oxygen-glucose deprivation (simulated ischaemia). There is marked neuronal loss in the CA1 subfield of the hippocampus [visualized with fluorescent tissue dye propidium iodide, which is only able to enter damaged cells with impaired membrane integrity]. The CA1 subfield (sometimes referred to as Sommer's sector) is also particularly susceptible to hypoxia and ischaemia in the human brain. From Sundstrom et al: Drug Discovery Today 2005;10(14), with permission.

medium. Preparations of this kind can remain viable for as long as six weeks, maintaining normal connectivity and activity (Fig. 10.18A). Cerebral ischaemia can be simulated by combined **oxygen–glucose deprivation**, producing reproducible lesions that compare well with their in vivo counterparts (Fig. 10.18B). Slice cultures therefore combine many of the positive characteristics of whole animal studies without the major drawbacks of dissociated cell cultures.

Neuroprotective agents

Many neuroprotective agents have been developed to block events in the ischaemic cascade (e.g. excitotoxicity, oxidative stress, calcium overload) and although they work very well in animal models, clinical trials have been uniformly disappointing for numerous reasons (discussed below).

Temporal factors

Most agents that work well in experimental animals target the early stages of the ischaemic cascade and many are given as **pre-treatment** (prior to ischaemia), but around 50% of patients do not reach hospital until at least 3 hours after stroke onset, missing a critical 'window of opportunity'.

Problems with animal models

Comparisons between laboratory animals and humans may not always be valid. In animals the lesion is strictly controlled and occurs in a uniform group of specially bred (genetically identical) animals. This ignores **genetic differences** between subjects and the contribution of other factors such as co-morbidity, age and extent of collateral blood supply. Cognitive and behavioural impairments are also difficult to model and assess in laboratory animals.

Outcome measures

Outcome measures used in preclinical trials may be inappropriate. Studies typically rely on **total lesion size** to measure stroke severity, but this may not be valid in humans (e.g. a substantial right frontal lobe lesion may be clinically silent, whereas a small internal capsule stroke might cause profound hemiplegia). Another potential problem is the experimental **end-point**. In animal models this is usually minutes or hours after the event, but in clinical trials it may be months or years.

Failure of drug delivery

Agents travelling in the bloodstream may not be able to reach the targeted area of the brain, either due to poor perfusion of ischaemic tissues or failure to cross the **blood–brain barrier** (see Ch. 5), but this is not relevant in many animal models. Furthermore, **side effects** of certain drugs can prevent administration of effective doses that are equivalent to those used in preclinical studies.

White matter ischaemia

Another source of difficulty is that the majority of basic science research focuses on protection and salvage of neurons in the **cortical grey matter**, but a significant burden of pathology following stroke is due to loss of white matter and axonal connections between cortical regions.

Key Points

- Numerous neuroprotective agents have been developed to block events in the ischaemic cascade (e.g. excitotoxicity, inflammation, oxidative stress, calcium overload) and although they work well in animal models, clinical trials have been uniformly disappointing.
- A key factor in the failure of neuroprotective agents is timescale because most drugs used in experimental animals target early post-ischaemic events that have ended by the time the patient reaches hospital (50% arriving more than three hours after stroke onset).
- Other factors that contribute to the failure of neuroprotective agents include problems with animal models of human disease, inappropriate outcome measures in clinical trials, drug toxicity or delivery failure, together with heterogeneity in genetic, constitutional and systemic factors.

Delayed neuronal cell death

In recent years, interest has shifted to the process of **delayed neuronal cell death**, by which the initial core lesion gradually expands into the ischaemic penumbra. Factors implicated in this process include reperfusion injury, nitric oxide release and delayed apoptosis.

Reperfusion injury

Natural thrombolytic mechanisms may re-open occluded blood vessels within 24 hours in up to a third of cases (spontaneous reperfusion). As the blood flow is restored, neuronal activity increases dramatically and **reactive oxygen species** are produced in large quantities. The sudden burst of free radicals overwhelms **scavenging mechanisms** and inactivates **complex I** of the mitochondrial respiratory chain. The resultant **oxidative stress** damages key cellular elements including mitochondria and a vicious cycle develops, leading to reperfusion-associated neuronal cell death. There is experimental and clinical evidence that **controlled cooling** may protect against reperfusion injury, lowering energy demands and reducing the rate of free radical formation.

Nitric oxide release

Nitric oxide is one of several **reactive oxygen species** released in the ischaemic brain and is generated in large quantities on reperfusion. It is synthesized from **L-arginine** (by inflammatory cells and ischaemic neurons) by various isoforms of **nitric oxide synthase** (**NOS**).

Synthesis by endothelial cells is neuroprotective, since it promotes vasodilation and inhibits platelet and leukocyte adhesion, improving cerebral blood flow. Production in neurons and microglial cells is stimulated by inflammatory cytokines and is strongly neurotoxic. Nitric oxide also generates the highly cytotoxic molecule **peroxynitrite, $ONOO^-$** by reacting with superoxide anion, which has been shown to promote apoptosis in the ischaemic penumbra. In keeping with this, inhibition of nitric oxide synthase is neuroprotective in animal models.

Delayed apoptosis

Although the majority of cell death following stroke is necrotic, up to a fifth may be due to **programmed cell death** (particularly in the ischaemic penumbra). **Apoptotic bodies** derived from dead neurons have been identified in the reperfused penumbra and inhibitors of apoptosis (e.g. **cyclosporin A**) are neuroprotective in animal models of stroke. Astrocytes also undergo apoptosis during reperfusion in response to a rise in intracellular calcium, reducing an important source of metabolic support for sublethally injured neurons.

Key Points

- Newer neuroprotective strategies are targeting the process of delayed neuronal cell death by which the core lesion expands into the ischaemic penumbra.
- Important contributors to this process include reperfusion-associated brain injury, the neurotoxic effect of released nitric oxide and delayed apoptosis.
- Reperfusion-associated brain injury can be reduced by controlled cooling. This lowers energy demands and reduces the rate of free radical formation when the bloodflow returns.

Chapter 11
Epilepsy

CHAPTER CONTENTS

The epilepsies are a group of disorders characterized by abnormal electrical activity in the brain. This leads to recurrent **unprovoked seizures** (Greek: epilēpsia, to seize) in which there are paroxysmal disturbances of movement, sensation or behaviour. The clinical features of a seizure (or 'ictus') reflect the location of the abnormal discharges and their extent of spread through the cerebral cortex.

Epilepsy is the most common serious neurological disorder worldwide, affecting up to 1% of the general population. A single seizure does not usually warrant a diagnosis of epilepsy; in most cases, this requires two or more unprovoked seizures separated by at least 24 hours. **Provoked seizures** are distinct from epilepsy and occur in up to 5% of people at some point in their lifetime; causes include head injury, stroke, infection, fever, alcohol withdrawal and metabolic derangements.

Types of seizure

The two main types of seizure are illustrated in Fig. 11.1. **Primary generalized seizures** diffusely involve both cerebral hemispheres at onset and consciousness is usually lost. **Partial (focal) seizures** have a discrete cortical origin and the clinical features reflect the function of the affected area. Abnormal electrical activity can often be recorded during a seizure using scalp electrodes (discussed below).

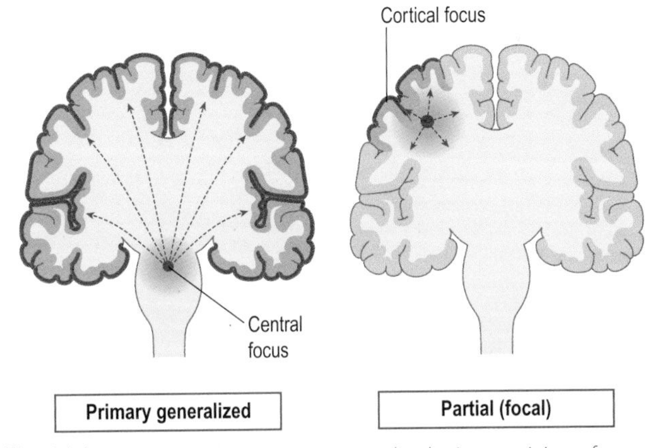

Fig. 11.1 **Types of seizure.** Primary generalized seizures originate from a central focus in the thalamus or brain stem and involve both cerebral hemispheres at onset. Partial (focal) seizures begin in a discrete cortical region and are due to an abnormality in the neighbouring grey or white matter. A focal seizure may spread to become secondarily generalized.

Primary generalized seizures

This type of seizure appears to originate from abnormal oscillations in **thalamocortical loops** (reciprocal connections between the thalamus and cerebral cortex). There may be convulsions as a result of the bilateral cortical involvement, but the clinical features are quite variable and there are several well-recognized patterns (e.g. absence, tonic, clonic, myoclonic, tonic-clonic and atonic). Usually it is not possible to identify a structural brain lesion in people with primary generalized epilepsy and most cases are classified as **idiopathic**. This means that the cause is not known, but there is assumed to be an underlying genetic basis.

Partial (focal) seizures

This type of seizure arises from a discrete focus such as a cortical malformation or tumour. In **simple partial seizures** there is a disturbance of motor, sensory, cognitive or autonomic function without loss of consciousness. In **complex partial seizures**, the focal symptoms are accompanied by disturbance of normal awareness or responsiveness. Complex partial seizures commonly originate in the temporal lobe. They are frequently preceded by an **aura** (Latin: breeze or soft wind) such as a strange sensation or an unpleasant smell.

A **secondarily generalized seizure** occurs when a partial seizure spreads to involve both cerebral hemispheres. This may be preceded by focal symptoms (e.g. involuntary limb movement or head turning), but these can be missed if generalization is rapid. The presence of localizing neurological signs after the seizure (such as weakness) provides an important clue that there is a discrete (focal) cortical origin.

General aspects

There are numerous epilepsy syndromes with differences in seizure type, age at onset, presumed aetiology and EEG findings (Clinical Box 11.1). They can be classified in different ways such as mode of onset (generalized versus focal) or age at presentation. Many epilepsy syndromes arise in childhood

Clinical Box 11.1: Electroencephalography (EEG)

Electrical recording from the scalp can be used to look for **epileptiform discharges** from the cerebral cortex to support a clinical diagnosis of epilepsy (Figs 11.2 & 11.3). An abnormal interictal trace is recorded in around 50% of people with clinically definite epilepsy, but the diagnostic yield can be increased to 80% by sleep deprivation, hyperventilation or intermittent **photic stimulation** (flickering light). In some cases it is not possible to record epileptiform discharges, even during a seizure (for instance, if the seizure focus is too deeply seated to be picked up by scalp electrodes). The false positive rate is 0.5% in adults and 4% in children.

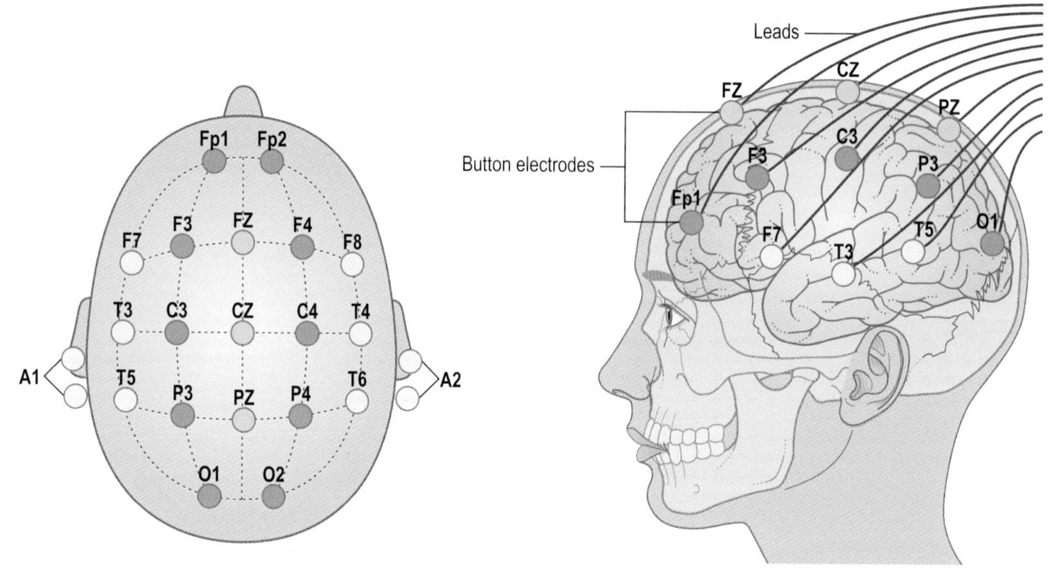

Fig. 11.2 **Placement of scalp electrodes for electroencephalography (EEG).** Electrodes are placed in standard positions for recording electrical traces from the surface of the brain [Fp, frontopolar; F, frontal; C, coronal; P, parietal; T, temporal; O, occipital; Z, midline; odd numbers, left; even numbers, right]. From Fitzgerald: Clinical Neuroanatomy and Neuroscience 5e (2006) with permission.

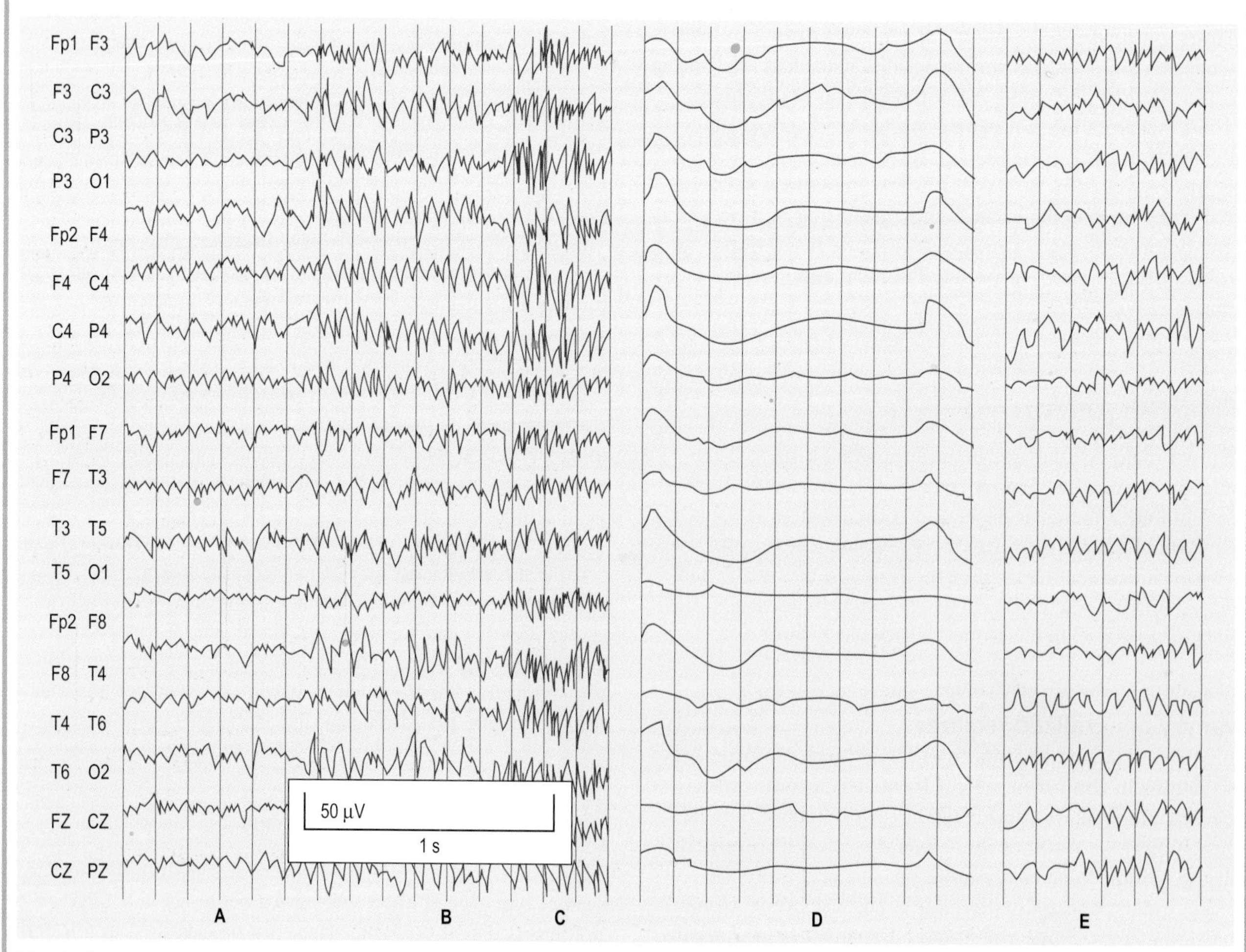

Fig. 11.3 **EEG trace during a generalized tonic-clonic (convulsive) seizure. (A)** Normal interictal recording; **(B)** Generalized seizure activity in all electrode positions; **(C)** Generalized convulsive (tonic-clonic) activity; **(D)** Immediate postictal period with slow waveform pattern throughout; **(E)** Resumption of normal waveforms. From Fitzgerald: Clinical Neuroanatomy and Neuroscience 5e (2006) with permission.

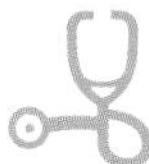

Clinical Box 11.2: Focal motor seizures

These are simple partial seizures that originate in the **primary motor cortex** and cause convulsions in the opposite half of the body. There is no loss of consciousness, by definition. The seizure typically begins with involuntary movements in one part of the body (e.g. the great toe, thumb or corner of the mouth). As the wave of abnormal electrical activity spreads across the motor strip, clonic (jerking) movements gradually progress to involve more of the body. This is called the **Jacksonian march**. After the seizure there may be contralateral weakness for up to 48 hours, referred to as **Todd's paresis**.

Clinical Box 11.3: Rolandic epilepsy

The commonest childhood epilepsy syndrome is **benign epilepsy with centrotemporal spikes**. The alternative term **Rolandic epilepsy** refers to the seizure focus in the region of the central sulcus, which was referred to historically as the fissure of Rolando. This syndrome is characterized by **focal motor seizures** (simple partial seizures) with **speech arrest** and **hypersalivation** (drooling), often with secondary generalization. Rolandic epilepsy usually presents below the age of ten and is regarded as benign since it often disappears during puberty.

Key Points

- The epilepsies are a group of neurological disorders caused by abnormal electrical activity in the brain. Epilepsy is the tendency to have recurrent, unprovoked seizures.
- Epilepsy is the most common serious neurological disorder worldwide, affecting 1% of the general population. Provoked seizures are distinct from epilepsy and occur in up to 5% of people.
- Seizures can be classified as partial (focal) or generalized. Partial seizures are further classified as simple or complex, depending on whether or not conscious awareness is altered.
- Primary generalized seizures are usually classified as idiopathic, meaning that the cause is unknown, but there is assumed to be an underlying genetic basis.
- Partial seizures arise from a discrete cortical focus such as a tumour or malformation. They may spread to involve both cerebral hemispheres and become secondarily generalized.
- An abnormal interictal EEG trace is found in approximately 50% of people with clinically definite epilepsy, rising to 80% with provocation (sleep deprivation, hyperventilation, etc).

and some have highly characteristic features (Clinical Boxes 11.2, 11.3 & 11.4).

Aetiology of epilepsy

Cases with a clear genetic, structural or metabolic cause are referred to as **symptomatic epilepsy**. The term **cryptogenic** is used when the aetiology is unknown but is assumed to be symptomatic (or **idiopathic** if a genetic cause is suspected). Adult-onset seizures are more likely to be symptomatic of a structural lesion (such as a vascular malformation, brain tumour, abscess or stroke) but anyone with focal-onset or drug-resistant epilepsy should have an MRI scan. The most common cause worldwide is **cysticercosis**, a parasitic brain infection caused by ingestion of eggs from the pork tapeworm, *Taenia solium*.

Clinical Box 11.4: West's syndrome

West's syndrome (or **infantile spasms**) is a seizure disorder with progressive cognitive decline that is associated with a specific interictal EEG pattern called **hypsarrhythmia** (consisting of random high-voltage spikes and waves). West's syndrome begins in the first year of life and is characterized by abrupt, shock-like episodes called **salaam attacks**, in which there is sudden flexion of the upper limbs, neck and hips with the knees drawn up against the body. It is frequently associated with a developmental or perinatal brain injury such as anoxia or encephalitis.

Common seizure patterns

Despite the large number of epilepsy syndromes, there are several commonly encountered types of seizure, each with distinctive **semiology** (clinical manifestations). An example of a simple partial seizure has been described in Clinical Box 11.2; in the following sections, typical features of a complex partial seizure and two very different forms of primary generalized seizure will be described.

Complex partial seizures

The most common partial epilepsy syndrome is **temporal lobe epilepsy** (TLE) which is characterized by simple and complex partial seizures of temporal lobe origin, often with secondary generalization. A typical complex partial seizure in temporal lobe epilepsy lasts less than two minutes and may begin with an **aura**. This may be a peculiar smell, reflecting the role of the mesial temporal lobe in olfaction, or a strange 'rising' sensation between the epigastrium and throat. As the seizure takes hold the patient stops what they are doing and enters a state of altered consciousness. They may feel a strong sense of familiarity (**déjà vu**) or a strange feeling of unfamiliarity (**jamais vu**). The experiences sometimes have religious or spiritual connotations and may be associated with euphoria. At this point it becomes impossible to converse with the patient and there may be repetitive, semi-purposeful actions such as chewing, lip-smacking, picking at clothing or aimless reaching. These behaviours are referred to as **automatisms** (automatic behaviours). The seizure is followed by a period of **postictal confusion** with little recollection of the episode.

Generalized tonic-clonic seizures

This is the convulsive type of seizure (formerly known as **grand mal**) that most people associate with the word epilepsy and is the most common form of seizure overall. There may be a **prodromal phase**, 24–48 hours before the attack. This is characterized by light-headedness, malaise or a sense that something is about to happen. The seizure may begin with an aura, followed by distinct **tonic** (rigid) and **clonic** (jerking) phases.

Tonic phase (30 seconds)

Intense neuronal discharges from the cerebral cortex cause the entire body to become rigid (Fig. 11.4A). Spasm of the

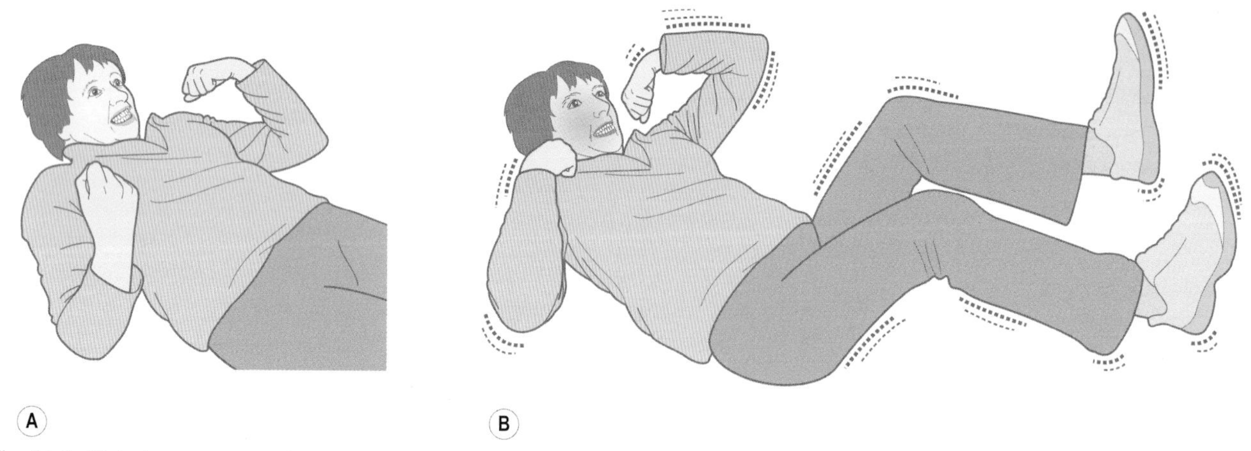

Fig. 11.4 **Clinical appearances of a generalized tonic-clonic seizure. (A)** The tonic phase lasts around 30 seconds. The entire body becomes rigid, respiration ceases and the patient becomes cyanotic; **(B)** The clonic (jerking) phase is characterized by violent symmetrical convulsions, often associated with laboured breathing and frothing at the mouth, typically lasting around 60 seconds.

laryngeal and respiratory muscles forces air out of the chest, often producing an **epileptic cry**. The eyes deviate upwards and the patient falls stiffly to the ground, remaining in a state of tonic muscular contraction. Breathing ceases temporarily, leading to **cyanosis**.

Clonic phase (60 seconds)
This is characterized by violent, symmetrical **convulsions**, with muscular contraction and relaxation (Fig. 11.4B). Breathing is noisy and poorly coordinated, with salivation that appears as 'frothing at the mouth'. The face may be pink and congested or cyanosis may persist if ventilation is poor. **Tongue biting** and other injuries sometimes occur and the patient may be incontinent of urine. As the clonic phase comes to an end the jerking movements gradually subside.

Postictal coma (up to 30 minutes)
As the seizure ends, breathing and colour return to normal but the patient remains unconscious. This is probably due to the large-scale release of neurochemicals during the seizure including **opiates** and the inhibitory neurotransmitter **GABA** (gamma-aminobutyric acid). On waking there may be **postictal confusion**, agitation or somnolence, together with muscular stiffness and headache.

Absence seizures

This is another type of primary generalized seizure (formerly known as **petit mal**) that commonly occurs in **childhood absence epilepsy**. Absences are characterized by brief (5–10-second) episodes in which the patient becomes unaware of their surroundings. These occur unpredictably, with abrupt onset and offset. During an absence the patient stops whatever he or she is doing and becomes unresponsive, but maintains normal posture and muscle tone. The expression is blank, sometimes with fine flickering of the eyelids or face. There is no aura or postictal confusion and patients are often unaware that anything has happened. Frequent absences may cause severe disruption to concentration and impaired school performance.

Genetic factors in epilepsy

The risk of epilepsy is 2–3 times greater in those with an affected parent, sibling or child and the concordance rates are significantly higher in identical twins. In most cases the heritable component is complex and **polygenetic**, involving multiple genes interacting with environmental variables, but single-gene disorders are also described.

Key Points

- Numerous epilepsy syndromes (e.g. benign Rolandic epilepsy, West's syndrome) can be recognized based upon differences in seizure type, age at onset, aetiology and EEG findings.
- Seizure disorders fall into three main aetiological groups: symptomatic (with a known structural, metabolic or genetic cause), idiopathic (probably genetic), and cryptogenic (probably symptomatic).
- The most common type of ictal event is a generalized tonic-clonic seizure, characterized by separate tonic (rigid) and clonic (jerking) phases followed by postictal coma.
- Complex partial seizures are common in temporal lobe epilepsy. They are often preceded by an aura and may be accompanied by automatic behaviours (automatisms).
- Absence seizures are a type of primary generalized seizure seen in childhood absence epilepsy and are characterized by 5–10-second periods of 'unresponsiveness' with abrupt onset and offset.

Inherited seizure disorders

Approximately 2% of epilepsy syndromes show a clear pattern of **Mendelian inheritance**. This is most often **autosomal dominant** with variable penetrance, but examples of autosomal recessive, X-linked and mitochondrial inheritance have also been described. Most known mutations affect ion channels (sodium, potassium, calcium or chloride) and these disorders are referred to as **channelopathies**. This is assumed to alter the balance of excitatory and inhibitory influences and may be associated with focal or generalized seizures.

There are very few single-gene conditions in which epilepsy is the main feature. An example is the syndrome of **benign familial neonatal seizures**, an autosomal dominant voltage-gated potassium channelopathy which tends to spontaneously remit in adulthood. Another is **autosomal dominant nocturnal frontal lobe epilepsy**, caused by mutations in the nicotinic acetylcholine receptor gene. A separate group of conditions cause a **progressive myoclonic epilepsy** syndrome, with shock-like **myoclonic jerks** and gradual intellectual decline.

Key Points

- The risk of epilepsy is 2–3 times higher in those with an affected parent, sibling or child and is also significantly more common in identical twin pairs.
- Inheritance is likely to be complex and polygenetic and most of the genes are unknown. Simple Mendelian forms of epilepsy do exist but are uncommon (less than 2% of cases).
- Some inherited forms of partial and generalized epilepsy are caused by abnormalities in ion channels for sodium, potassium, calcium or chloride (ion channelopathies).

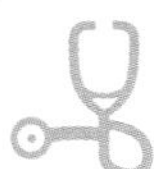

Clinical Box 11.5: Vagus nerve stimulation

Some patients with epilepsy may benefit from stimulation of the tenth cranial nerve. A **vagus nerve stimulator** is implanted under general anaesthetic in the neck region and is attached to a subcutaneous pacemaker unit in the upper chest. This is usually carried out in people with pharmacoresistant seizures, halving seizure frequency in up to 50% of patients, but the exact mechanism of action is not known.

Diagnosis and management

The diagnosis of epilepsy is clinical and requires a detailed eyewitness account of the episodes. If EEG is performed, this may provide evidence to support the clinical diagnosis. Video recording combined with EEG (referred to as **telemetry**) may be particularly helpful in difficult cases (Fig. 11.5). Epilepsy can usually be managed pharmacologically, but a neurosurgical procedure may be suitable in a minority of cases. In some patients, the less invasive option of a **vagus nerve stimulator** may be considered (Clinical Box 11.5).

Anti-epileptic drugs (AEDs)

Two thirds of patients can be managed effectively with anti-epileptic drugs and adequate control is usually achieved with a single agent (**monotherapy**). Some of the important side effects of anti-epileptic drugs are discussed in Clinical Box 11.6.

Mechanisms of action

A minority of anti-epileptic agents are the product of **rational drug design**, based upon knowledge of cellular events in epileptogenesis. Most are discovered fortuitously or by **systematic screening** of a large number of candidate compounds in an animal model of epilepsy. For this reason the mode of action is not always clear, but most agents fall into one of four main categories (discussed below).

Sodium channel antagonists

Inhibition of **voltage-gated sodium channels** is the most common mechanism. This interferes with the depolarization phase of the action potential, which is mediated by a fast inward sodium (Na^+) current. Many agents prolong channel inactivation by preferentially binding to sodium channels in their inactivated state. This increases the **refractory period** of the neuronal membrane (see Ch. 6). Repetitive neuronal firing at high frequencies is specifically reduced

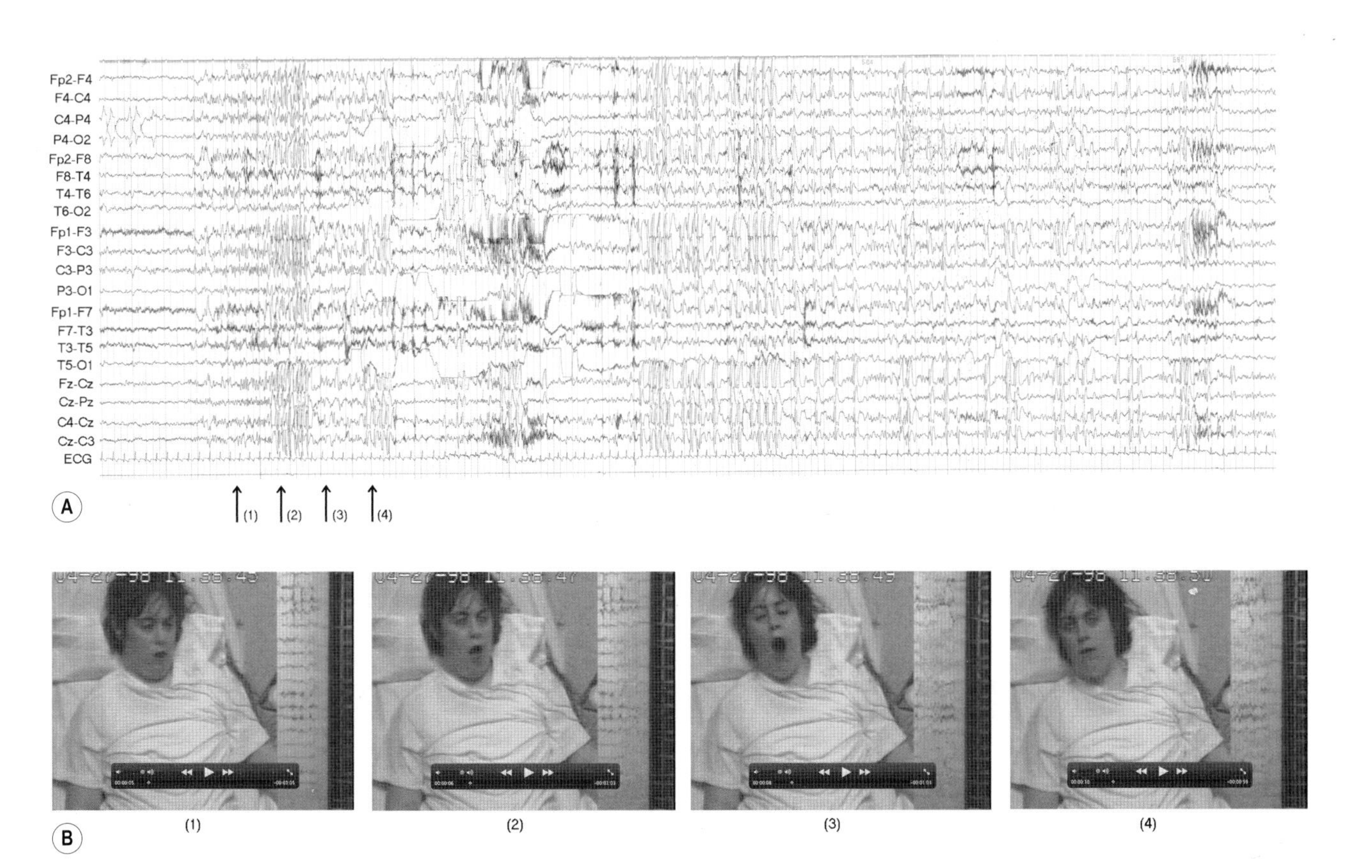

Fig. 11.5 **Patient undergoing video telemetry in epilepsy.** The EEG trace **(A)** and video sequence **(B)** capture an ictal event, characterized by involuntary orofacial movements. From Specchio, N et al: Epilepsy and Behavior: Ictal yawning in a patient with drug-resistant focal epilepsy: Video/EEG documentation and review of literature reports. Epilep Behav 2011 Nov; 22(3):602–605 with permission.

Clinical Box 11.6: AED side effects

Some common and important side effects of anti-epileptic drugs are illustrated in Fig. 11.6. Most are central nervous system depressants, so they tend to cause **drowsiness** and **impaired concentration**. Many have a toxic effect on the cerebellum, especially when serum levels are high, causing **dysarthria** (slurred speech), **diplopia** (double vision) and **ataxia** (incoordination). Other agents have specific side effects including allergic reactions, skin rashes, gum hypertrophy, acne or hirsuitism. As a group, anti-epileptic agents are known to be **teratogenic** (Greek: teras, monster) increasing the risk of birth defects from 2% to 6%. **Sodium valproate** carries the greatest risk, but teratogenicity is also increased in patients receiving more than one anti-epileptic agent **(polytherapy)**.

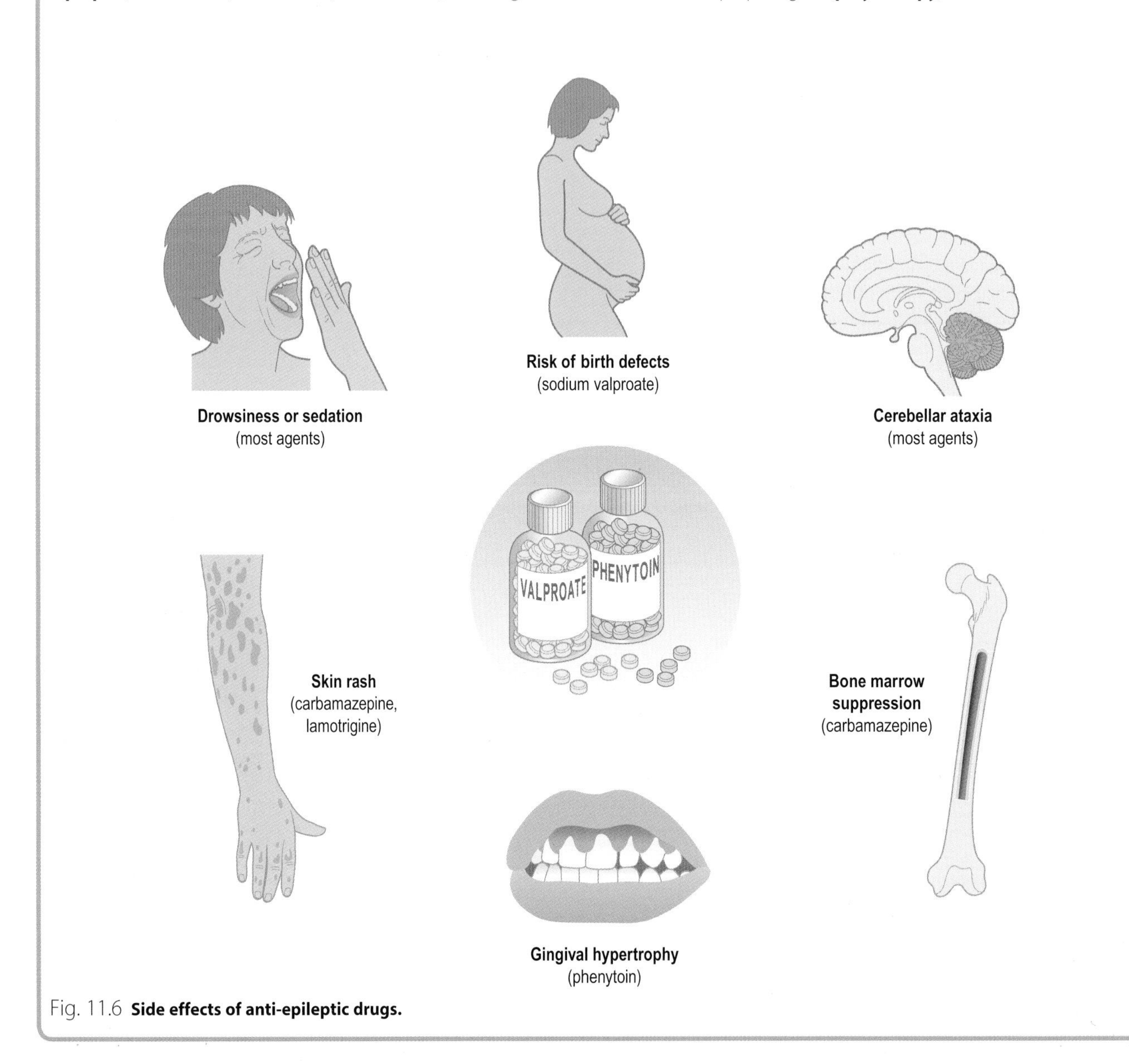

Fig. 11.6 **Side effects of anti-epileptic drugs.**

(**activity-dependence**), minimizing interference with normal brain activity. Examples of agents that block sodium channels include: phenytoin, carbamazepine, sodium valproate and lamotrigine.

Calcium channel antagonists

These agents inhibit **voltage-gated calcium channels**, which contribute to membrane depolarization and action potential generation (in the neuronal cell body) and transmitter release (at the axon terminal). Calcium channels also act as **pacemakers**, supporting oscillating patterns of activity between the cortex and thalamus. This is important in the generation of absence seizures, for which the calcium channel antagonist **ethosuximide** is effective. Drugs which antagonize calcium channels include: sodium valproate, gabapentin, phenytoin and lamotrigine.

GABA potentiators

These drugs increase activity at inhibitory synapses (see Ch. 7). Some act via **post-synaptic $GABA_A$ receptors** which are linked to a chloride ion channel; this stabilizes the neuronal membrane via an inward chloride (Cl^-) current. These include (i) **benzodiazepines** (e.g. clonazepam, diazepam) which increase the *frequency* of channel opening and (ii) **barbiturates** (e.g. primidone, phenobarbital) which increase the *duration* of channel opening. Others act at **metabotropic (G-protein-coupled) $GABA_B$** receptors which influence **second messenger cascades**; this causes

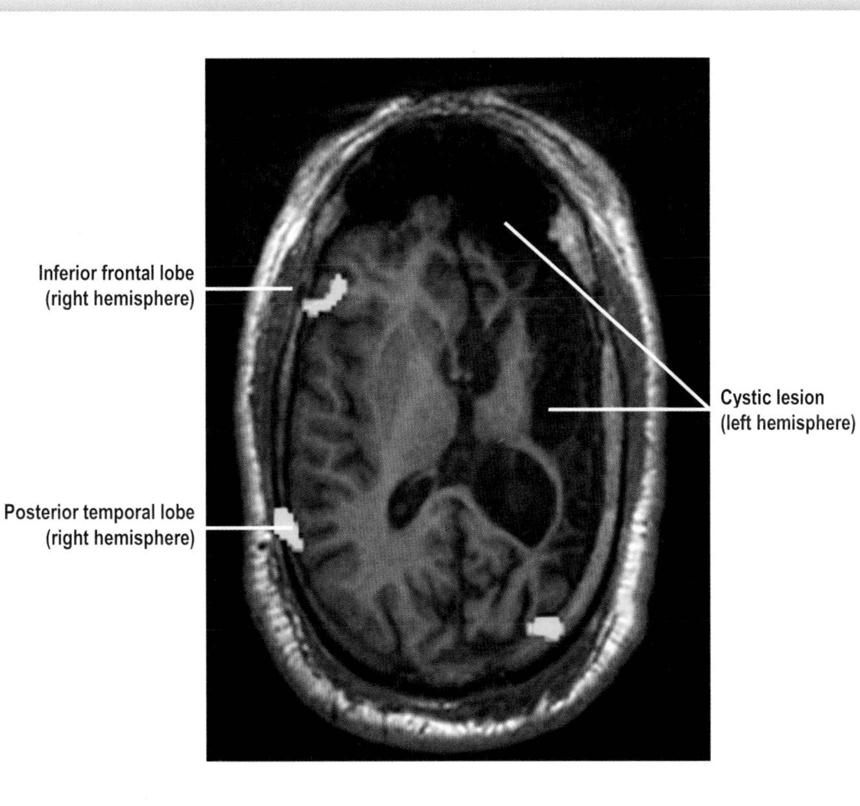

Fig. 11.7 **Preoperative assessment prior to epilepsy surgery.** This patient has a large cystic lesion in the left cerebral hemisphere. The image shows a functional MRI (fMRI) scan in the axial plane during a word generation task used to determine if radical epilepsy surgery is likely to lead to post-operative language impairment. There is increased regional cerebral blood flow in the inferior frontal and posterior temporal regions in the right cerebral hemisphere suggestive of language reorganization to the unaffected (right) side of the brain in this patient which predicts a more favourable outcome following surgery (NB language is normally represented in the left cerebral hemisphere in 95% of right-handed people and 70% of those who are left-handed; see Ch. 3). From Bargalló, Núria: Eur J Radiol 2008 67(3): 401–408 with permission.

longer-lasting hyperpolarization of the neuronal membrane by opening potassium channels. Several anti-epileptic agents increase the amount of GABA available by modulating its synthesis (sodium valproate), reuptake (tiagabine), release (gabapentin) or breakdown (vigabatrin).

Glutamate modulators

Glutamate receptor antagonists have a powerful anti-epileptic effect in animal models, but are not suitable for clinical use. This is because of the unacceptable side effects that would be caused by widespread interference with excitatory neurotransmission. Nevertheless, several well-established anti-epileptic drugs have some effect on the synthesis, release, reuptake or degradation of glutamate (e.g. topiramate, felbamate, lamotrigine).

Failure of anti-epileptic drugs

Seizure control is inadequate in 30% of patients. An important factor is **non-compliance** and large studies in the UK and USA have shown that two thirds of patients regularly fail to take their medication. This can be improved by patient education and modified-release (once daily) preparations.

Pharmacoresistance

Focal (partial) seizures are more likely to be drug resistant, especially in **temporal lobe epilepsy**. Resistance may develop with progression of the underlying disease or as a result of alterations in ion channels and receptors. Another cause is upregulation of **multi-drug transporter proteins** which are present at the blood–brain barrier and eject **lipophilic molecules** from the brain. A similar mechanism underlies resistance to chemotherapeutic agents in certain cancers. One of the best known drug resistance proteins is **p-glycoprotein**; others include the multi-drug-resistance-associated proteins (MRPs) and breast cancer resistance protein (BCRP).

Surgery in epilepsy

Approximately 10% of patients with drug-resistant focal epilepsy might benefit from a neurosurgical procedure. Before any surgical intervention, detailed **preoperative assessment** is carried out including **psychometric testing** and **functional brain imaging**, to assess the potential impact of surgery on memory, language and intellect (Fig. 11.7).

Types of procedure

The aim of surgery in epilepsy is usually to (i) remove a causative lesion or (ii) interrupt white matter pathways to prevent seizures from spreading.

Partial or complete removal of a lobe (**lobectomy**) may be appropriate for a focal lesion. The most commonly performed procedure is **temporal lobectomy** with **hippocampectomy**, in order to treat drug-resistant temporal lobe epilepsy.

Division of the corpus callosum (**callosotomy**) can be used to prevent interhemispheric spread of seizures. Resection of an entire cerebral hemisphere (**hemispherectomy**) or surgical 'disconnection' of the cerebral cortex (**functional hemispherotomy**) is occasionally performed for severe unilateral disease (Clinical Box 11.7).

The outcome of surgery is excellent in three quarters of cases and up to 70% of patients with well-circumscribed lesions can expect to be left seizure free. In the small number of cases requiring hemispherectomy the cure rate may be as high as 95%.

Neuropathology of epilepsy

There are no specific pathological features in primary generalized epilepsy. In **focal epilepsy** the three common findings are: hippocampal sclerosis, cortical malformations and benign tumours.

Clinical Box 11.7: Rasmussen's encephalitis

This is a very rare inflammatory brain disease of childhood that is characterized by severe, **unilateral seizures** with progressive intellectual decline. Contralateral **hemiplegia** and **hemianopia** develop over a number of years as one hemisphere is progressively destroyed (Fig. 11.8). The aetiology is uncertain, but is thought to be **autoimmune** in origin. Anti-epileptic drugs are ineffective and surgical resection of the affected hemisphere is often the only option.

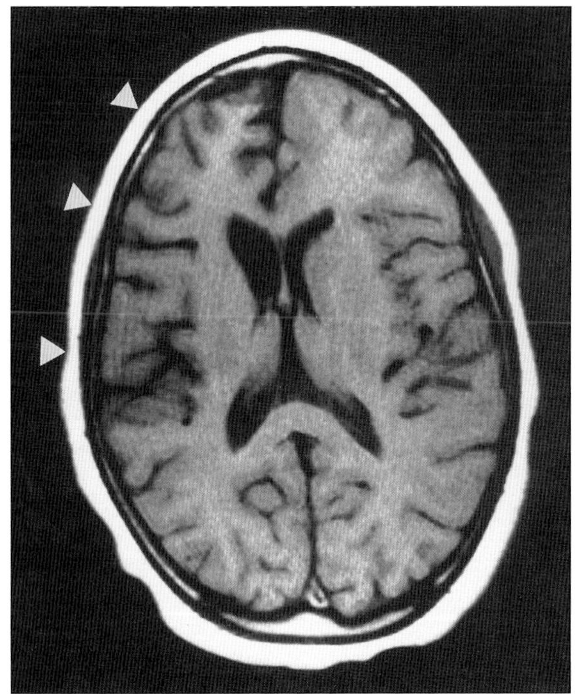

Fig. 11.8 **Rasmussen's encephalitis.** T1-weighted axial MRI scan showing marked unilateral atrophy which is particularly prominent in the frontal lobe. From Gibbs, JW et al: Physiological analysis of Rasmussen's encephalitis: patch clamp recordings of altered inhibitory neurotransmitter function in resected frontal cortical tissue. Epilep Res 1998 June; 31(1):13–27 with permission.

Key Points

- Two thirds of patients can be managed effectively with anti-epileptic drugs (AEDs) and in most cases this can be achieved with a single agent (monotherapy).
- The major types of AED are: sodium channel antagonists (e.g. phenytoin, sodium valproate); calcium channel antagonists (e.g. ethosuximide); and GABA potentiating agents (e.g. benzodiazepines, barbiturates). Some agents also modulate glutamate neurotransmission.
- Anti-epileptic drugs have a number of side effects including drowsiness, reduced concentration and cerebellar ataxia. Incidence of birth defects is also increased, particularly with sodium valproate.
- Seizure control is inadequate in 30% of patients. This may reflect pharmacoresistance in some cases, but an important contributing factor is non-compliance.
- Approximately 10% of drug-resistant focal epilepsy might benefit from a surgical procedure to remove a causative lesion or prevent the spread of seizure activity.

Hippocampal sclerosis

Hippocampal sclerosis is the most common pathological finding in focal epilepsy, accounting for 65% of cases. The typical MRI findings are unilateral volume loss on T1-weighted images and increased signal (**hyperintensity**) on T2-weighted images (Fig. 11.9). Resected surgical specimens usually appear shrunken and may feel firm or **sclerotic** when they are sliced (Greek: sklerōs, hard).

Microscopic features

Examination of the specimen under the microscope shows marked loss of neurons in the pyramidal cell layer of the hippocampus, accompanied by glial scarring (Fig. 11.10). Neuronal loss is most pronounced in the **CA1 subfield**, a region that is **selectively vulnerable** to a range of pathological processes including hypoxia, ischaemia and excitotoxic injury (see Ch. 8). In severe cases there may be widespread loss of hippocampal neurons, but those within the CA2 subfield and dentate gyrus tend to be resistant.

Another common finding is **granule cell dispersion**. The granule cell layer is thicker than usual and its normally rounded neurons become spindle-shaped, reminiscent of migrating nerve cells. This is thought to be due to the birth and migration of new neurons, triggered by seizure activity. Changes in hippocampal connectivity (in particular, a phenomenon called **mossy fibre sprouting**) are discussed below in the context of partial seizure mechanisms. In 10% of cases a second lesion such as a malformation or tumour is also found ('dual pathology').

Aetiology of hippocampal sclerosis

Retrospective studies in adults with hippocampal sclerosis have identified an **initial precipitating insult** (during childhood) in up to 90% of cases. This is most often a **febrile convulsion**, a fever-associated seizure that occurs in up to 5% of normal children under the age of 5 years (with no further problems in the vast majority of cases). In a small proportion of children, regular spontaneous seizures develop after a variable **latent**

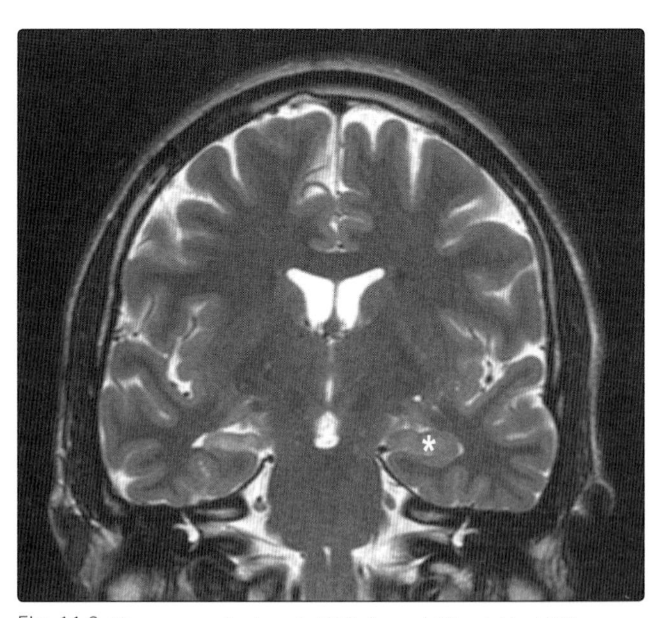

Fig. 11.9 **Hippocampal sclerosis (HS).** Coronal, T2-weighted MRI scan showing unilateral volume loss and T2 hyperintensity in comparison to the normal hippocampus (*) with associated enlargement of the lateral ventricle. Courtesy of Dr Andrew MacKinnon.

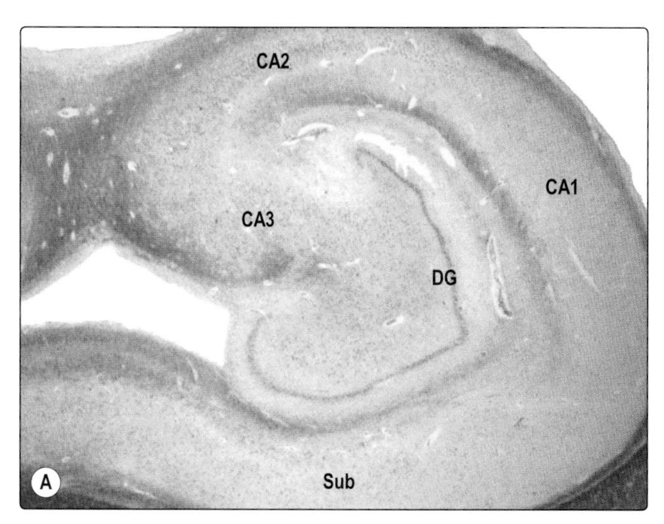

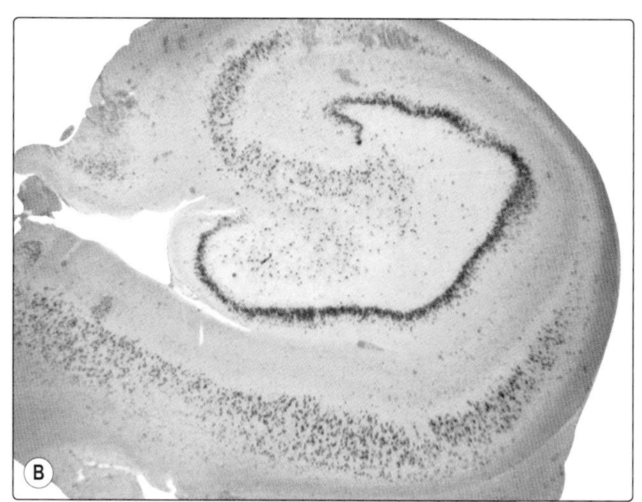

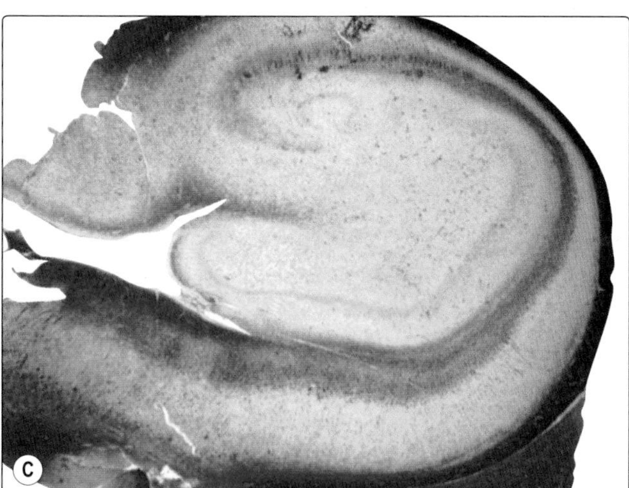

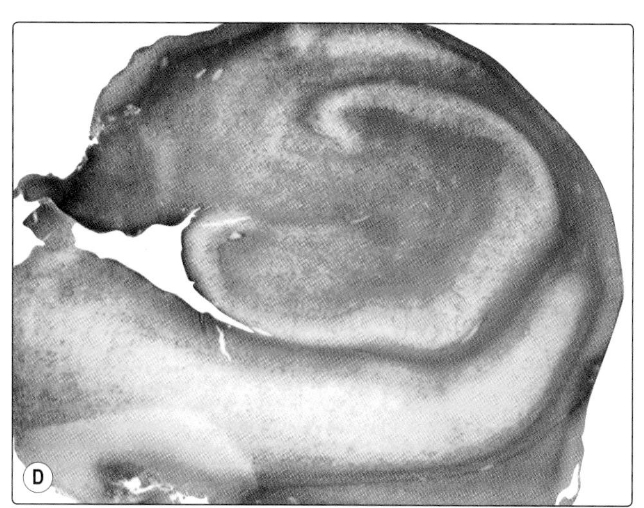

Fig. 11.10 **Pathological features of hippocampal sclerosis. (A)** Micrograph of a normal human hippocampus (stained with Luxol fast blue/cresyl violet) showing the main anatomical structures [DG = dentate gyrus; CA1-3 = subfields of Ammon's horn; Sub = subiculum]; **(B)** Immunohistochemistry for the neuronal marker NeuN in a patient with hippocampal sclerosis showing neuronal loss in the CA1 subregion; **(C)** The same specimen stained with Luxol fast blue (a myelin stain) which shows collapse of the CA1 subfield; **(D)** Astrogliosis (glial 'scarring') in the same case, which is most obvious in CA1, demonstrated using antibody-labelling for the astrocytic marker GFAP (glial fibrillary acidic protein).

period (usually <10 years). The phenomenon has been replicated in animal models, providing evidence that temporal lobe epilepsy might be caused by damage to the immature brain (the concept that 'seizures beget seizures').

Another possibility is that a pre-existing **developmental abnormality** of the hippocampus is responsible for both the febrile convulsions in childhood and the development of epilepsy in later life. This idea is supported by the finding of subtle hippocampal abnormalities in relatives of people with hippocampal sclerosis (who do not have epilepsy themselves).

Malformations of cortical development

This is a group of neuronal migration disorders characterized by abnormal development of the cerebral cortex, termed **cortical dysplasia**. This accounts for approximately 20% of cases in epilepsy surgical specimens and is an important cause of pharmacoresistant partial seizures. There are several types (some of which are discussed in Clinical Box 11.8) but the most common form is **focal cortical dysplasia**.

Focal cortical dysplasia (FCD)

In this condition the affection region of the cerebral cortex is thickened and the junction with the subcortical white matter is blurred (Fig. 11.11A). The microscopic structure of the cortex is disturbed, with malorientated neurons and abnormal cell types (Fig. 11.11B):

- **Balloon cells** are large, rounded cells with intermediate features between neurons and glia; the presence of balloon cells is diagnostic of focal cortical dysplasia.

> ### *Clinical Box 11.8: Cortical migration disorders*
>
> This group of disorders is characterized by abnormal lamination and folding of the cerebral cortex. The pattern of surface convolutions is simplified and the cortex is abnormally thick. The most severe form is **lissencephaly** in which the surface of the brain is smooth (Greek: lissos, smooth). Two thirds of cases are caused by mutations or deletions affecting the **LIS1** or **XLIS** (**DCX**) genes on chromosomes 17p and Xq respectively, which are involved in microtubule binding and cell motility. In **subcortical band heterotopia** (or **double cortex syndrome**) a thick band of abnormal grey matter is found beneath the cerebral cortex. This is caused by germline deletions in the DCX/XLIS gene and occurs almost exclusively in females. Cortical migration disorders are often associated with epilepsy and cognitive impairment.

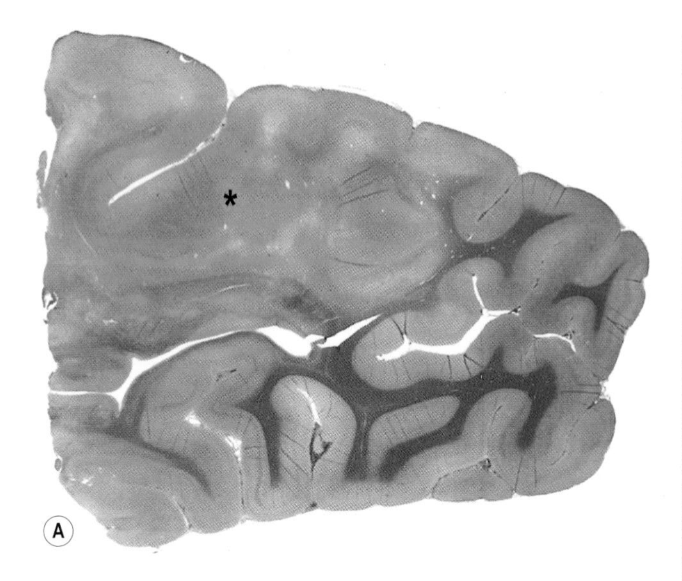

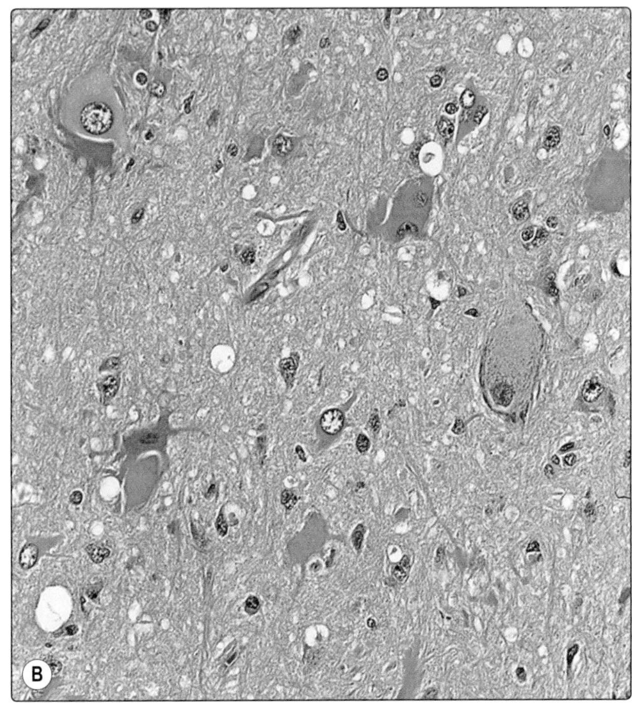

Fig. 11.11 **Focal cortical dysplasia (FCD). (A)** Brain specimen showing an area of abnormal cortical architecture (*) with blurring of the normally sharp boundary between the cerebral cortex (stained pink) and subcortical white matter (stained blue). This is a combined preparation using haematoxylin and eosin with Luxol fast blue; **(B)** Micrograph of FCD (routine haematoxylin and eosin staining) showing the disorganized cortical structure with abnormal (dysplastic) cells. The presence of balloon cells is best confirmed with immunohistochemistry (antibody labelling) by demonstrating large, swollen cells that express both neuronal and glial proteins. From Burger: Surgical Pathology of the Nervous System and its Coverings 4e (Churchill Livingstone 2002) with permission.

- **Dysplastic neurons** have abnormal, bizarrely shaped cell bodies and dendrites, in addition to abnormal orientation and positioning within cortical laminae.
- **Giant neurons** are large pyramidal cells with an otherwise normal morphology. They can be found throughout the dysplastic cortex.

Epileptiform discharges have been obtained in electrode recordings from dysplastic cortex in human surgical specimens and appear to arise from abnormal neurons. Interestingly, the foci of dysplasia are indistinguishable from cortical 'tubers' in **tuberous sclerosis** (Clinical Box 11.9).

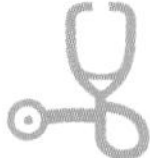

Clinical Box 11.9: Tuberous sclerosis

This is an autosomal dominant condition affecting 1 in 6000 live births. There are two causative genes, **TSC1** and **TSC2** (located on chromosomes 9 and 16 respectively), which take part in cytoplasmic signalling pathways involved in cell growth and development. Features of tuberous sclerosis include epilepsy and developmental delay together with characteristic skin lesions (Fig. 11.12). The risk of certain cardiac, renal and glial tumours is also increased. Brain imaging shows multiple cortical **tubers** which represent areas of focal cortical dysplasia.

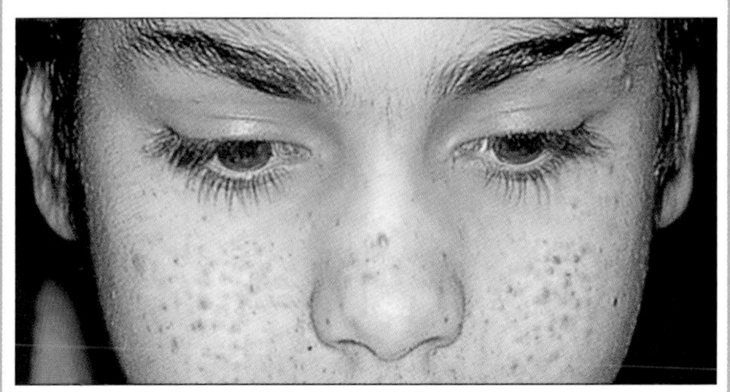

Fig. 11.12 **Facial angiofibromas ('adenoma sebaceum') in a patient with tuberous sclerosis.** This is one of many neurocutaneous syndromes with manifestations in both the skin and nervous system. From McIntosh, N et al: Forfar and Arneil's Textbook of Pediatrics 7e (Churchill-Livingstone 2008) with permission.

Glioneuronal tumours

Two tumours with a predilection for the mesial temporal lobe commonly cause drug-resistant focal epilepsy: **dysembryoplastic neuroepithelial tumour (DNT)** and **ganglioglioma**. These are both classified as 'low-grade' tumours, meaning that they are benign and slow-growing (see Ch. 5).

Microscopic examination shows a mixture of immature neurons and glial cells. In DNT, the main glial component consists of **oligodendroglia-like cells (OLCs)** (Fig. 11.13). The characteristic elements in ganglioglioma are **ganglion cells**, large neurons with rounded cell bodies and large nuclei. In 50% of cases **binucleate ganglion cells** can be found. Epileptiform discharges sometimes originate from abnormal

Key Points

- There are no specific pathological features in primary generalized epilepsy. In focal epilepsy the three common findings are: hippocampal sclerosis, cortical malformations and benign tumours (such as DNT and ganglioglioma).
- Hippocampal sclerosis is the most common pathology encountered in epilepsy surgical specimens, accounting for 65% of cases. There is neuronal loss and gliosis in Ammon's horn (particularly the CA1 subfield) accompanied by mossy fibre sprouting and granule cell dispersion.
- In 90% of cases of HS there is evidence of an initial precipitating insult (e.g. a febrile convulsion) with a variable latent interval before seizure onset (usually <10 years).
- It is not clear if the early-life event damages the hippocampus or if a pre-existing developmental abnormality is responsible for both the febrile convulsions and the subsequent epilepsy.

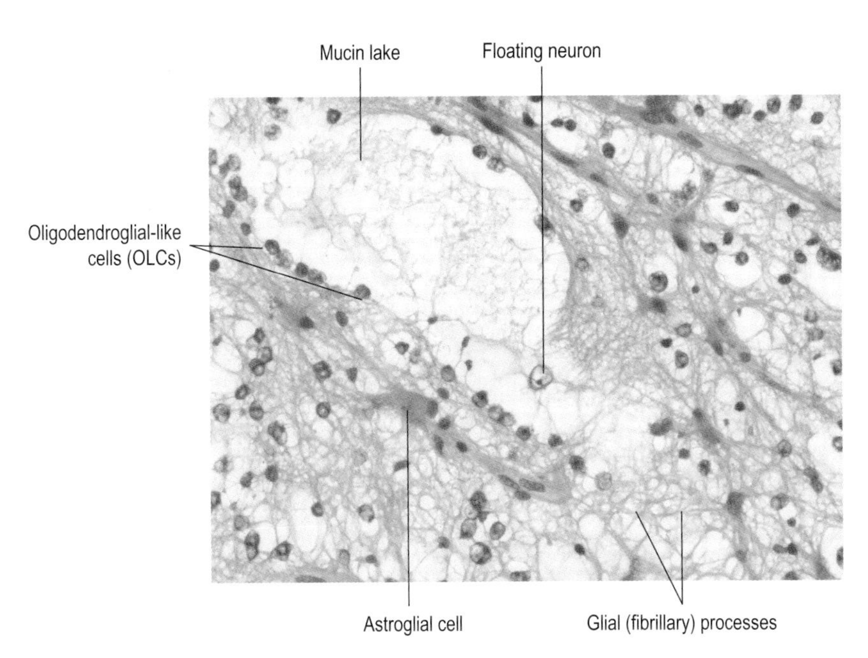

Fig. 11.13 **Microscopic appearances of dysembryoplastic neuroepithelial tumour (DNT).** Rows of cells with round nuclei (oligodendroglia-like cells or OLCs) can be seen lining up on either side of a large, mucin-filled lake. A 'floating neuron' with a large nucleus and prominent nucleolus is present with the mucin lake. Astrocytic cells (with a spidery appearance) can also be identified. This overall pattern is referred to as the 'specific glioneuronal element' and is diagnostic of DNT. (Routine haematoxylin and eosin staining.)

neurons within the tumour itself and in other cases result from disturbance to the **perilesional cortex**, which is often removed together with the tumour.

Partial seizure mechanisms

It was traditionally assumed that epilepsy resulted from a simple imbalance between excitatory and inhibitory influences in the brain (Fig. 11.14). It is now regarded as a **network phenomenon** that arises from abnormal **synchronized discharges** in large neuronal assemblies. Reseach (in animal models) has shown associated changes in connectivity, receptors and ion channels.

> ### *Clinical Box 11.10: Status epilepticus*
>
> A patient is said to be in **status epilepticus** if seizure activity persists for more than 30 minutes. This may be the result of a single prolonged seizure or **serial seizures** with no intervening recovery of consciousness. The seizures may be of any type. **Complex partial status epilepticus** (or **epilepsia partialis continua**) sometimes presents with bizarre behavioural disturbances that may mimic a psychiatric disorder. **Generalized convulsive status epilepticus** is a medical emergency with a mortality of 10–20%. This may be due to hyperthermia, metabolic derangement, prolonged hypoxia or acute brain injury. If seizure control cannot be gained with intravenous anticonvulsant agents then general anaesthesia may be required.

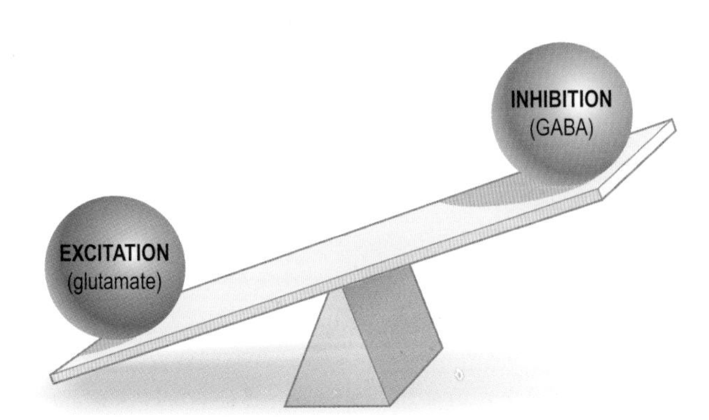

Fig. 11.14 **The classical concept that epilepsy results from an imbalance between excitatory and inhibitory influences is now known to be a gross over-simplification.**

Animal models of epilepsy

Experimental models of epilepsy are extremely important for the development and screening of novel anti-epileptic drugs and for the investigation of partial seizure mechanisms.

Acute seizure models

There are a number of acute models that can be used to induce seizures in non-epileptic experimental animals. One option is to use a **chemoconvulsant substance** (e.g. picrotoxin, kainic acid, pilocarpine, strychnine, penicillin or pentylenetetrazole) which can be administered in different ways such as subcutaneous injection or direct application to the cortical surface. Another is to use focal electrical stimulation, such as the **maximal electroshock (MES)** method in which mice or rats receive an electrical stimulus that is just strong enough to cause maximal seizure activity. This is widely used in the screening and assessment of potential anti-epileptic drugs.

Acute seizure models are used to simulate a range of epilepsies including generalized tonic-clonic, myoclonic and absence seizures. Prolonged stimulation (e.g. with pilocarpine) may induce **status epilepticus** (seizure activity lasting more than 30 minutes; see Clinical Box 11.10). This leads to changes in the medial temporal lobe that are similar to those seen in human **temporal lobe epilepsy**.

Chronic seizure models

Chronic seizure models are useful not only to investigate the acute events involved in seizure onset and termination, but also the **interictal** events, including long-term changes in synaptic connections, receptor subunit composition and peptide expression.

A popular animal model of temporal lobe epilepsy is called **kindling**, which alludes to the process of starting a fire. In this method, an electrode is used to deliver a repetitive, low-frequency electrical stimulation to the **medial temporal region** of a rodent (e.g. within the amygdala or hippocampus; see Ch. 3). The current is not sufficient to cause a seizure, but sustained electrical stimulation over a period of time eventually leads to epileptiform discharges, together with a long-lasting susceptibility to further stimulation or even **spontaneous seizures**. It is thought that repetitive stimulation leads to abnormal recruitment of synaptic strengthening mechanisms (**long-term potentiation** or **LTP**) that are involved in learning and memory (see Ch. 7).

Genetic seizure models

A number of genetic models of chronic epilepsy also exist. These include naturally occurring animals that are genetically predisposed to epileptic seizures: either spontaneously or as a result of various types of stimulation (e.g. **audiogenic epilepsy**, which is triggered by sudden loud noises). These are available in numerous species including mice, rats, gerbils and dogs and the range of seizure types is wide. There are also various **transgenic** or **genetic knockout** mice models of epilepsy (e.g. inhibitory neuropeptide 'knockout' mice that have spontaneous epileptic seizures).

Electrical basis of epilepsy

Electrical recordings in animal models of epilepsy have identified abrupt shifts in the resting membrane potential of hippocampal neurons: the **paroxysmal depolarization shift (PDS)**. An inward sodium current (mediated by voltage-gated ion channels) is followed by a prolonged, **calcium-dependent depolarization**. The PDS lasts ten times longer than a normal action potential and is associated with an intense burst of nerve impulses. It is terminated by calcium-sensitive potassium channels which repolarize the neuronal membrane. A prolonged period of **after-hyperpolarization** then follows (see Ch. 6). When a paroxysmal depolarization shift occurs simultaneously in several million cortical neurons it can be detected by scalp electrodes as an **interictal spike**. If the abnormal activity spreads over a large enough cortical area (more than a few centimetres in the human brain) it may develop into a seizure.

Key Points

- Experimental models of epilepsy are important for the development and screening of new anti-epileptic drugs and for investigating partial seizure mechanisms.
- Acute seizure models (e.g. using chemoconvulsant agents or maximal electroshock stimulation) can be used to induce seizures in non-epileptic experimental animals.
- Chronic seizure models (e.g. the kindling model of temporal lobe epilepsy) allow the study of interictal events and long-term changes in neurons, synapses and receptors.
- Genetic epilepsy models are available in a range of species, some of which are naturally occurring and others that have been specially bred (e.g. transgenic mice).
- Recordings in animal models of epilepsy show that interictal spikes are associated with calcium-mediated paroxysmal depolarization shifts in the neuronal membrane.

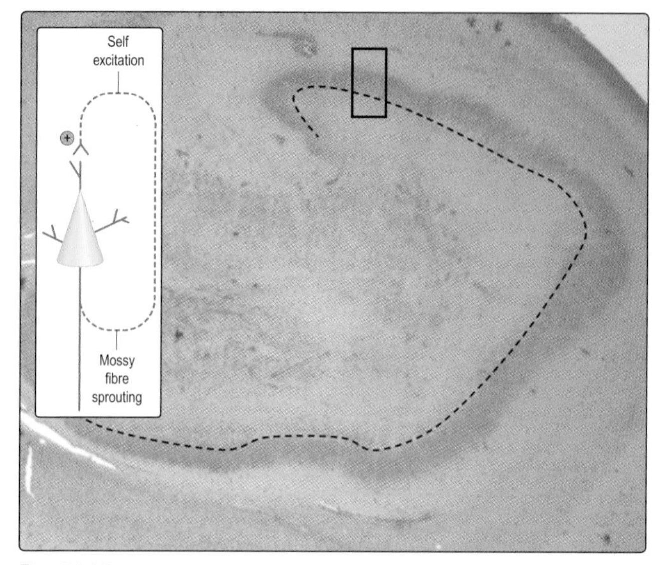

Fig. 11.15 **Mossy fibre sprouting in hippocampal sclerosis.** Immunohistochemistry for the neuropeptide dynorphin shows newly sprouted mossy fibres emerging from the granule cell layer (dashed line). These may form aberrant, self-excitatory connections (inset).

Pathophysiology of epilepsy

Much of the experimental work on **epileptogenesis** has focused on the mesial temporal region, from which 60% of seizures originate. The main contributing factors are discussed in the following sections.

Increased excitation/decreased inhibition

Seizures can be provoked in animal models by blocking inhibitory (GABAergic) neurotransmission and in 80% of cases the abnormal discharges originate in the **hippocampus**. Loss of inhibition may therefore contribute to temporal lobe epilepsy in humans.

The activity of hippocampal neurons within the dentate gyrus is normally restrained by a population of inhibitory interneurons called **basket cells**. Basket cells are in turn excited by **mossy cells**, located in the hilum of the dentate gyrus. A proposed mechanism contributing to temporal lobe epilepsy is the selective death of **hilar mossy cells**, reducing excitatory drive to basket cells and releasing hippocampal neurons from their normal state of inhibition: the **dormant basket cell hypothesis**.

Alterations in connectivity

The axons of dentate granule cells (**mossy fibres**) normally extend into the hilum of the dentate gyrus and synapse on CA3 pyramidal neurons. In hippocampal sclerosis new axons arise from the granule cell layer in a process referred to as **mossy fibre sprouting**. Importantly, these new processes form aberrant, potentially self-excitatory connections within the granule cell layer that may promote seizure activity (Fig. 11.15). Abnormal connectivity of inhibitory interneurons might also contribute to epileptogenesis by encouraging **synchronized bursting** in groups of excitatory neurons (Fig. 11.16). This might help to explain why powerful inhibitory agents exacerbate some forms of epilepsy.

Changes in receptors and ion channels

A number of seizure-associated alterations have been observed at the neuronal cell and receptor level, including changes in the pattern of action potential firing. This has led to the concept of the **epileptic (bursting) neuron**. It appears that

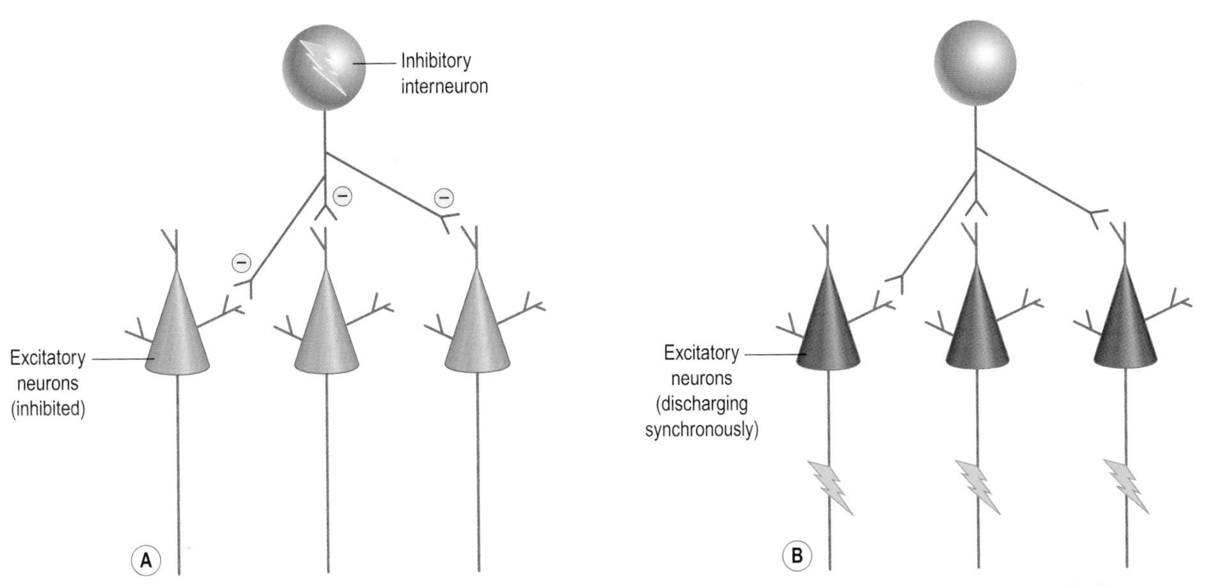

Fig. 11.16 **Abnormal synchronization may be triggered by inhibitory neurons.** Powerful activity in an inhibitory interneuron with divergent projections may inhibit several excitatory neurons simultaneously **(A)** leading to synchronous discharge as they all recover at the same moment **(B)**.

previously normal pyramidal neurons can change their behaviour during epileptogenesis to become 'bursters'. This probably results from alterations within ion channels (or changes in their subunit composition) in the neuronal cell body. Synchronization can also be facilitated by the addition or strengthening of direct intercellular bridges between neurons called **gap junctions** (see Ch. 7).

Changes in inhibitory peptides

The hippocampus is richly supplied by axon terminals releasing **inhibitory neuropeptides** including neuropeptide Y, somatostatin, enkephalins and dynorphin. These are co-released with classical neurotransmitters and have powerful anti-convulsant properties. This is mediated by changes in **second messenger cascades** and increase or decrease in cytosolic substrates such as cyclic AMP (cAMP). Genetically engineered 'knockout' animals with reduced or absent expression of inhibitory peptides show markedly **reduced seizure threshold** or spontaneous seizures and there is evidence for alterations in neuropeptide expression in human epilepsy.

The role of astrocytes

Astrocytes may play a direct role in epileptogenesis, contributing to the generation of brief, high-frequency discharges called **very fast oscillations** (**VFOs**). This is thought to depend upon the presence of **gap junctions** between astrocytes. These allow depolarizing currents to pass freely between cells, generating oscillations at frequencies of 80–200 Hz. These oscillations (also called **ripples**) are normal in the hippocampus, but pathological in the neocortex and have been detected prior to focal seizure activity. Oscillations have also been recorded in human brain tissue removed during epilepsy surgery and **gap junction inhibitors** have been shown to possess anti-convulsant properties in animal models.

> **Key Points**
>
> - Epilepsy is a 'network phenomenon', caused by abnormally synchronized electrical discharges originating in interconnected groups or assemblies of cortical neurons.
> - Epileptogenic networks show many pathological changes including: increased excitation, decreased inhibition, changes in receptors and ion channels or loss of peptide inhibition.
> - Astrocytes may play a direct roll in epileptogenesis, contributing to the development of very fast oscillations or ripples (80–200 Hz) mediated by gap junctions.

Mechanism of absence seizures

Unlike most forms of primary generalized epilepsy, the mechanism in absence seizures is well understood. It is due to derangement of a rhythmic pattern of oscillations that normally occurs between the cortex and thalamus during sleep. This creates the typical **spike and wave discharge** seen on the EEG (Fig. 11.17).

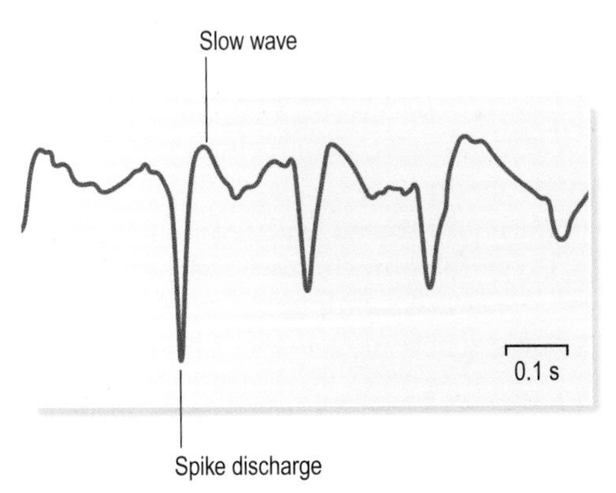

Fig. 11.17 **Spike and wave discharges in absence seizures.** The abnormal discharges emerge from a normal background EEG trace at a typical frequency of 3 Hz (cycles per second).

The thalamic relay and sleep

The thalamus acts as the 'gateway' to the cerebral cortex and contains specific thalamocortical relay nuclei for all sensory modalities apart from olfaction (see Ch. 3). **Thalamocortical neurons** projecting to the primary sensory areas of the cortex can be said to operate in two modes:

- **During wakefulness** (Fig. 11.18A) they are tonically active, transmitting sensory information to the cortex.

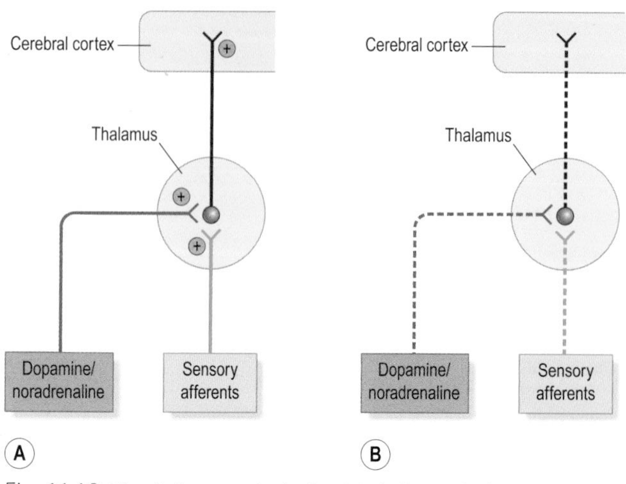

Fig. 11.18 **The thalamocortical relay (A) during wakefulness and (B) during sleep.**

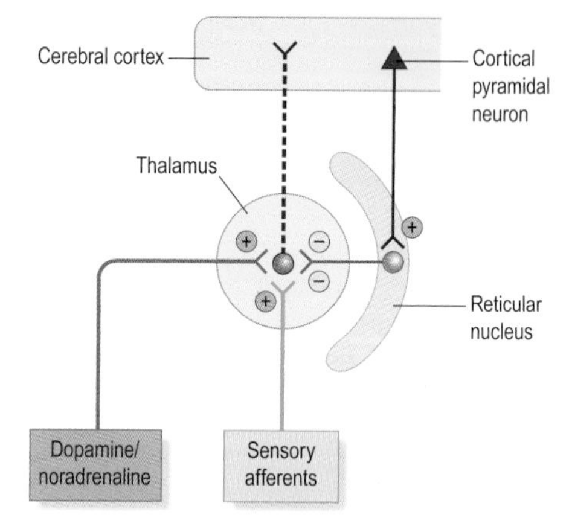

Fig. 11.19 **Mechanism of absence seizures.** It is thought that the inhibitory reticular nucleus may be stimulated by a hyperexcitable focus in the primary sensory cortex. This powerfully inhibits the thalamus and triggers the sleep spindle oscillations inappropriately in the waking state.

Excitatory noradrenergic and cholinergic projections from the **diffuse neurochemical systems** of the brain stem (see Ch. 1) contribute to their excitation.

- **During sleep** (Fig. 11.18B) thalamocortical sensory relay neurons are quiescent. This is due to reduced peripheral afferents (in a dark, quiet environment) and decreased activity in the diffuse projections from the brain stem.

Sleep-associated **hyperpolarization** (inhibition) of thalamocortical neurons triggers a rhythmic pattern of oscillations between thalamus and cortex. This normally appears on the EEG as the **sleep spindle**, characterized by regular bursts of activity at a frequency of 12–14 Hz (cycles per second).

Origin of thalamic bursting

The sleep spindle depends upon a **hyperpolarization-dependent cation channel** which is expressed by thalamocortical neurons. The resting membrane potential for thalamocortical neurons is −60 mV and the reversal potential (see Ch. 6) for the hyperpolarization-dependent channel is −30 mV. Opening of the hyperpolarization-dependent channel therefore causes **depolarization** of thalamocortical cells (from −60 mV to −30 mV).

Co-recruitment of a second hyperpolarization-dependent channel, a **T-type calcium channel**, enables calcium as well as sodium to enter thalamocortical neurons. This triggers a burst of action potentials both in the thalamic neurons and in the cortical regions to which they project. Once the membrane of the thalamocortical neuron is fully depolarized (to −30 mV) both hyperpolarization-dependent channels close. The membrane is then repolarized to its resting value of −60 mV (by a calcium-sensitive potassium channel) and the oscillating cycle of depolarization and repolarization begins again.

Origin of absences

In absence seizures, inappropriate activation of the sleep spindle mechanism is believed to occur when thalamocortical relay neurons are **hyperpolarized** in the waking state (thereby triggering the hyperpolarization-dependent channels). This creates a burst of thalamocortical oscillating activity that blocks transmission of information to the cerebral cortex, since the thalamic 'gateway' is temporarily closed. The cortex is therefore briefly deprived of peripheral sensory input, manifesting as an 'absence'.

Inhibition comes from the **reticular nucleus** of the thalamus which utilizes the inhibitory neurotransmitter GABA (Fig. 11.19). This nucleus appears to be stimulated by a hyperexcitable focus in the **primary somatosensory cortex**. In keeping with this idea, absence seizures can be triggered by cortical excitation in animal models, but only if thalamocortical connections are intact. This also explains why the calcium-channel antagonist **ethosuximide** is effective in the treatment of absence seizures.

Key Points

- Childhood absence seizures are a form of primary generalized epilepsy characterized by spike and wave discharges on the EEG at a frequency of 3 Hz.
- Absence seizures are thought to represent inappropriate activation of the sleep spindle in the waking state, triggered by hyperpolarization of thalamocortical relay neurons.
- This leads to activation of two hyperpolarization-dependent channels in the thalamus (a cation channel and a T-type calcium channel) which sets off the abnormal thalamocortical oscillations.
- Inhibition (hyperpolarization) comes from the reticular nucleus of the thalamus which may in turn by activated by discharge from a hyperexcitable region in the primary sensory cortex.
- The thalamocortical model of absence seizures explains many of the key features, including the effectiveness of the calcium-channel antagonist ethosuximide.

Sudden death in epilepsy

The overall mortality rate in people with epilepsy is 2–3 times higher than that of the general population. In some cases this is due to progression of an underlying disease process (such as a brain tumour) but may also be the result of accidental injury, drowning or suicide.

Seizures are not generally life-threatening, provided that the airway is protected and that oxygenation is adequate. However, the risk of sudden death is 20–30 times higher than in non-epileptic controls and there is a well-recognized syndrome of **sudden unexpected death in epilepsy**

(**SUDEP**). This excludes deaths due to **status epilepticus** (see Clinical Box 11.10) and can only be diagnosed when the following criteria are met (see also Fig. 11.20):

- Sudden unexpected death in a person known to have epilepsy.
- No evidence of accidental injury or drowning.
- No alternative cause of death identified at autopsy.

SUDEP is most commonly seen in young adults with poorly controlled tonic-clonic seizures. It is more common in males and is associated with the use of multiple anti-epileptic drugs, poor compliance and alcohol misuse.

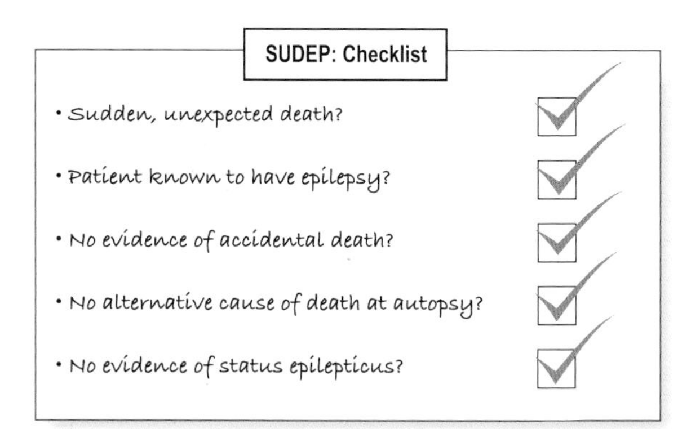

Fig. 11.20 **Sudden unexpected death in epilepsy (SUDEP): checklist for diagnosis.**

Cause of death

The mechanism of death in SUDEP is uncertain, but cardiorespiratory abnormalities are known to occur in temporal lobe epilepsy, including: **cardiac dysrhythmias** (disturbances of heart rhythm), **apnoea** (cessation of respiration) and **hypoxaemia** (low blood oxygen levels). In particular, there is evidence that seizures originating from the **insula** and **amygdala** (which have powerful visceral and autonomic projections; see Ch. 3) may lead to episodes of **asystole** (cardiac standstill).

Key Points

- The mortality rate in people with epilepsy is 2–3 times higher than that of the general population, attributable to accidental deaths, underlying disease processes, status epilepticus and SUDEP.
- Status epilepticus is a continuous state of seizure activity that lasts for at least 30 minutes without recovery of consciousness. Convulsive status epilepticus is a medical emergency with a mortality of 10–20%.
- Diagnosis of SUDEP requires a post-mortem examination (showing no alternative cause of death) and excludes accidental death and status epilepticus.
- The cause of death in SUDEP is uncertain but may reflect inhibition or disturbance of brain stem cardiac or respiratory centres, leading to respiratory or cardiac arrest.

Psychological aspects

The differential diagnosis for epileptic seizures is wide (Fig. 11.21) and includes **non-epileptic attacks** of psychological origin (Clinical Box 11.11). There are a number of other psychological aspects to consider in patients with epilepsy, including a significant impact on leisure activities and occupation and an association with psychiatric illness.

Climbing, swimming and other outdoor pursuits may be extremely hazardous without proper supervision and in the UK and USA there are strict **driving restrictions** (Clinical Box 11.12). Occupational restrictions also apply for pilots, train drivers and members of the armed forces and emergency services.

- Syncope (fainting attacks)
- Cardiac dysrhythmia
- Hyperventilation/panic attacks
- Vestibular disorders
- Non-epileptic pseudoseizures
- Transient ischaemic attacks
- Narcolepsy
- Hypoglycaemia
- Migraine

Fig. 11.21 **Differential diagnosis of epileptic seizures.** Pseudoseizures are now more commonly referred to as psychogenic non-epileptic attacks.

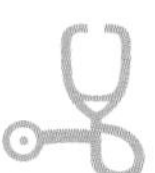

Clinical Box 11.11: Psychogenic (non-epileptic) attacks

Some patients have non-epileptic attacks that resemble epileptic seizures, but are psychological in origin ('pseudoseizures'). This is referred to as **psychogenic non-epileptic attack disorder**. Episodes of this type are more likely in people with a history of psychiatric illness or self-injury. It is usually possible to distinguish them from epileptic seizures by the presence of the following features:

- Non-random occurrence (e.g. frequently in the presence of medical staff).
- Bizarre, asymmetric thrashing movements or pelvic thrusting.
- Quiet breathing and normal blood oxygenation (pink face).
- Absence of tongue-biting.
- Normal EEG during the episode.
- Failure to respond to anti-epileptic medication.

Despite these clues, it can be difficult to make the distinction, particularly since both types of event may occur in some patients and non-epileptic attacks often signify an underlying psychiatric disorder. Video telemetry can be very helpful in making the diagnosis.

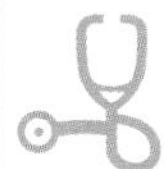

Clinical Box 11.12: Epilepsy and driving

In the UK, people with active epilepsy are not allowed to drive and it is the responsibility of the patient to inform the **Driver and Vehicle Licensing Agency** (**DVLA**) of the diagnosis. This rule may not apply in **nocturnal epilepsy** (if seizures have occurred exclusively during sleep for at least three years) or in some types of partial seizure. For ordinary drivers, a licence may be reinstated after a seizure-free period of 12 months, but limitations are more stringent for heavy goods and public service vehicles.

Association with psychiatric illness

Most people with epilepsy are of normal intelligence and do not have psychiatric illness, but there is an increased risk of anxiety, depression and suicide. There is also a more specific association between temporal lobe epilepsy and psychosis.

Mood disorders in epilepsy

The incidence of **depression** and **anxiety** is increased in people with epilepsy. A relatively high proportion of patients suffer from phobic states or major depression and the **suicide risk** is three times higher than that of the general population. This may in part be a reaction to the diagnosis of a chronic disorder that places restrictions on lifestyle and occupation, but is also likely to be related to the underlying brain abnormality or seizure activity in some patients.

Psychosis in temporal lobe epilepsy

The **psychoses** (such as schizophrenia) are a group of psychiatric disorders characterized by delusions and hallucinations. **Delusions** are strongly held (fixed) beliefs that are not acquired by normal rational means and are highly resistant to counter-evidence. They are frequently bizarre and may be contradictory. **Hallucinations** are sensory experiences (e.g. voices, sounds, images) that do not relate to objects or events in the real world. In temporal lobe epilepsy, psychosis may be postictal (after a seizure) or interictal (between seizures).

Postictal psychosis

Postictal psychosis occurs in up to 10% of patients with temporal lobe epilepsy. It typically emerges within a few hours of a seizure or cluster of seizures (following a 'lucid interval') but occasionally occurs up to 48 hours later. It is characterized by an abrupt alteration of the mental state with hallucinations and delusions (often with strong religious features) but little or no confusion, together with mixed mood disturbance that may include intense anxiety. This is to be distinguished from **postictal confusion** that occurs just after a seizure and generally lasts no more than 30 minutes.

Interictal psychosis

Up to a third of patients with temporal lobe epilepsy exhibit psychotic symptoms between seizures. This is termed **interictal psychosis**. The features differ from those of schizophrenia in that they lack **negative symptoms** such as social withdrawal and self-neglect. In addition, the mood state tends to be elevated rather than depressed.

Seizures and psychosis

There appears to be a reciprocal relationship between seizure activity and psychosis. This is demonstrated by the fact that drug-resistant psychotic states can be treated by deliberately inducing a convulsive seizure (**electroconvulsive therapy** or **ECT**).

Conversely, in some patients with epilepsy, most often with seizures of temporal lobe origin, abrupt suppression of epileptiform activity with anti-convulsant agents ('**forced normalization**' of the EEG) can lead to acute psychosis, usually after a delay of around 24 hours. Upon withdrawal of the anti-epileptic medication, psychotic features tend to resolve as the EEG returns to its interictal state.

Key Points

- Most people with epilepsy are of normal intelligence and do not have psychiatric illness, but there is an increased risk of anxiety, depression and suicide.
- There is a more specific association between temporal lobe epilepsy and psychosis, which may be postictal (following seizures) or interictal (between seizures).
- Other psychological factors to consider in patients with epilepsy include restrictions on lifestyle, driving and occupation.

Chapter 12
Dementia

CHAPTER CONTENTS

Dementia (from the Latin, meaning loss of mind) is characterized by a marked decline in memory, intellect or personality that is severe enough to interfere with daily life or work. It is a clinical syndrome with many underlying causes rather than a specific diagnosis, but almost two-thirds of cases are due to **Alzheimer's disease**. Reversible confusional states such as delirium are specifically excluded and most cases are chronic, progressive and incurable.

General aspects

Dementia is predominantly a sporadic disease of old age. The prevalence is about 1% in people over 60, rising exponentially to affect more than 20% of those aged 85 and above. Although the risk increases with advancing years, dementia is not a normal part of the ageing process and there are a number of early-onset forms that are more likely to be inherited.

Clinical features

In most cases of dementia, such as Alzheimer's disease, memory loss is a prominent and early component, but in certain types (e.g. **frontotemporal dementia**, discussed below) it is relatively spared. Loss of memory is usually accompanied by a marked decline in **higher cognitive functions** such as reasoning, visuospatial ability and language, together with changes in mood, behaviour and personality. The specific profile of higher cognitive deficits depends on the extent and distribution of pathology in the **cerebral cortex** (Fig. 12.1).

In some cases the clinical picture is dominated by a generalized slowing of thought, termed **bradyphrenia** or 'subcortical-type' dementia (Greek: bradys, slow). A hallmark of **subcortical dementia** is that responses to questions are generally accurate but take a long time to be produced. There may also be a general impairment of reasoning, planning and decision-making. This type of dementia is commonly associated with cerebrovascular disease.

Assessment and diagnosis

The diagnosis of dementia is primarily clinical. A useful tool in the assessment of a person with suspected cognitive decline is the **mini mental state examination** (**MMSE**) which is a basic test of orientation, memory, attention, language and visuospatial ability. A score below 25 out of 30 points is suggestive of dementia and individuals with Alzheimer's disease typically decline at a rate of 2–4 points per year. Information from relatives can be used to assess dementia severity using questionnaires such as the **Clinical Dementia Rating** (**CDR**) scale. More formal testing can be carried out by clinical psychologists.

Psychometric testing

A widely used measure of cognitive ability is the **intelligence quotient** (**IQ**) which is a detailed assessment of reasoning, language and memory. Scores are standardized and age-corrected so that the average IQ is 100 and 95% of individuals score between 70 and 130 (Fig. 12.2). Repeated testing can be used to show changes in cognitive ability over time.

An estimate of **premorbid intelligence** can be obtained using the **National Adult Reading Test** (**NART**). This uses 50 irregularly spelled words of decreasing lexical frequency (e.g. debt, epitome, impugn). Pronunciation of previously familiar words is maintained in the early stages of dementia and performance correlates well with premorbid verbal IQ.

Types of dementia

The main types of dementia are discussed below. The most common cause is **Alzheimer's disease**, accounting for around 65% of cases. **Dementia with Lewy bodies** (**DLB**) represents a further 20% and **vascular dementia** is responsible for 10% of cases. The remaining 5% include the **frontotemporal dementias**, which are an important cause of cognitive decline in people under the age of 60 (accounting for nearly half of cases in this age group, after Alzheimer's disease). It should be noted that some patients have less severe cognitive impairment that falls short of the criteria for dementia (Clinical Box 12.1).

Reversible causes

Some forms of cognitive impairment are potentially treatable and should be excluded in the investigation of a patient with suspected dementia. These include **nutritional deficiencies** (e.g. vitamin B_{12}, folate), **endocrine disturbances** (such as hypothyroidism), **alcohol-related dementia** (reversible with abstinence), **syphilis** (now rare in the developed world), **depressive pseudodementia** (treatable with antidepressant drugs) and **normal pressure hydrocephalus** (see Clinical Box 12.2). A 'routine dementia screen' therefore includes a range of blood tests and urinalysis, together with an MRI scan of the brain.

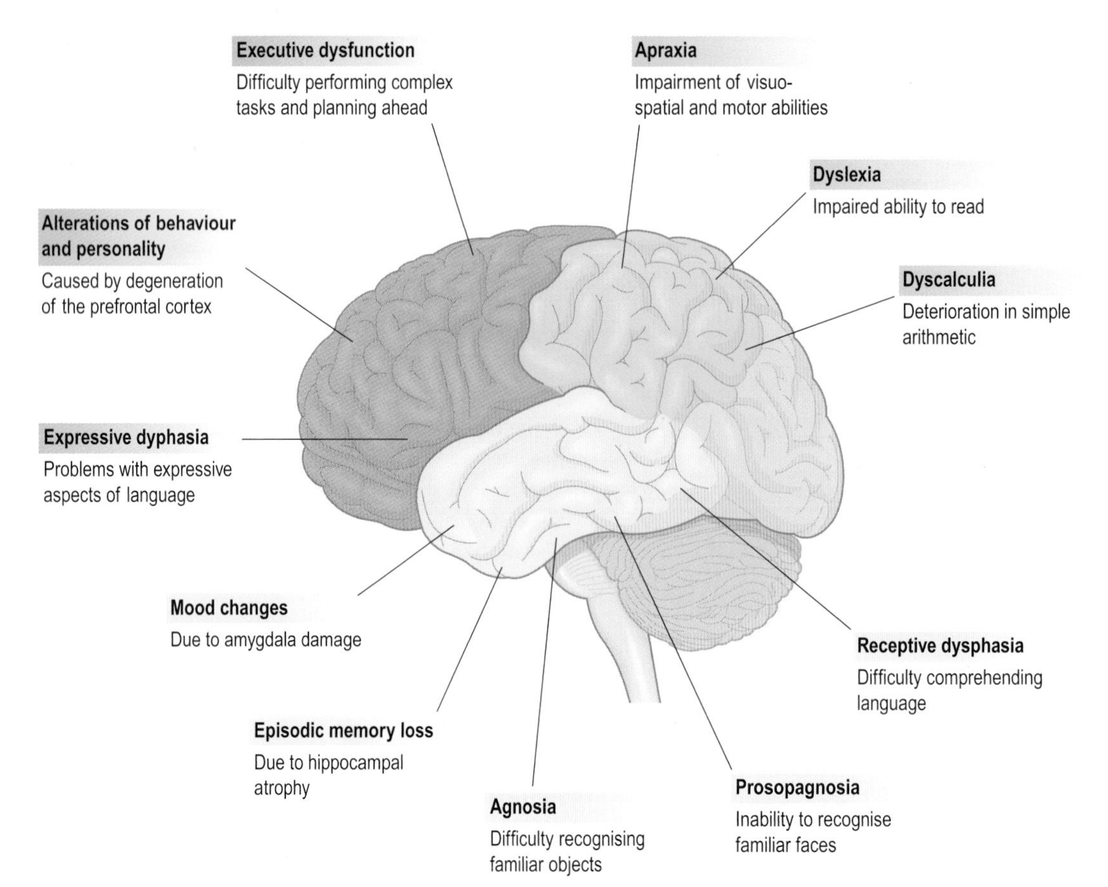

Fig. 12.1 **Clinical features of dementia.** This figure shows some of the common features of dementia that are caused by degenerative changes in different parts of the cerebral cortex (frontal lobe = red, parietal lobe = blue, temporal lobe = yellow). The clinical picture in a particular person depends upon the distribution and severity of the changes.

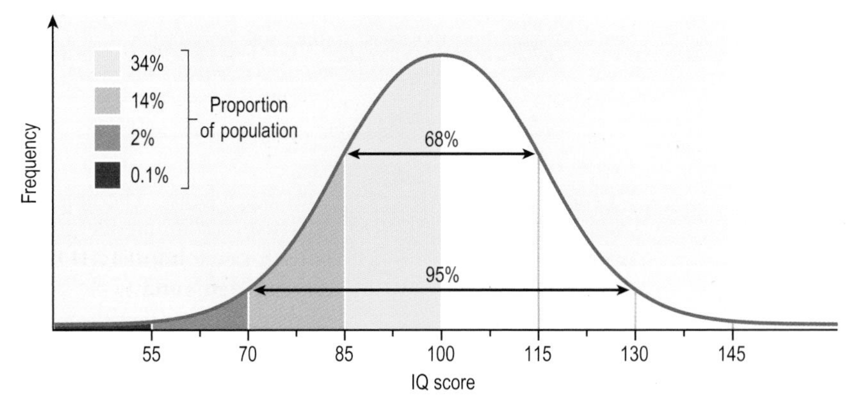

Fig. 12.2 **Distribution of IQ scores in the general population.** Intelligence in the general population has a normal distribution, meaning that scores fall on a symmetrical bell curve. The mean IQ is 100 and the standard deviation is 15, such that 95% of scores fall between 70 and 130.

Clinical Box 12.1: Mild cognitive impairment

Some patients present with mild cognitive impairment (MCI) that is confirmed on objective testing, but is not severe enough to interfere with daily life or work (and therefore does not meet the criteria for dementia). MCI is not a specific diagnosis and it may not be progressive, although a proportion of patients will eventually develop Alzheimer's disease or another form of dementia. The prevalence of mild cognitive impairment may be up to 25% in people over 75.

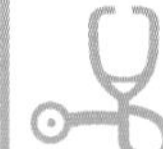

Clinical Box 12.2: Normal pressure hydrocephalus

Normal pressure hydrocephalus affects 1 in 200 people over the age of 65 and presents with a triad of **dementia**, **gait disturbance** and **urinary incontinence**. The cerebral ventricles are enlarged, but the CSF pressure is usually normal, although longer-term recording has revealed periodic pressure elevations in some people (hence the alternative term, **intermittently raised pressure hydrocephalus**). Up to 50% of patients show dramatic improvement after surgical implantation of a **shunt** to divert excess CSF to the abdomen (see Ch. 2, Clinical Box 2.2).

Key Points

- Dementia is characterized by a marked decline in mental faculties (such as memory, intellect or personality) that is severe enough to interfere with daily life or work.
- It is a syndrome rather than a specific diagnosis with many underlying causes, but by far the most common is Alzheimer's disease, accounting for 65% of cases.
- Dementia is not part of the normal ageing process, but risk increases exponentially beyond the sixth decade, with a prevalence of at least 20% in people over the age of 85.
- Memory loss is a core feature in most types of dementia, together with deterioration in higher cognitive functions including reasoning, visuospatial ability and language.
- Mild cognitive impairment (MCI) is present in up to 25% of people over the age of 75. It is not a specific diagnosis and does not always progress to dementia.

Alzheimer's disease

Alzheimer's disease is the leading cause of dementia in all age groups. The vast majority of cases appear to be sporadic, but 5% are clearly inherited in an autosomal dominant manner.

Clinical aspects

The diagnosis of Alzheimer's disease is predominantly clinical and post-mortem studies suggest that it is correct in at least 80% of cases. Two variants of Alzheimer's disease that might cause diagnostic confusion are discussed in Clinical Box 12.3.

Memory loss

Loss of **short-term memory** is a prominent, early feature. Patients may ask the same question repeatedly or forget recent conversations and events. The ability to take in new information is affected first, with relative preservation of long-term memories and knowledge. Recollection of personal experiences (**episodic memory**) is particularly affected. Since the onset is insidious, this may initially be mistaken for normal age-related forgetfulness. As the disease progresses, earlier memories are gradually eroded and ultimately patients are unable to recall key details of their own lives.

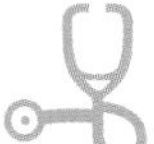

Clinical Box 12.3: Alzheimer's disease variants

In the **frontal variant** of Alzheimer's disease there are prominent changes in personality and behaviour, with disturbance of frontal **executive function** (organizing, planning, decision-making) and **expressive language**. This presentation of Alzheimer's disease (which is rare) is usually misdiagnosed as frontotemporal dementia. In **posterior cortical atrophy** the parietal lobes are particularly affected, leading to severe visuospatial and perceptual problems, with relative preservation of expressive language and memory. There may also be difficulty recognizing people and objects (particularly from unusual angles) or judging distance and speed (e.g. of approaching cars). Other common features in posterior cortical atrophy are **dyslexia** (difficulty reading and spelling) and **dyscalculia** (problems with simple arithmetic).

Visuospatial problems

Patients with Alzheimer's disease often get lost in familiar places and may forget where they have left things. These features, together with impaired recall of daily events, reflect severe pathology in the medial temporal lobe. This involves structures such as the **entorhinal cortex** and **hippocampus** that are involved in **spatial navigation** and formation of **episodic memories** (see Ch. 3).

Other visuospatial problems are due to abnormalities of the temporal and parietal association areas. **Parietal lobe pathology** may interfere with the ability to understand **spatial relationships** and manipulate objects, making it difficult to carry out ordinary daily tasks like getting dressed. Degeneration of the **temporal neocortex** may affect visual recognition of objects and people (including close friends and family members).

Reasoning and language

As with most forms of dementia, there is a general decline in **problem-solving ability** and **abstract reasoning** which impairs decision-making and judgement. This affects the capacity to manage personal affairs without supervision and interferes with ordinary daily activities such as shopping, cooking and paying bills. Language problems are very common, with **word-finding difficulties** and reduced verbal fluency in the initial stages, sometimes progressing to almost complete loss of verbal communication in advanced dementia.

Psychiatric features

Early in the course of the disease, patients tend to become withdrawn and may experience **depression** or **anxiety**. There may be **disinhibition**, with inappropriate or child-like behaviour. Awareness of declining intellectual ability and loss of independence may lead to frustration and irritability, with mood swings or angry outbursts. As time passes, **apathy** is more common, with reduced interest in activities that were previously enjoyable. Delusions, hallucinations and paranoia sometimes occur in the very late stages.

Neuroimaging

Functional brain imaging in early Alzheimer's disease may show **reduced blood flow** and **glucose metabolism** in the posterior temporo-parietal regions and hippocampus (Fig. 12.3), before obvious structural changes are evident on MRI. Over time there is progressive **brain atrophy**, with **ventricular dilatation**, **cortical thinning** and **hippocampal atrophy**. Longitudinal studies show that people with Alzheimer's disease lose brain tissue at a rate of 2% per year on average (up to 5% per year in the hippocampus), which is four times higher than in age-matched controls (Fig. 12.4).

Progression and death

The rate of progression is highly variable, with typical disease duration ranging from 5 to 15 years. Patients may initially be able to remain at home, but will require assistance with day-to-day activities and become increasingly dependent on carers. Ultimately, supervision is required for all **activities of daily living** including bathing and toileting. At some point specialized institutional care is usually most appropriate, particularly if the primary carers are themselves elderly. In the advanced stages of dementia, most sufferers tend to be become bed-bound and mute. Death is often due to a complication of immobility such as pneumonia.

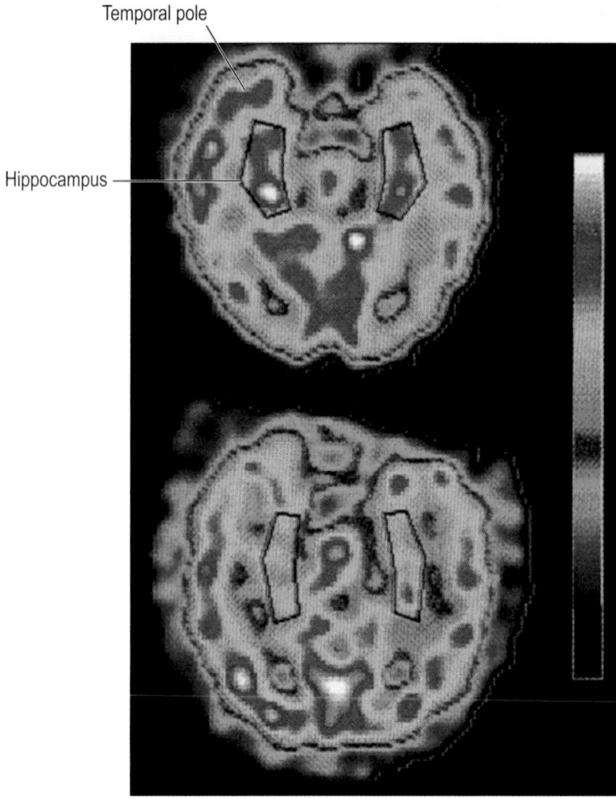

Fig. 12.3 **Reduced hippocampal blood flow in early Alzheimer's disease.** These images were obtained via single photon emission computer tomography (SPECT) scanning using a radioactive tracer and show regional cerebral blood flow. The upper image is a normal control subject and the lower image is from a patient with early Alzheimer's disease. The sections are in the axial (horizontal) plane and pass through the temporal lobe. The black box shows the position of the hippocampus in the medial temporal lobe. From Rodriguez, G. et al.: Hippocampal perfusion in mild Alzheimer's disease. Psychiatry Research: Neuroimaging (2000, pp. 65–74) with permission.

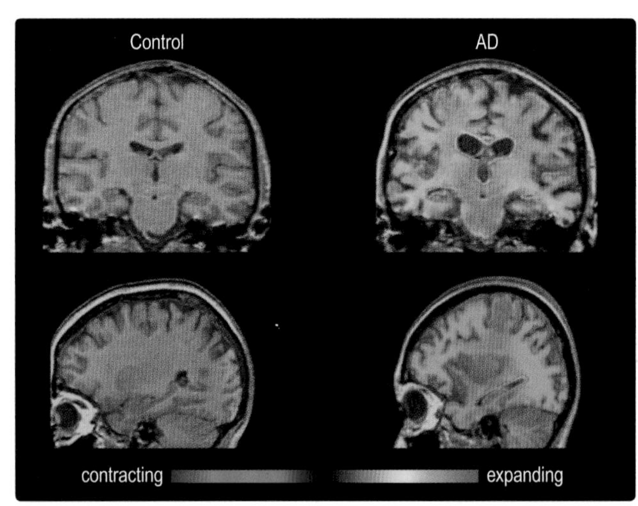

Fig. 12.4 **Neuroimaging showing progressive brain atrophy in Alzheimer's disease (AD) in comparison to an age-matched control.** These are fluid-registered volumetric MRI scans from a 60-year-old patient with Alzheimer's disease [right] and a normal age-matched control [left]. In each case, two MRI scans were acquired one year apart and have been registered together. Regions of brain loss are shown as blue-green; increases in CSF spaces are shown as red-yellow. In the patient with Alzheimer's disease, there is marked volume loss in the hippocampi and temporal lobes, with widespread symmetrical atrophy in other parts of the cerebral hemispheres and dilation of the ventricles. The control shows normal age-related atrophy. Courtesy of Professor Nick Fox.

Key Points

- Alzheimer's disease is the leading cause of dementia in all age groups. Early features include (i) marked loss of episodic memory and (ii) spatial disorientation (both reflecting severe medial temporal lobe degeneration).
- As the disease progresses there is a gradual decline in all aspects of cognitive ability over a variable period of around 5–15 years, together with changes in mood, personality and behaviour.
- The frontal variant of Alzheimer's disease is characterized by striking personality and behavioural changes. In posterior cortical atrophy the clinical picture is dominated by visuospatial problems, with relative preservation of memory and language.

Risk factors

The most important risk factor for Alzheimer's disease, apart from advancing age, is possession of a particular variant of the **Apolipoprotein E gene** (*APOE*) on chromosome 19 (discussed below). It is also more common in people with **ischaemic heart disease**, in those with limited educational attainments or lower socioeconomic status – and in association with previous head injury (Clinical Box 12.4).

Familial clustering of *APOE* alleles, together with a large number of unknown **susceptibility genes**, may help to explain the observation that Alzheimer's disease is more common in people with an affected parent or sibling and that concordance rates are significantly higher in identical twins.

Apolipoprotein E

There are three common ***APOE* alleles**: epsilon-2 (*APOE2*), epsilon-3 (*APOE3*) and epsilon-4 (*APOE4*). These encode a lipoprotein that is involved in plasma lipid transport, including the uptake and distribution of cholesterol. ***APOE4*** is associated with a higher incidence of sporadic Alzheimer's disease, such that two copies of the allele increase risk approximately 20-fold and more than 50% of patients with Alzheimer's disease have at least one copy. In contrast, ***APOE2*** appears to be protective. The role of **Apolipoprotein E** in the pathogenesis of Alzheimer's disease is incompletely understood, but it has been shown to bind to and influence the removal of **amyloid beta peptide** from the brain, accumulation of which is a key event in the pathogenesis of Alzheimer's disease (discussed below).

Other genetic factors

Possession of a rare variant of the ***TREM2*** gene (triggering receptor expressed on myeloid cells 2) on chromosome 6 is associated with a three-fold increase in Alzheimer's disease risk. The mechanism is uncertain at present, but the gene is involved in **microglial activation** and **brain inflammation**, providing an important clue to pathogenesis in sporadic disease.

Genome-wide analysis has revealed **single nucleotide polymorphisms** or **SNPs** ('snips') in three genes that may be associated with modestly increased risk of Alzheimer's disease: ***CLU*** (clusterin or Apolipoprotein J); ***PICALM*** (phosphatidylinositol-binding clathrin assembly protein); and ***CR1*** (complement component 3b/4b receptor 1).

The associations of these SNPs are much weaker than for *APOE* but are most significant for the related gene *CLU*. Both encode apolipoprotein molecules that bind amyloid beta and are involved in its clearance from the brain: **ApoE** protein promotes amyloid beta clearance, whereas

ApoJ is involved in its uptake into the brain from the bloodstream.

Protective factors

Alzheimer's disease is more common in females, even after accounting for greater longevity, and **hormone-replacement therapy** (**HRT**) may be protective in post-menopausal women. Moderate consumption of alcohol also appears to be beneficial, together with regular mental, physical and social activities. It has been claimed that use of **non-steroidal anti-inflammatory drugs** (**NSAIDs**) is associated with a reduced risk, but clinical trials have failed to show a protective effect.

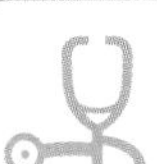

Clinical Box 12.4: Dementia pugilistica

Dementia pugilistica or '**punch drunk**' **syndrome** is a form of acquired cognitive impairment that occurs in up to a fifth of professional boxers (Latin: pugilator, boxer). It also occurs in other sports in which there may be mild head trauma, such as football and horse racing. The microscopic features are similar to Alzheimer's disease, but the anatomical distribution is different. Pathology is often found in the **substantia nigra** of the midbrain and cognitive decline may be combined with features of **Parkinson's disease** (in which nigral degeneration is a key pathological feature; see Ch. 13).

Key Points

- The most important risk factor for Alzheimer's disease (apart from advancing age) is possession of one or more copies of the *APOE4* allele, which is present in more than 50% of patients.
- Alzheimer's disease is also more common in people with ischaemic heart disease, in those with limited educational attainments, lower socioeconomic status or a history of head injury.
- It is more common in females and hormone-replacement may be beneficial in post-menopausal women. The positive effect of anti-inflammatory drugs is unproven.
- Moderate consumption of alcohol may also be beneficial, together with regular mental, physical and social activities.

Pathological features

Post-mortem examination of the brain in Alzheimer's disease shows reduced brain weight, with **cortical atrophy** and **enlarged ventricles**. Loss of brain tissue is often particularly obvious in the medial temporal lobes and hippocampi and there may be marked thinning of the cerebral cortex with widening of the sulci. Microscopic examination shows characteristic 'plaques' and 'tangles'.

Plaques (Fig. 12.5)

A pathological hallmark of Alzheimer's disease is the presence of **plaques** in the cerebral cortex, consisting of insoluble protein aggregates. Plaques are found in the extracellular space (between neurons) and are predominantly composed of **amyloid beta peptide** (**Aβ**). Like all forms of amyloid, the deposits take up the tissue stain **Congo red** and show apple-green birefringence under polarized light (see Ch. 8). Plaques can be identified using silver staining, but are best demonstrated using **immunohistochemistry** (antibody labelling).

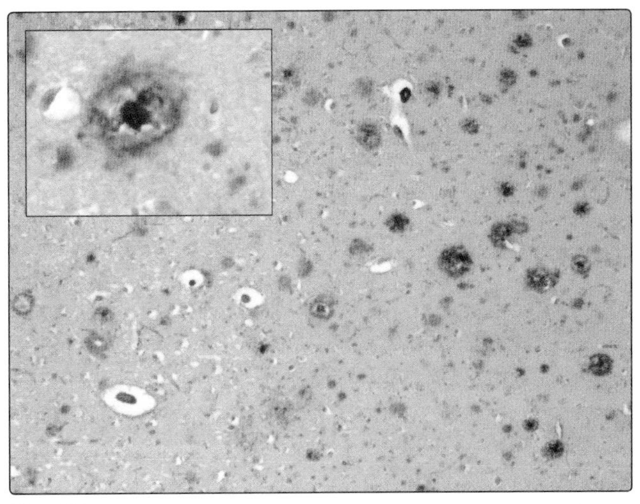

Fig. 12.5 **Cortical plaques in Alzheimer's disease.** This micrograph demonstrates extensive amyloid beta deposits (amyloid plaques) in the cerebral cortex of a person who died of Alzheimer's disease. *Inset*: a single 'cored plaque' with a dense central core of amyloid is shown at higher magnification [immunohistochemical preparation for Aβ peptide].

Although widespread, plaques are most common in the **hippocampus**, **entorhinal cortex** and **amygdala**. They are found in moderate numbers in frontal, parietal and temporal **association cortices**, but are uncommon in the primary sensory and motor areas. There are two main types:

- **Diffuse plaques** are composed of amyloid beta peptide in a non-fibrillary (non-amyloid) form and may be numerous in older people who do not have dementia.
- **Neuritic plaques** are surrounded by abnormal dystrophic neurites (thickened, tortuous neuronal processes) and sometimes have a dense, central core of amyloid ('cored plaques'; see Fig. 12.5).

Unlike diffuse plaques, neuritic plaques are strongly associated with cognitive decline. Aβ is also deposited in the walls of blood vessels, leading to **cerebral amyloid angiopathy** (Clinical Box 12.5).

Neurofibrillary tangles (Fig. 12.6)

The second major pathological finding in Alzheimer's disease is the **neurofibrillary tangle** (**NFT**). This is a **filamentous inclusion** composed of the microtubule-associated protein **tau**, which is normally present in axons (see Ch.5).

Tangles are best demonstrated by immunohistochemistry for tau. They are found in the cytoplasm of surviving neurons and may persist after a neuron has died to form a **ghost**

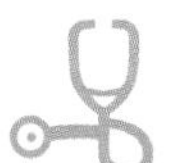

Clinical Box 12.5: Cerebral amyloid angiopathy

Aβ is deposited in cortical blood vessels in 90% of patients with Alzheimer's disease, which is termed **cerebral amyloid angiopathy** (**CAA**) (see Ch. 8, Fig. 8.14). Amyloid deposition leads to degeneration of vascular smooth muscle, weakening the vessel wall and predisposing to **microinfarctions** and **intracerebral haemorrhage** (see Ch. 10, Fig. 10.2B). CAA can occur in the absence of dementia and accounts for a quarter of intracerebral haemorrhages in the elderly. The bleeding is superficial or 'cortical' rather than deep (in contrast to hypertension-related haemorrhages, which frequently occur in the region of the basal ganglia).

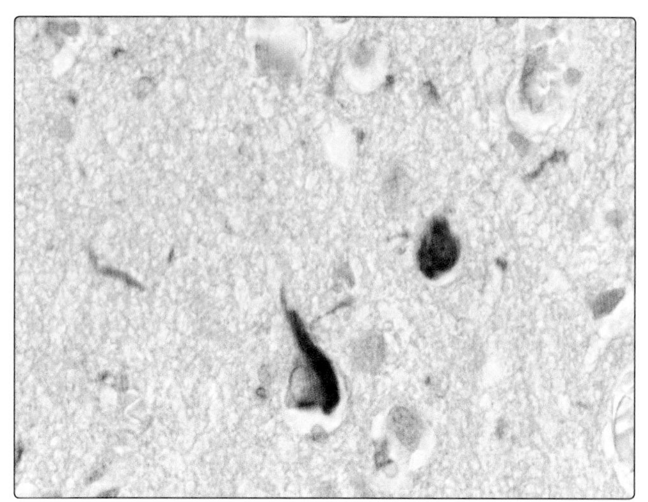

Fig. 12.6 **Neurofibrillary tangles in Alzheimer's disease.** Micrograph showing two cortical neurons containing neurofibrillary tangles. The small, rounded inclusion (right) is a 'globose' tangle whilst the larger, more pyramidal-shaped inclusion (left) is a 'flame' tangle. The different appearances of the pathological inclusions reflect the shape of the neuronal cell body, which is filled with abnormal tau protein. A few fine 'neuropil threads' can also be seen, representing neuronal processes filled with tau [immunohistochemistry for hyperphosphorylated tau protein].

tangle in the extracellular space. Tau-positive inclusions are also found in dystrophic neurites (in 'neuritic' plaques) and in other abnormal neuronal processes, as **neuropil threads**.

Tau is a **phosphoprotein** with 79 serine and threonine phosphorylation sites, less than half of which are normally phosphorylated. Neurofibrillary tangles contain hyperphosphorylated tau in the form of **paired helical filaments** (**PHFs**) that resemble twisted ribbons (Fig. 12.7).

Neuronal and synaptic loss

Quantitative post-mortem studies in patients with Alzheimer's disease have shown significant neuronal loss in the hippocampus and medial temporal lobe. The **entorhinal cortex** is particularly affected, with more than 90% neuronal loss in advanced Alzheimer's disease. This area gives rise to the **perforant path** (a major afferent projection to the hippocampus, see Ch. 3), meaning that the hippocampus is effectively 'disconnected' from the neocortex in Alzheimer's disease.

More widespread loss of nerve cells and synaptic connections is found throughout the cerebral cortex and there is a reduction in the number of **dendritic spines** (see Ch. 5). Cell death also occurs in the brain stem, including the noradrenergic **loci coerulei** (singular: locus coeruleus) in the pons, which are normally pigmented but appear pale in Alzheimer's disease.

Profound neuronal loss occurs in **Meynert's nucleus**, a large cholinergic nucleus in the base of each cerebral hemisphere which contributes to the diffuse neurochemical system for **acetylcholine** (see Ch. 1). Degeneration of this projection (which diffusely innervates the neocortex and hippocampus) has a negative impact on memory, attention and cognition. For this reason, agents that potentiate cholinergic neurotransmission may improve symptoms in Alzheimer's disease (see below).

Pathogenesis of Alzheimer's disease

Accumulation of **amyloid beta** is widely believed to be a key initiating event in the development of Alzheimer's disease.

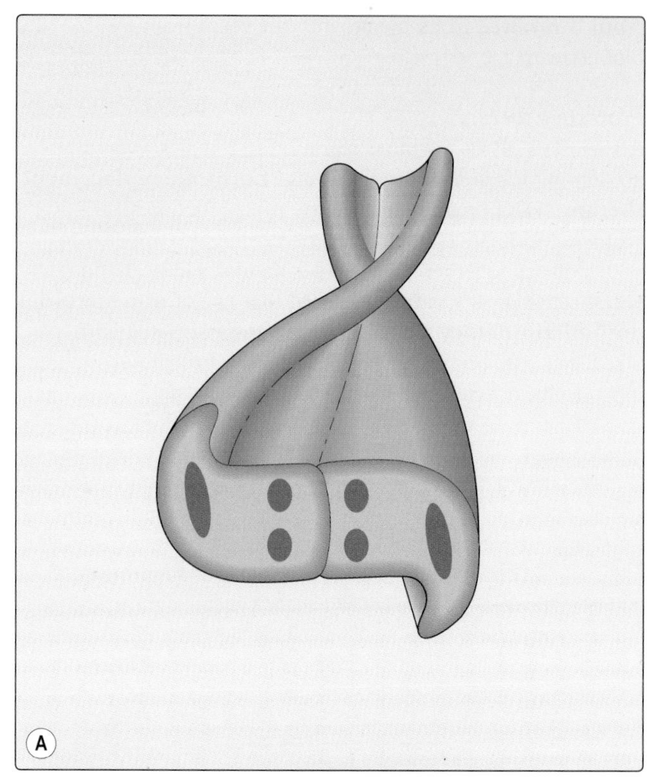

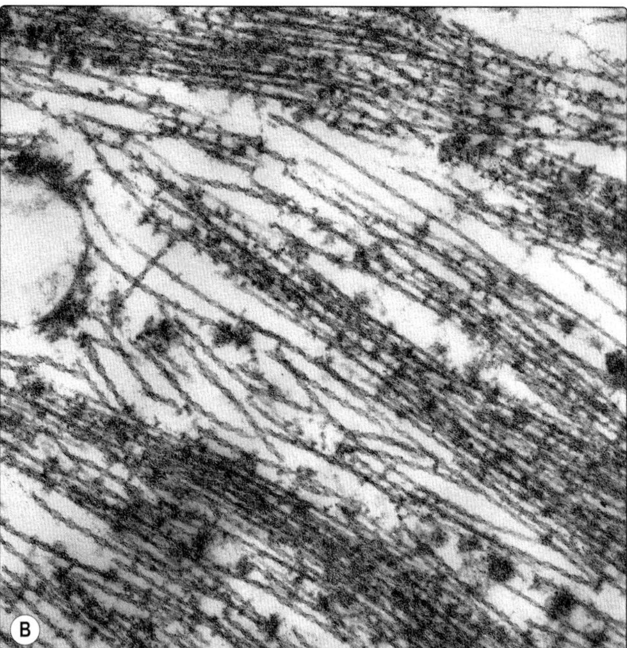

Fig. 12.7 **Paired helical filament (PHF) tau forms neuronal inclusions in Alzheimer's disease and other neurodegenerative conditions.** **(A)** Illustration showing the twisted structure of PHF-tau, which has a diameter of 22 nm and a periodicity of 80 nm; **(B)** An electron micrograph showing paired helical filament tau. From Ellison and Love: Neuropathology 2e (Mosby 2003) with permission.

This appears to trigger a cascade of pathological events in the neuron, leading to tau hyperphosphorylation and tangle formation: the **amyloid cascade hypothesis**. Neuronal injury is thought to be mediated by a combination of cytopathic mechanisms including oxidative stress, excitotoxicity and inflammation, culminating in programmed cell death (see Ch. 8).

Formation of amyloid beta

Amyloid beta is a soluble peptide of 40 or 42 amino acids (Aβ40, Aβ42). It is produced by proteolytic cleavage of

amyloid precursor protein (**APP**) (Fig. 12.8A). This is a large transmembrane protein that appears to be involved in synaptic plasticity and learning. There are six isoforms of APP in the human brain, composed of 695–770 amino acids (depending on alternative splicing). It has a single intramembranous portion, a large extracellular domain and a short cytoplasmic tail. The Aβ sequence is partly contained in the intramembranous portion.

Key Points

- Pathological changes in Alzheimer's disease include brain atrophy, ventricular enlargement and cortical thinning. Microscopic examination shows plaques and tangles in the cortex.
- Diffuse and neuritic plaques are composed of Aβ, which is deposited in the extracellular compartment (between nerve cells) as insoluble aggregates.
- Neurofibrillary tangles occupy the neuronal cytoplasm and are composed of insoluble filamentous aggregates of hyperphosphorylated tau protein, arranged as paired helical filaments.
- The cortex shows widespread loss of neurons, synapses and dendritic spines and a global reduction in cholinergic neurotransmission (due to severe degeneration of Meynert's nucleus).
- More than 90% of patients with Alzheimer's disease also have deposition of amyloid beta in cortical blood vessels, leading to cerebral amyloid angiopathy (CAA).

Amyloid processing

There are two APP processing pathways (Fig. 12.9) mediated by a family of proteolytic enzymes called **secretases** (see also Fig. 12.8B). The pathogenic Aβ fragment is released from APP by sequential beta and gamma secretase cleavage. The C-terminal fragment is released into the cytoplasm and is involved in nuclear signalling. APP is encoded on chromosome 21, which accounts for the high incidence of Alzheimer-type changes in people with **Down's syndrome** (trisomy 21) who have an extra copy of the chromosome. This leads to increased production of Aβ, associated with a greater than 50% chance that the brain will contain plaques and tangles by early middle age.

Primary (alpha) pathway

The **primary pathway** for APP processing involves sequential activity of **alpha** and **gamma secretase** (Fig. 12.9A). Alpha secretase releases a large **soluble APP fragment** into the extracellular fluid. This is followed by gamma secretase cleavage, which acts on the intramembranous portion of APP. The cleavage point of alpha secretase falls in the middle of the Aβ sequence, thereby destroying the pathogenic peptide. The primary pathway is therefore **non-amyloidogenic** and since it is dominant, very little Aβ is normally produced in the brain.

Alternative (beta) pathway

This pathway involves the sequential action of **beta** and **gamma secretases**. It liberates amyloid beta from APP and is therefore potentially amyloidogenic (Fig. 12.9B). **Beta-secretase** cleaves APP at the distal end of the Aβ sequence and gamma secretase acts at the proximal end (within the plasma membrane). The alternative pathway releases either a 40 or 42 amino acid species of amyloid beta.

Ratio of Aβ40 to Aβ42

This is determined by the multi-protein **gamma-secretase complex** that includes the enzymes **presenilin-1** and **presenilin-2** (**PS-1** and **PS-2**) and affects the pattern and distribution of the pathological changes. Aβ42 tends to form plaques in the cerebral cortex and is more associated with dementia. The more soluble Aβ40 fragment is frequently deposited in blood vessels, causing **cerebral amyloid angiopathy**. Several inherited forms of Alzheimer's

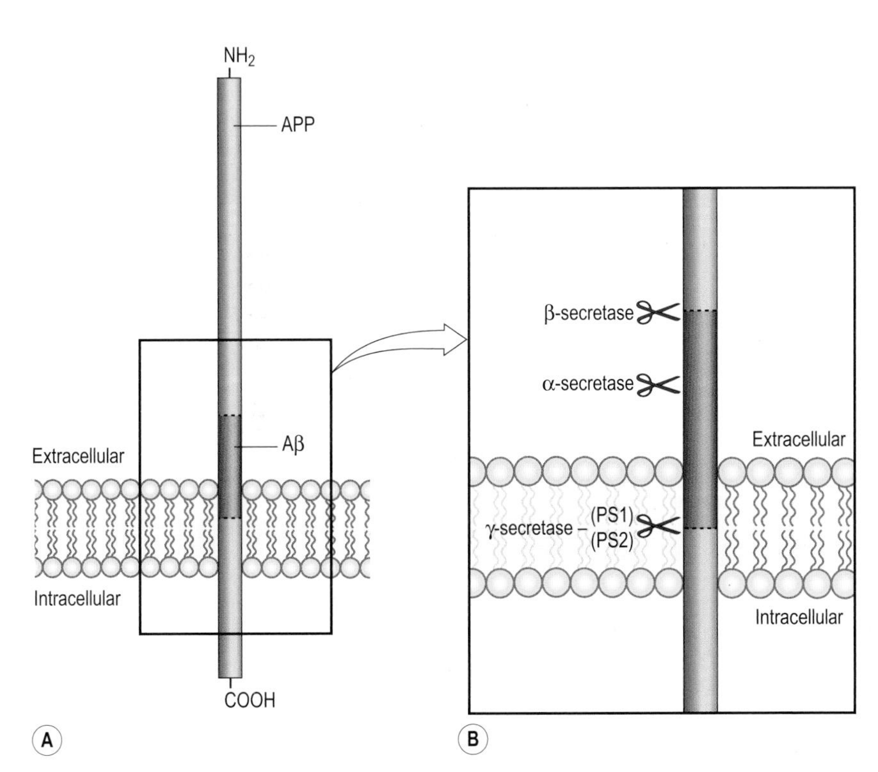

Fig. 12.8 **Amyloid precursor protein (APP). (A)** The sequence corresponding to the amyloid beta peptide (Aβ) is shown in red, partially embedded in the neuronal plasma membrane; **(B)** A closer view, showing the sites of action of the main APP processing enzymes. Gamma-secretase is a multi-subunit integral membrane protein that includes the enzymes presenilin-1 and presenilin-2 (PS1/PS2).

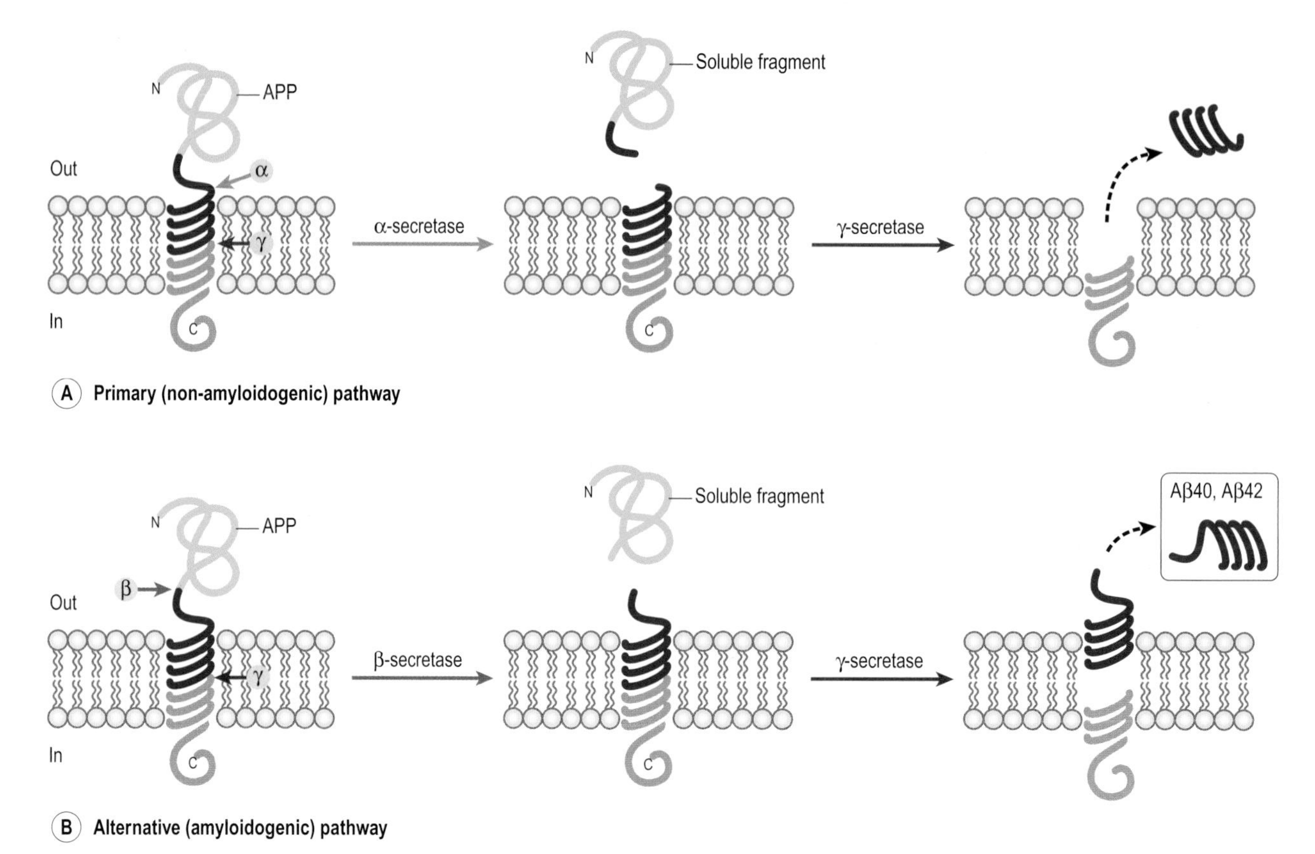

Fig. 12.9 **Processing of amyloid precursor protein. (A)** The primary (alpha) pathway involves sequential cleavage by alpha and gamma secretases, which destroys the pathogenic (Aβ) fragment and is therefore non-amyloidogenic; **(B)** The alternative (beta) pathway involves sequential cleavage by beta and gamma secretases, which releases the pathogenic Aβ species. The alternative pathway is therefore potentially amyloidogenic.

Key Points

- Deposition of Aβ in the cerebral cortex is believed to be a key initiating event in the development of Alzheimer's disease, leading to tau hyperphosphorylation and tangle formation within neurons (the 'amyloid cascade hypothesis').
- Aβ is produced by proteolytic cleavage of the precursor molecule APP. Processing via the primary (alpha secretase) pathway is dominant and does not lead to Aβ release.
- Processing via the alternative (beta secretase) pathway releases soluble Aβ peptide. The ratio of Aβ40:Aβ42 is determined by the gamma secretase complex.
- The less soluble Aβ42 tends to form cortical plaques and is more associated with dementia, whereas Aβ40 deposition in blood vessels leads to cerebral amyloid angiopathy.

disease involve mutations in genes concerned with **APP processing** that increase the amount of Aβ (or Aβ42) (Clinical Box 12.6).

Formation of neurofibrillary tangles

The next step in the 'amyloid cascade' is abnormal phosphorylation of the microtubule-associated protein **tau.** This normally binds to (and stabilizes) axonal microtubules, but in its hyperphosphorylated form, tau dissociates from microtubules and tends to self-aggregate (Fig. 12.10). This may reflect excessive activity in **tau kinases** (which add phosphate groups to proteins) such as **glycogen synthase kinase 3-beta (GSK-3β)** and **cyclin-dependent kinase 5 (CDK5)** but the mechanism is not certain.

Clinical Box 12.6: Familial Alzheimer's disease

Familial Alzheimer's disease (FAD) accounts for only 5% of cases, but has provided invaluable insights into the pathogenesis of sporadic disease. All forms show **autosomal dominant** inheritance with a high degree of penetrance. Presentation is usually below the age of 65 and the term **early-onset Alzheimer's disease** is therefore used. Most cases of familial Alzheimer's disease are due to mutations in one of the three main genes involved in amyloid processing:

- ***APP***, on chromosome 21, which encodes amyloid precursor protein.
- ***PSEN1***, on chromosome 14, which encodes presenilin-1 (PS-1).
- ***PSEN2***, on chromosome 1, which encodes presenilin-2 (PS-2).

Mutations in the genes for PS-1 or PS-2 account for nearly half of familial Alzheimer's disease cases. There is usually increased Aβ production, with alteration of the **Aβ40:Aβ42 ratio**, so that more of the plaque-forming **Aβ42** species is produced. In many FAD families with known mutations in the *APP* gene, the region of the protein flanking the amyloid beta sequence is affected, which is also associated with increased Aβ42 production. This is in contrast to mutations affecting the central portion of the amyloid sequence, which are more likely to cause cerebral amyloid angiopathy.

Once dissociated from microtubules, monomers of phosphorylated tau aggregate into **protofilaments (oligomers)** and then **filaments**, eventually forming mature neurofibrillary tangles. The spread of tangle pathology through the brain follows six **Braak stages**, which can be divided into early, intermediate and late phases (Fig. 12.11).

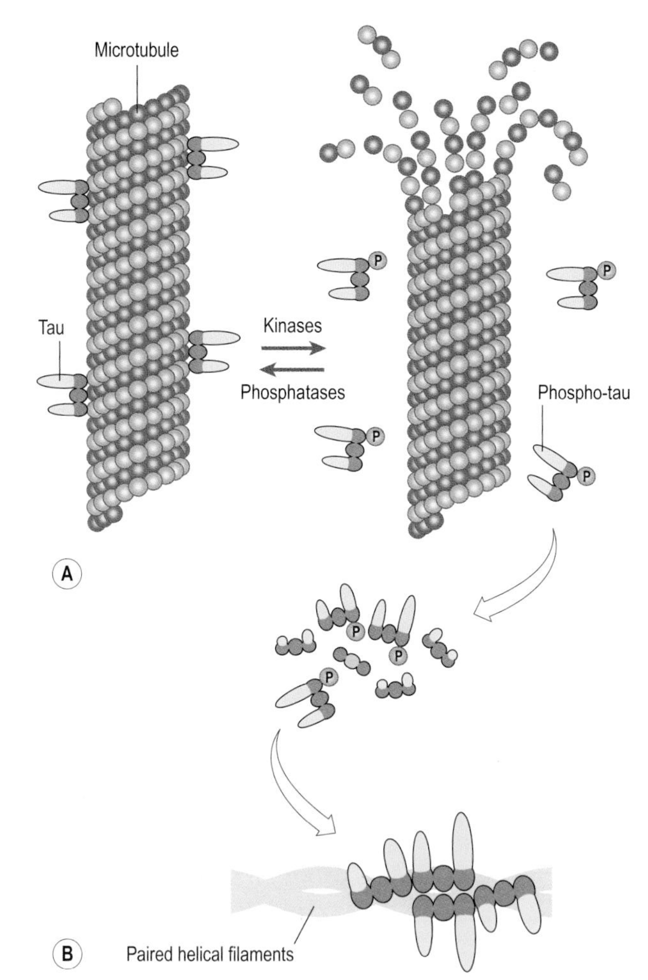

Fig. 12.10 **Tau is a microtubule-associated protein (MAP) that is normally found predominantly in axons. (A)** In its unphosphorylated state, tau binds to microtubules and helps to stabilize them. Phosphorylation is regulated by the activity of kinases (which add phosphate groups) and phosphatases (which remove them); **(B)** Hyperphosphorylated tau monomers dissociate from microtubules and, at sufficient concentrations, tend to self-aggregate to form paired helical filament tau (the main constituent of neurofibrillary tangles).

Tangles first appear in the **entorhinal cortex** and **hippocampus** (Braak stages I–II) during the presymptomatic phase of the disease. Pathology gradually spreads to involve more of the **limbic lobe**, **amygdala** and neighbouring **fusiform gyrus** in the intermediate phase (Braak stages III–IV). This is likely to correspond to incipient dementia or mild cognitive impairment. Clinical dementia appears as tangle pathology extends to the **association areas** of the neocortex (Braak stage V) and finally to the **primary sensory** and **motor areas** (Braak stage VI).

Amyloid beta clearance

In normal individuals, small amounts of Aβ are continuously produced and eliminated. Abnormal build-up of Aβ may therefore reflect increased production, decreased elimination or some alteration in the balance between these two processes. Excessive production of Aβ is implicated in a small minority of cases (e.g. in **Down's syndrome** and in **familial Alzheimer's disease** associated with mutations of *PSEN1*, *PSEN2* or *APP*) but in the vast majority of sporadic disease, failure of Aβ clearance appears to be the most important factor.

Key Points

- Mutations in the presenilin or APP genes are responsible for most inherited (autosomal dominant) early-onset forms of Alzheimer's disease. In all cases there is excessive Aβ production.
- Deposition of Aβ in the cerebral cortex (particularly Aβ42) appears to trigger a cascade of events within neurons, leading to the accumulation of hyperphosphorylated tau.
- Tau hyperphosphorylation is thought to be mediated by an imbalance between phosphatases and kinases, with excessive activity of tau kinases such as CDK5 and GSK-3β.
- Neurofibrillary tangles first appear in the medial temporal lobe (hippocampus, entorhinal cortex) and spread progressively throughout the limbic lobe and neocortex in six Braak stages.

Mechanisms for Aβ removal

Several enzymes have been identified in the brain and within the walls of arteries that contribute to the elimination of amyloid beta, including **neprilysin** and **insulin-degrading enzyme** (**IDE**). Many other enzymes are capable of degrading Aβ and may contribute to its clearance, including some that are typically associated with other roles (e.g. angiotensin converting enzyme). Export of Aβ from the brain, across the blood–brain barrier, is mediated by a **low-density lipoprotein-receptor-related protein** (**LRP-1**) in the endothelium of cerebral blood vessels.

The efficacy of enzyme degradation and export to the bloodstream declines in the elderly, in whom the much slower process of **perivascular drainage** may be more important. This is less effective in stiff, **arteriosclerotic** blood vessels (since there is reduced transmission of arterial pulsations that encourage bulk flow of perivascular fluid) which helps to explain the association between dementia and ischaemic heart disease.

Pathological effects of amyloid beta

The degree of cognitive decline correlates poorly with the amount of insoluble (plaque-associated) Aβ deposited in the cerebral cortex, but is strongly associated with (i) the extent of **tangle pathology** and (ii) the **soluble Aβ fraction**. This raises the possibility that a **prefibrillar species** of amyloid (contained in the soluble fraction) may be primarily responsible for neurotoxicity in Alzheimer's disease, leading to the formation of neurofibrillary tangles. This raises the possibility that amyloid plaques may therefore be protective rather than harmful, representing an attempt by the cell to 'trap' potentially neurotoxic components as insoluble aggregates.

Toxic oligomeric species

Soluble Aβ monomers self-aggregate to form **oligomers** which associate with the cell membrane and form ring-like arrangements with an aqueous pore. This is similar to the **membrane attack complex** of the complement cascade. Pore formation compromises the neuronal plasma membrane, admitting sodium, water and free calcium ions, which damage the cell. Excessive influx of calcium, in particular, is known to be a final common pathway in many forms of neuronal cell death. There is also evidence that Aβ oligomers: (i) are toxic to mitochondria, increasing **oxidative stress** and lowering the threshold for **apoptosis**; (ii) may contribute to the formation of neurofibrillary tangles within nerve cells, by promoting **hyperphosphorylation of tau**; and (iii) appear to cause **synaptic dysfunction** and loss.

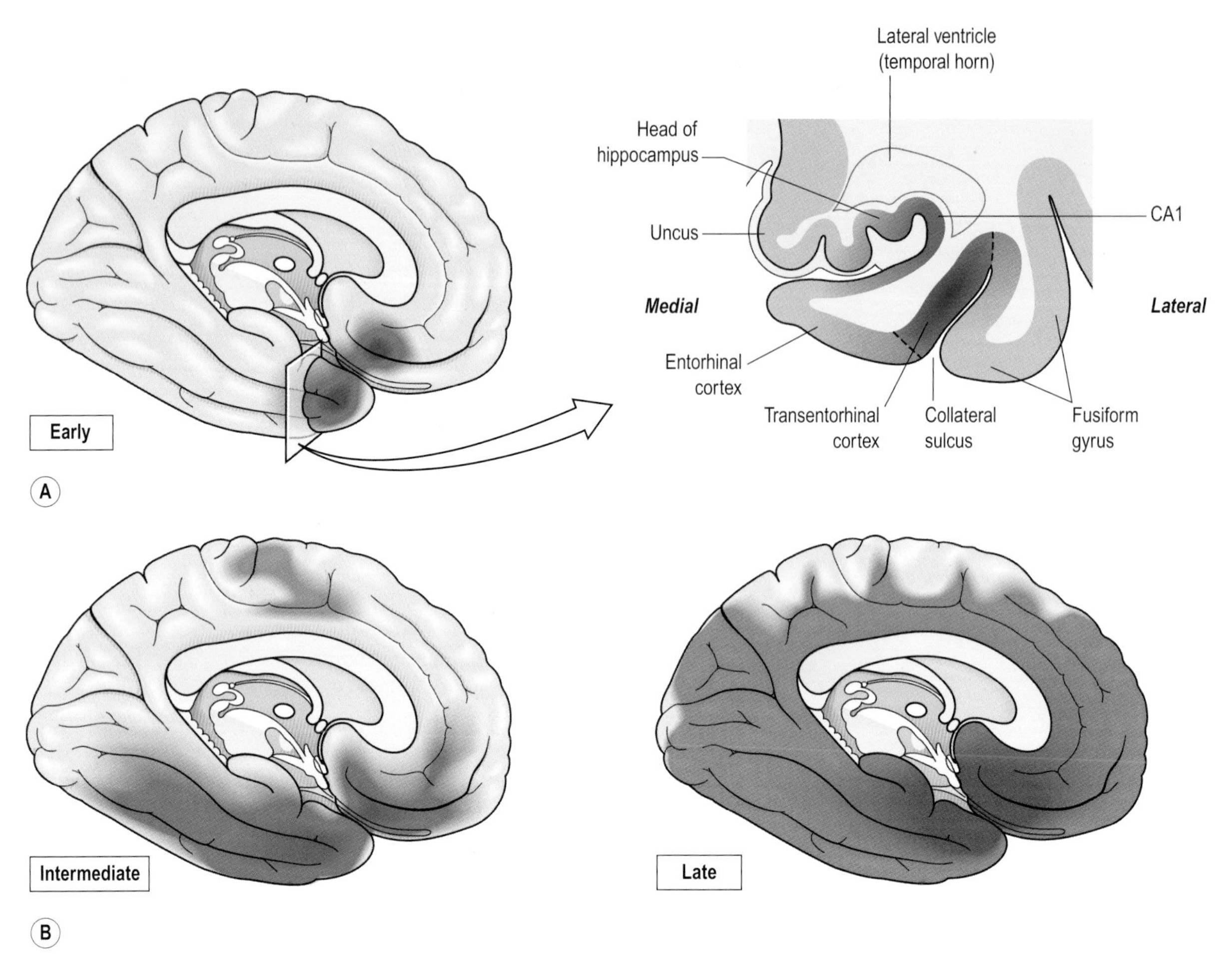

Fig. 12.11 **Progression of tangle pathology in Alzheimer's disease. (A)** Coronal section through the temporal lobe showing the distribution of tangle pathology in early (Braak I–II) Alzheimer's disease. The earliest and most severely affected area (between the dashed lines) is the transentorhinal cortex; **(B)** Progression of tangle pathology in the intermediate (Braak III–IV) and late (Braak V–VI) stages.

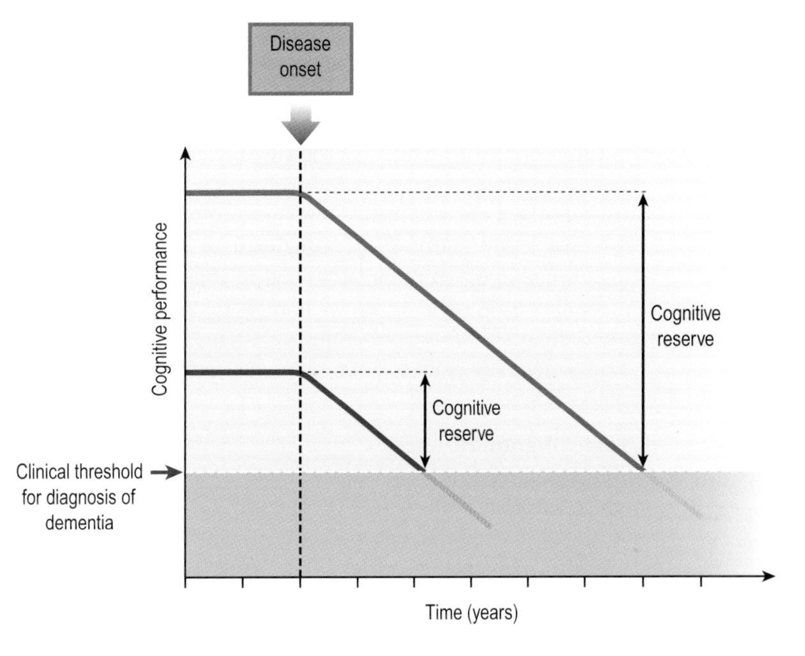

Fig. 12.12 **The concept of cognitive reserve.** Individuals of average intelligence (red line) may show clinical signs of dementia much earlier after disease onset than people with a higher degree of premorbid intelligence or education (purple line), assuming that the rate of progression is similar.

Pathological ageing and cognitive reserve

Post-mortem studies have shown that the typical pathological changes of Alzheimer's disease are present to a greater or lesser extent in many elderly people with no history of dementia. This is referred to as **pathological ageing**. In some cases the pathology is advanced, despite no evidence of cognitive decline during life. This is thought to reflect greater **cognitive reserve** capacity in some people, due to higher levels of premorbid intelligence or education (Fig. 12.12).

Treatment of Alzheimer's disease

No agents are currently available that can reverse or halt the progression of Alzheimer's disease. Treatment is therefore limited to symptomatic and supportive measures.

> *Key Points*
> - In normal individuals a small amount of Aβ is continuously produced and eliminated.
> - Mechanisms for removal include enzymatic degradation and active transport into the bloodstream (which decline with age) and perivascular drainage (which also declines with age and is less effective in people with cerebrovascular disease).
> - The mechanism by which Aβ damages neurons is not entirely certain, but Aβ oligomers are known to be associated with neuronal membranes and form pore-like structures (similar to those of the membrane attack complex) which admit sodium, water and calcium into the cell.
> - Other potential mechanisms of Aβ toxicity include mitochondrial dysfunction, oxidative stress, promotion of tau hyperphosphorylation and disruption of synapses.
> - Alzheimer-type changes are present to a variable extent in many cognitively normal older people, which is thought to reflect greater cognitive reserve capacity.

Pharmacological agents

The cholinergic deficit in Alzheimer's disease contributes to memory impairment and can be improved to some degree by **cholinesterase inhibitors** (e.g. donepezil, rivastigmine, galantamine). These drugs potentiate cholinergic transmission by inhibiting acetylcholine degradation in the synaptic cleft. Modest benefit is seen in at least 50% of patients with mild to moderate dementia, but the improvement usually lasts less than 12 months. Side effects include diarrhoea, nausea and vomiting.

A second agent used in patients with Alzheimer's disease is **memantine**, an NMDA receptor antagonist that inhibits glutamatergic neurotransmission (see Ch. 7). The mechanism is uncertain, but may include protection against neuronal calcium overload. Clinical trials have shown some benefit in patients with moderate dementia, but not in those with mild cognitive decline.

Disease-modifying agents

A number of potential **disease-modifying agents** are currently in clinical trials, most of which aim to interfere with amyloid processing or tangle formation; strategies include:

- **Immunotherapy** (**Aβ vaccination**) to trigger an active immune response that will remove deposits of amyloid beta peptide from the brain (see below).
- **Passive immunization with anti-Aβ antibodies**, which also aims to remove amyloid deposits from the brain, but does not generate a lasting immunological response.
- **Inhibition of beta-secretase**, to block processing of APP in the alternative (amyloidogenic) pathway and therefore reduce Aβ production.
- **Inhibition of amyloid fibril formation**, preventing the molecular progression of the disease or blocking formation of a toxic prefibrillary species.
- **Inhibition of tau aggregation**, e.g. by the experimental agent methylthioninium chloride (methylene blue) which has shown encouraging results in clinical trials.
- **Inhibition/modulation of gamma-secretase** (e.g. PS-1/PS-2 inhibitors) altering the ratio of Aβ40 to Aβ42 so that less pathogenic (plaque-forming) Aβ42 is produced.

One of the most promising approaches to date has been **Aβ vaccination**, which has achieved almost complete plaque clearance in mouse models. Follow-up post-mortem studies in patients with Alzheimer's disease have confirmed some degree of plaque clearance, but: (i) only 20% of patients generate anti-Aβ antibodies; (ii) the improvement in cognitive state is minimal; and (iii) severe **meningoencephalitis** (inflammation of the brain and its coverings) occurs in 1 in 20 people. Theoretical concerns have also been raised that disrupting plaques may release harmful oligomeric species.

> *Key Points*
> - No disease-modifying treatments are currently available for Alzheimer's disease, but some symptomatic improvement can be gained using cholinesterase inhibitors or memantine.
> - Potential disease-modifying strategies include: (i) inhibition of beta secretase to reduce Aβ production; (ii) interference with amyloid fibril formation/maturation; and (iii) inhibition/modulation of gamma secretase to alter the ratio of Aβ40 to Aβ42.
> - Active immunotherapy (Aβ vaccination) has been very successful in animal models (achieving almost complete amyloid plaque clearance) but clinical trials have been disappointing.

Dementia with Lewy bodies

Dementia with Lewy bodies (DLB) is the second most common type of dementia after Alzheimer's disease, accounting for 20% of cases. It is predominantly sporadic, but rare familial forms with autosomal dominant inheritance have been described.

Clinical features

The three core elements of dementia with Lewy bodies (in addition to cognitive decline) are: (i) **visual hallucinations**; (ii) **fluctuation** in cognitive performance; and (iii) features of **parkinsonism**, such as tremor, rigidity and bradykinesia (see Ch. 13). Additional findings in support of the diagnosis include reduced dopamine levels in the basal ganglia or a **sleep disorder** (Clinical Box 12.7).

Around 50% of patients with DLB are highly sensitive to **neuroleptics** (antipsychotic agents) which act by antagonizing central dopamine receptors; this leads to severe muscular rigidity with immobility and confusion. Another common feature in patients with DLB is **autonomic dysfunction** including **postural hypotension** with fainting and falls. A proportion of patients exhibit frankly **psychotic features**, with hallucinations and delusions.

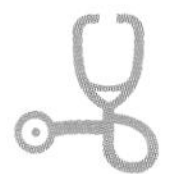

> *Clinical Box 12.7: Sleep disorders in DLB*
>
> Dementia with Lewy bodies may be associated with a number of sleep disorders including vivid dreams and nightmares. A characteristic feature occurs during **rapid eye movement** (**REM**) sleep, the phase during which dreaming is most likely to take place. This is called **REM sleep behaviour disorder** and is characterized by 'acting out' dreams or sleepwalking. It is thought to be due to interference with the normal brain stem mechanisms that ensure paralysis during sleep.

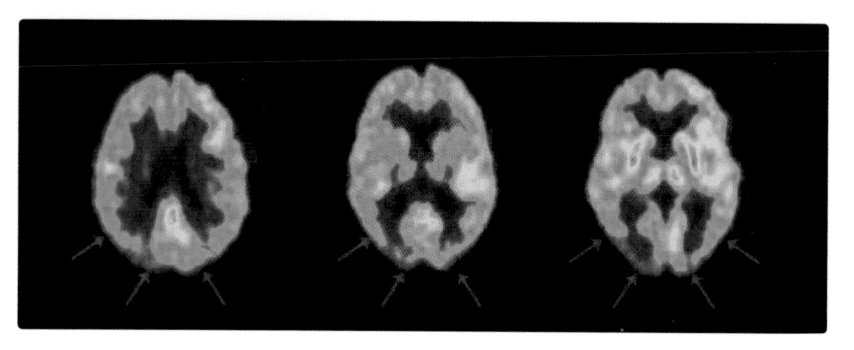

Fig. 12.13 **Functional neuroimaging in dementia with Lewy bodies (DLB).** Functional brain imaging in patients with DLB may show reduced glucose consumption (metabolism) in the occipital and posterior temporoparietal regions, as in this case. [The image was obtained by positron-emission tomography (PET) scanning, using ^{18}F-FDG, a positron-emitting isotope of glucose]. From Silverman, D et al: Positron emission tomography scans obtained for the evaluation of cognitive dysfunction. Seminars in Nuclear Medicine. Neuronuclear Imaging (2008, pp. 251–261) with permission.

Psychological testing and neuroimaging

Neuropsychological testing typically shows deficits in **attention** and frontal lobe **executive function** (such as planning, organizing and decision-making) and difficulty with **visuospatial tasks**. It may also confirm **fluctuation in cognitive performance** and attention. In contrast to Alzheimer's disease, there tends to be relative preservation of episodic memory.

Functional brain imaging often shows **reduced metabolism** and **cerebral blood flow** in the occipital and posterior temporoparietal regions (Fig. 12.13). This is in contrast to other forms of dementia in which the posterior hemisphere tends to be spared and may account for the prominent visual hallucinations in DLB.

> *Key Points*
>
> - DLB is the second most common type of dementia after Alzheimer's disease, accounting for around 20% of cases.
> - The core features, in addition to cognitive decline, are: visual hallucinations, fluctuation in cognitive performance and parkinsonism.
> - Up to 50% of patients show neuroleptic sensitivity and there may be autonomic dysfunction or sleep disorders including REM sleep behaviour disorder.

Pathological features

Macroscopic examination of the brain is often unremarkable but there may be generalized atrophy and dilation of the ventricles, with pallor of the substantia nigra (see Ch. 13, Fig. 13.5) and locus coeruleus (see Ch. 1). The microscopic features are indistinguishable from **Parkinson's disease with dementia** (**PDD**) and the distinction between PDD and DLB is purely clinical (see Ch. 13, Clinical Box 13.1).

Lewy bodies

Microscopic examination of the brain shows **pathological inclusions** (abnormal protein aggregates) in the cytoplasm of surviving neurons. These rounded intraneuronal structures, called **Lewy bodies**, appear bright pink on standard histological preparations (since they take up the red tissue dye **eosin**) and are often surrounded by a pale halo (Fig. 12.14A). Lewy bodies are best demonstrated by immunohistochemistry for **alpha-synuclein** protein, which is the major constituent (Fig. 12.14B). **Cortical Lewy bodies** are similar to those found in the brain stem, but lack a halo and are best seen on immunohistochemistry (Fig. 12.14C). Many patients also have some degree of Alzheimer's disease pathology (Fig. 12.14D) and there may be a **synergistic interaction** between alpha-synuclein and Aβ.

Progression of pathology

The pathological changes spread through the brain in a predictable fashion, analogous to the orderly progression of tangles in Alzheimer's disease (Fig. 12.15). Six **Braak stages** are described, which are the same as those in idiopathic Parkinson's disease (see also Ch. 13, Fig. 13.7). Synuclein-positive inclusions appear first in the **olfactory bulb** and **medulla** (**stage I**), before progressing to the **pons** (**stage II**) and **midbrain** (**stage III**). The first three stages are thus largely confined to the brain stem. Inclusions are next encountered in the limbic lobe, including the **entorhinal cortex** and **amygdala** (**stage IV**). The last two stages are neocortical, with inclusions in the higher-order **association cortices** (**stage V**) and finally in the **primary sensory** and **motor areas** (**stage VI**). The pathology and pathogenesis of the synuclein-related disorders (or **synucleinopathies**) is discussed further in Chapter 13.

> *Key Points*
>
> - The pathological features in dementia with Lewy bodies are indistinguishable from Parkinson's disease dementia, including widespread Lewy bodies (composed of alpha-synuclein protein).
> - Lewy bodies first appear in the olfactory bulb and medulla before progressively spreading to involve the midbrain, pons, limbic lobe, amygdala and neocortex (in six Braak stages).
> - Many patients also have variable Alzheimer-type changes and there appears to be a synergistic interaction between Aβ and alpha-synuclein.

Vascular dementia

Vascular dementia is the third most common cause of acquired cognitive decline in older people, accounting for approximately 10% of cases. The risk factors are the same as those for ischaemic heart disease and stroke (Fig. 12.16). The term **vascular cognitive impairment** is used to describe a non-progressive decline in intellectual ability with a vascular aetiology.

Clinical features

People with vascular dementia may show a step-wise loss of cognitive ability consistent with a series of strokes, referred to

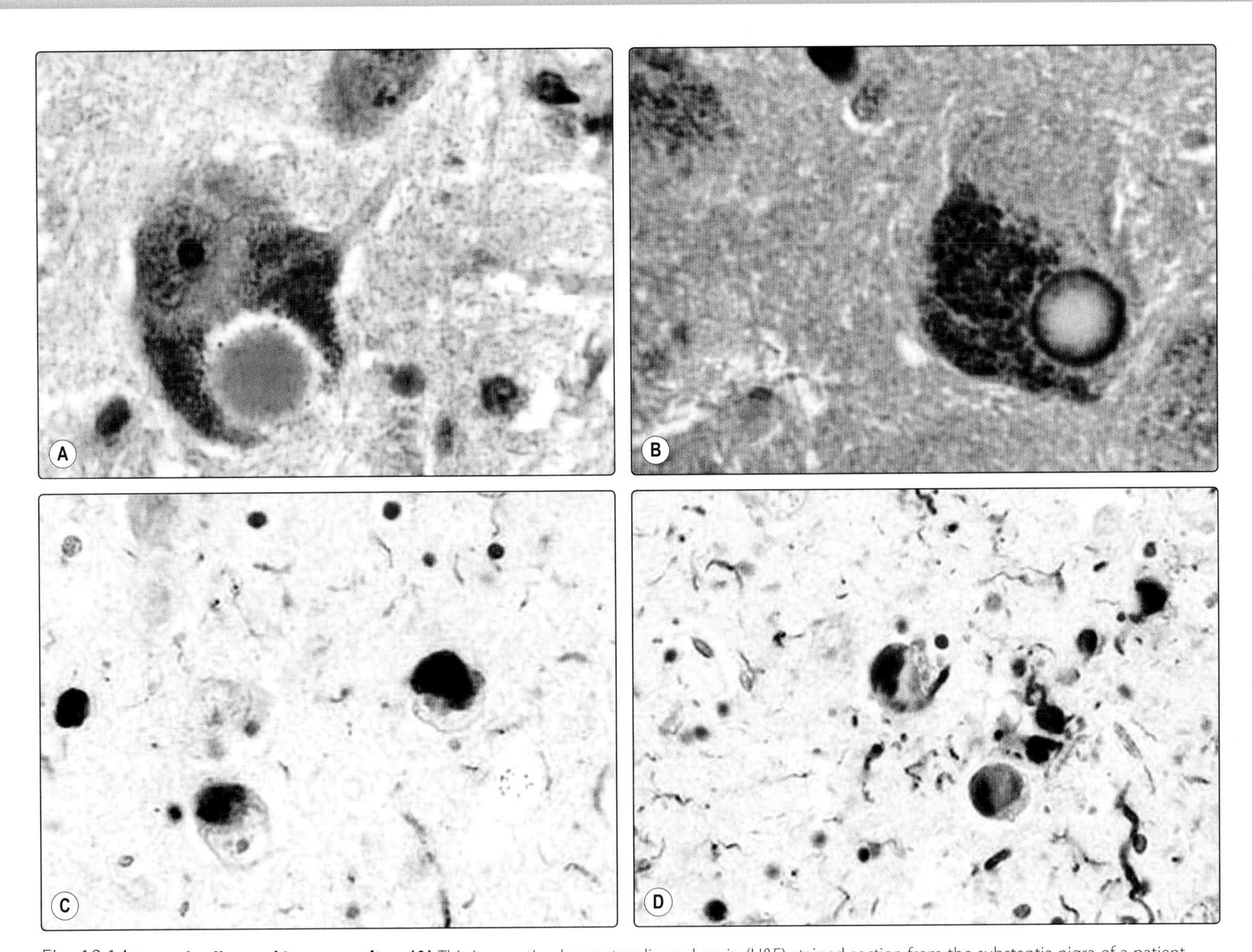

Fig. 12.14 **Lewy bodies and Lewy neurites. (A)** This is a routine haematoxylin and eosin (H&E)-stained section from the substantia nigra of a patient who had dementia with Lewy bodies (DLB). It shows a bright pink Lewy body in the neuronal cytoplasm, surrounded by brown neuromelanin pigment; **(B)** Lewy bodies can be demonstrated using immunohistochemistry (antibody labelling) for alpha-synuclein, which is the main protein constituent; **(C)** Cortical Lewy bodies are best detected by immunostaining for alpha-synuclein, in this case in the temporal lobe of a patient with DLB; **(D)** Immunohistochemistry for alpha-synuclein in a patient with Alzheimer's disease showing co-existing Lewy bodies and Lewy neurites in the temporal lobe. From Popescu, A and Lippa, CF: Parkinsonian syndromes: Parkinson's disease dementia, dementia with Lewy bodies and progressive supranuclear palsy. Clinical Neuroscience Research, Non-Alzheimer's Disease Dementias (2004, pp. 461–468) with permission.

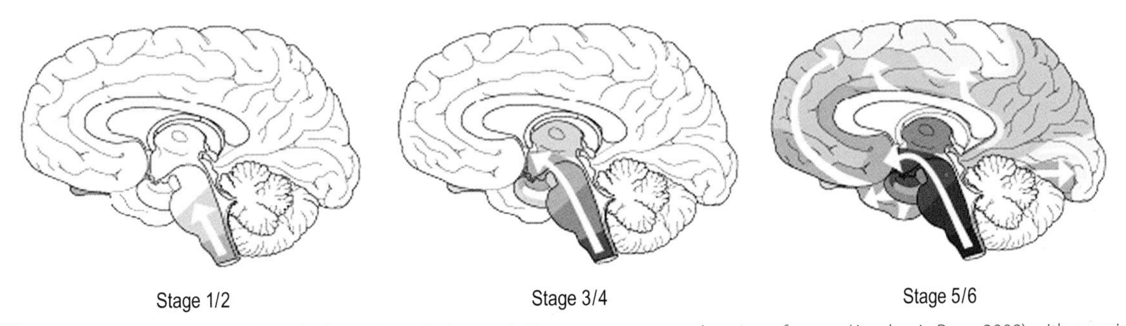

Fig. 12.15 **Progression of Lewy body pathology.** From Basbaum, A: The senses: a comprehensive reference (Academic Press 2008) with permission.

as **multi-infarct dementia** (Fig. 12.17). In others, the decline is more gradual and is dominated by generalized slowing of cognition with disturbed frontal executive function (i.e. bradyphrenia or 'subcortical-type' dementia). This is often due to **diffuse white matter disease**, sometimes referred to as Binswanger's encephalopathy (pronounced: BINSE-vangers).

Distinction from Alzheimer's disease

Distinguishing between Alzheimer's disease and vascular dementia may not be straightforward and the two often co-exist, but certain clinical features (discussed below) are more suggestive of vascular dementia.

In contrast to Alzheimer's disease, the course is more likely to fluctuate, with 'good and bad days' and the profile of deficits on neuropsychological testing may be more patchy. Mood changes such as anxiety, depression or **emotional incontinence** (inappropriate laughter or tearfulness) are also more prominent and symptoms tend to be worse in the evenings, called **sundowning**. The degree of memory loss is variable, but can be less obvious than in Alzheimer's disease.

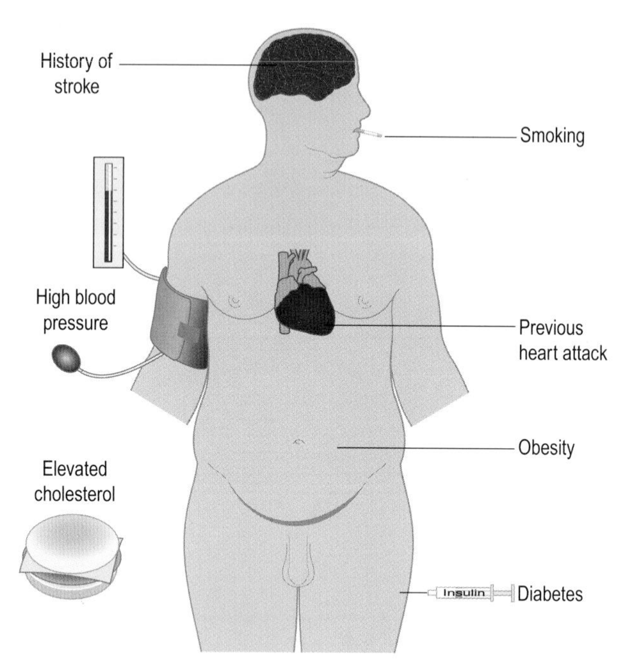

Fig. 12.16 **The risk factors for vascular dementia are the same as those for ischaemic heart disease.**

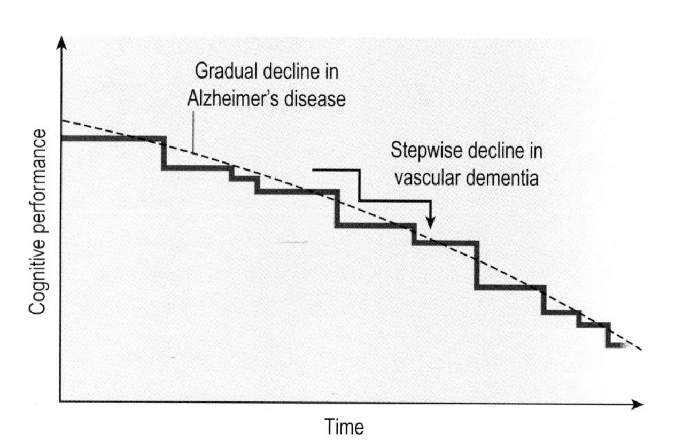

Fig. 12.17 **Multi-infarct dementia.** Progression is classically said to occur in a step-wise fashion consistent with a series of small strokes, in contrast to the gradual decline seen in Alzheimer's disease.

Associated damage to the basal ganglia sometimes leads to a pseudo-parkinsonian gait with short, shuffling steps: the **marche à petit pas** (French: walking with small steps) and there may be focal neurological signs consistent with one or more previous strokes. The typical imaging appearances are shown in Figure 12.18.

Pathological features

Vascular dementia may be caused by: (i) **small vessel disease**; (ii) **large vessel disease**; or (iii) a combination of the two. The term **mixed dementia** is used if there are co-existent features of Alzheimer's disease or another dementia. A rare inherited form of vascular dementia is discussed in Clinical Box 12.8.

Small vessel disease

This is the most common finding in patients with vascular dementia. It is frequently associated with **arterial hypertension**, diabetes and other vascular risk factors. High blood pressure damages the walls of small and medium-sized

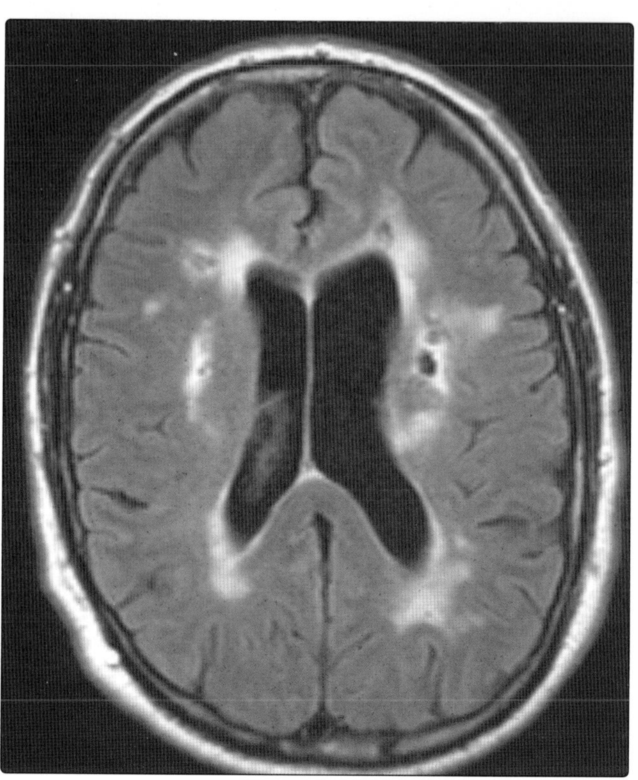

Fig. 12.18 **Axial MRI scan showing the typical imaging features of cerebral small vessel disease.** There is confluent hyperintensity in the periventricular white matter and patches of hyperintensity in the deep and subcortical white matter. Additionally, there are several small focal cavities (with the same signal intensity as CSF) which are typical of 'old' lacunar infarcts [T2-weighted MRI with CSF suppression: fluid-attenuation inversion recovery or 'FLAIR' sequence]. Courtesy of Dr Andrew MacKinnon.

Clinical Box 12.8: CADASIL

Cerebral autosomal dominant arteriopathy with subcortical infarcts and leukoencephalopathy is a rare **autosomal dominant** disorder that classically presents in young females who have a history of migraine with aura. It is characterized by multiple strokes affecting the subcortical white matter (Greek: leukos, white) leading to progressive dementia with psychiatric features. It is caused by mutation of the ***NOTCH3* gene** on chromosome 19, the same locus that is responsible for **familial hemiplegic migraine**. Electron microscopy shows deposits of **granular material** in the walls of small blood vessels which include part of the extracellular domain of the **notch3 receptor**.

blood vessels, leading to replacement of smooth muscle by collagen. This gives an amorphous or 'hyaline' (Greek: glassy) appearance under the microscope, termed **hyaline arteriosclerosis** (Fig. 12.19A). Some vessels show more striking wall destruction with replacement of smooth muscle by lipid-laden foam cells, termed **lipohyalinosis**.

Both types of small vessel pathology contribute to 'hardening' of the arteries and arterioles, referred to as **arteriosclerosis** and **arteriolar sclerosis** respectively (Greek: sklerōs, hard). Normally distensible blood vessels are thus converted into rigid pipes with limited ability to dilate in response to fluctuations in blood pressure. This leads to small strokes (less than 1 cm in diameter) called **lacunar infarcts** (Latin: lacūna, hole or gap) (Fig. 12.19B). There may also be a

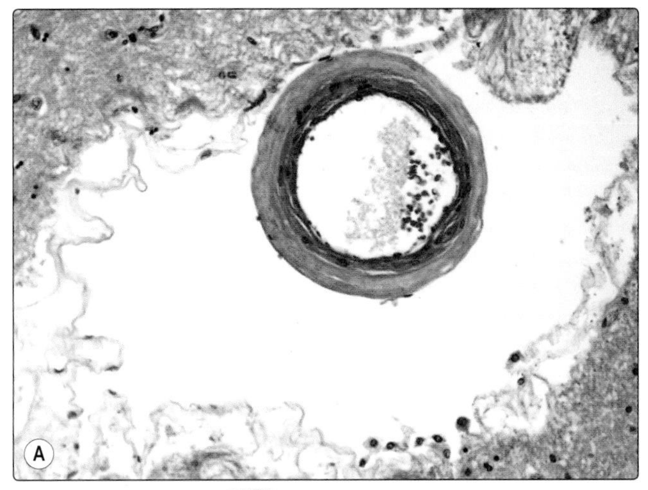

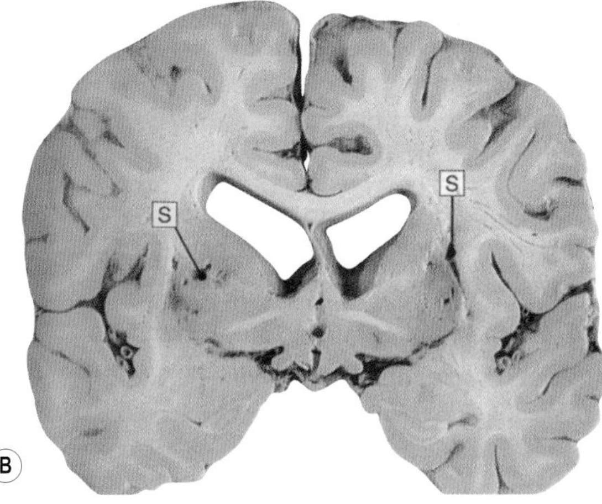

Fig. 12.19 **Pathological features of small vessel disease.** **(A)** Micrograph of a deep hemispheric blood vessel showing replacement of vascular smooth muscle by (pink) hyaline material. There is also marked enlargement of the perivascular space. From Prayson, R: Neuropathology 1e (Churchill Livingstone 2005) with permission; **(B)** Photograph of a coronal brain section showing multiple lacunar infarcts in the basal ganglia as a result of small vessel disease (including prominent slit-like spaces, labelled "S"). From Stevens and Lowe: Pathology 2e (Mosby 2000) with permission.

more general attenuation of the subcortical white matter with expansion of perivascular spaces, creating a 'moth-eaten' appearance.

Large vessel disease

Some patients develop dementia after a series of strokes, having lost a critical volume of brain tissue (usually at least 50–100 mL). In some cases a so-called **strategic infarct** may lead to 'single-stroke dementia'. This more abrupt decline is caused by damage to an area that is critical for memory such as the **hippocampus** or **anteromedial thalamus**.

Frontotemporal dementia

Frontotemporal dementia (FTD) is a clinical term for a group of conditions in which there is selective degeneration of the frontal and temporal lobes (Fig. 12.20). The lifetime prevalence is 1 in 6000 and it is equally common in males and females. FTD accounts for less than 5% of dementia overall, but is the second most common cause in people under 60 (after Alzheimer's disease). Onset is typically in middle age, with an average survival of around 6–8 years. A family history is present in 40% of cases.

Key Points

- Vascular dementia is the third most common type of acquired cognitive decline in later life (following Alzheimer's disease and dementia with Lewy bodies). It accounts for 10% of cases.
- It may present with a stepwise loss of cognitive ability (consistent with a series of small strokes) or a gradual decline (more in keeping with diffuse white matter or small vessel disease).
- Clinical features suggestive of vascular dementia rather than Alzheimer's disease include a fluctuating course and patchy cognitive profile, 'emotional incontinence' and sundowning. There may also be parkinsonian features or neurological signs consistent with one or more strokes.
- The most common pathological finding is small vessel disease (hyaline arteriosclerosis and lipohyalinosis) often in association with arterial hypertension and other vascular risk factors.
- Other pathological features include lacunar infarcts, generalized attenuation of the subcortical white matter and enlargement of the perivascular spaces.
- Regional infarcts may also be present. In some patients a 'strategic infarct' in an area critical for memory (e.g. the hippocampus or anteromedial thalamus) leads to an abrupt decline in cognitive ability, referred to as 'single-stroke dementia'.

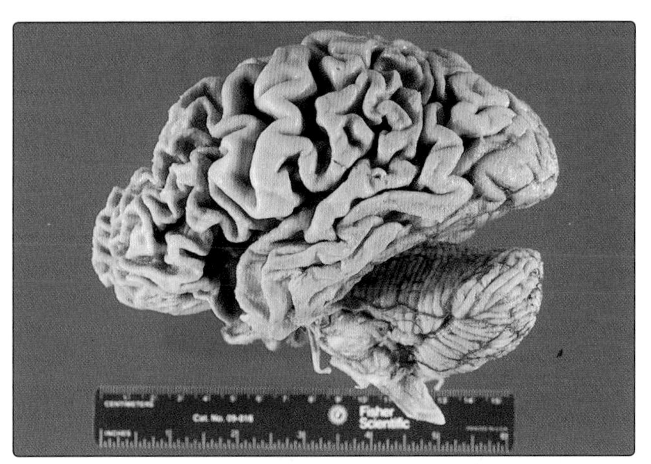

Fig. 12.20 **Post-mortem photograph of the brain in a case of frontotemporal dementia (FTD).** Macroscopic photograph showing selective degeneration of the frontal and temporal lobes. The primary sensory and motor areas are spared. From Prayson, R: Neuropathology 1e (Churchill Livingstone 2005) with permission.

Clinical features

Selective degeneration of the frontal and temporal lobes leads to a progressive deterioration in behaviour, personality and language. In difficult cases, specialized neuroimaging techniques may be helpful in distinguishing between FTD and Alzheimer's disease (Clinical Box 12.9).

Frontotemporal dementia subtypes

There are three main clinical patterns of frontotemporal dementia, sometimes with additional features of Parkinson's disease or motor neuron disease.

Behavioural variant of FTD

The **behavioural variant** of frontotemporal dementia accounts for 50% of cases. It is characterized by striking **personality change** with relative preservation of memory and language. Common features include **disinhibition** (e.g. inappropriate comments, reduced tact, self-centred behaviour) and **emotional blunting** (apathy, emotional

Clinical Box 12.9: Neuroimaging in frontotemporal dementia

A soluble amyloid-binding molecule has been developed that is able to cross the blood–brain barrier, called **Pittsburgh interesting compound B**. This can be radioactively labelled and used to demonstrate deposition of amyloid beta peptide in the brains of living people (called **PIB scanning**). A potential clinical application of this technique is in the differentiation between patients with frontotemporal dementia and Alzheimer's disease with prominent involvement of the frontal and temporal lobes (Fig. 12.21).

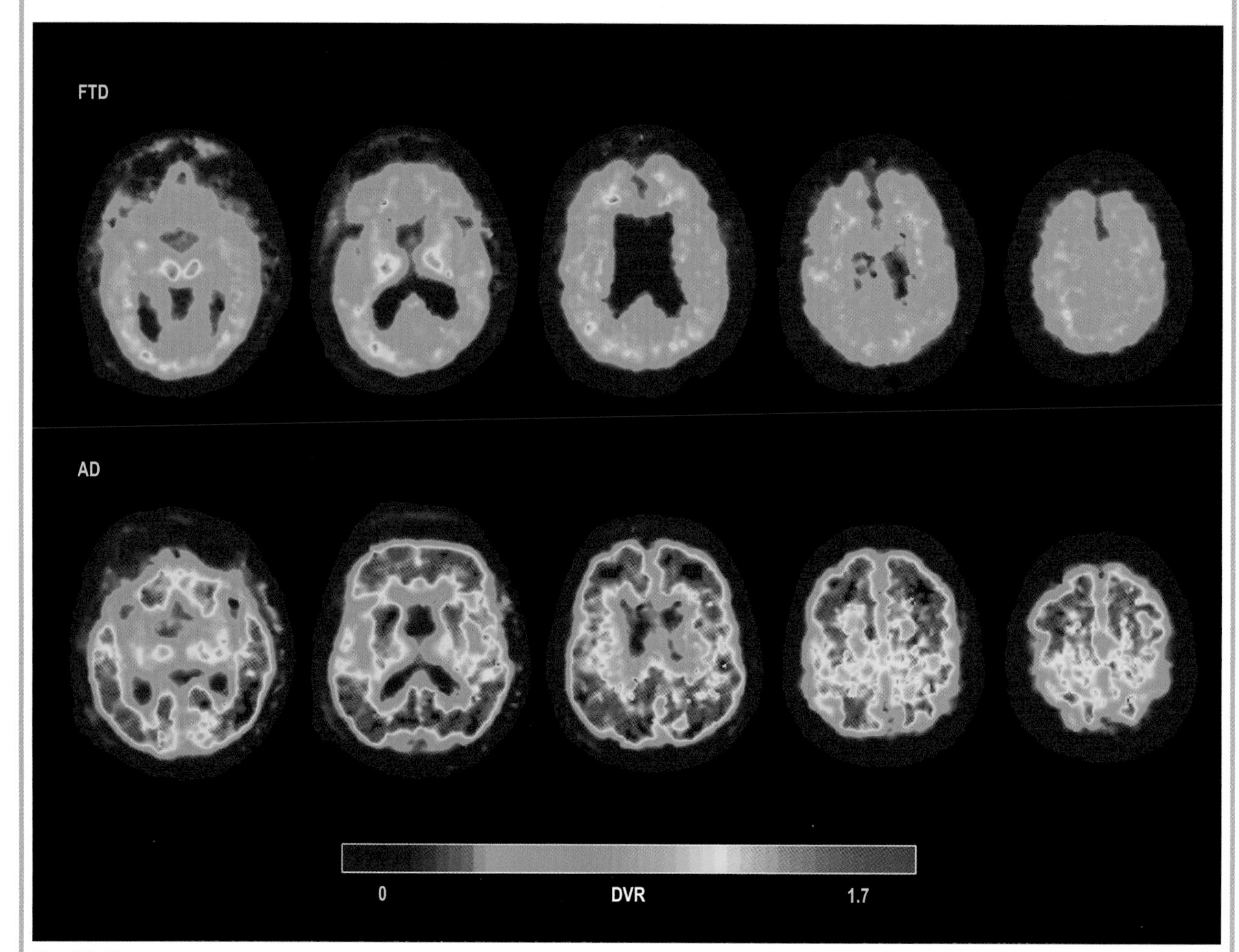

Fig. 12.21 **Positron emission tomography (PET) with the beta-amyloid specific radiotracer carbon-11 labelled Pittsburgh Compound B (^{11}C-PIB) in patients with frontotemporal dementia (FTD, top row) and Alzheimer's disease (AD, bottom row).** PIB-PET imaging in the patient with Alzheimer's disease reveals diffuse cortical binding of amyloid beta, in contrast to non-specific white matter labelling in the patient with FTD. In both cases, pathological confirmation of the diagnosis was subsequently obtained at post-mortem examination. Axial distribution volume ratio (DVR) images provided courtesy of Dr Gil Rabinovici.

coldness or loss of empathy). Many patients have elements of **obsessive-compulsive disorder** (**OCD**) (see Ch. 3, Clinical Box 3.10) and there may be altered eating habits with weight gain and a **craving for sweet foods**. Neuroimaging typically shows bilateral frontal (especially orbitofrontal) atrophy which is often worse on the non-dominant side (Fig. 12.22A). Many of these cases were formally referred to as 'Pick's disease' (Clinical Box 12.10).

Semantic dementia

In **semantic dementia** the ability to understand the meaning of words and concepts is gradually lost. Inability to name objects (**anomia**) is an early feature and there is gradual erosion of **semantic categories** used to classify people and objects. In the early stages this may lead to naming errors (e.g. referring to a bus as a car). Later, more general categories are used to describe particular objects (e.g. apples, oranges and bananas are all described as 'fruit'). In advanced stages, semantic categories are lost altogether (e.g. living versus non-living, plant versus animal) and everyday objects may appear strange or frightening. Neuroimaging shows severe bilateral temporal lobe atrophy (Fig. 12.22B).

Clinical Box 12.10: Pick's disease

All frontal-predominant dementias with marked behavioural changes were historically grouped together using the term Pick's disease. Most of these conditions would now be regarded as a form of **frontotemporal dementia**. In current usage the term **Pick's disease** (**PiD**) is restricted to an extremely rare entity characterized by rounded tau-positive inclusions in the neuronal cytoplasm called **Pick bodies**.

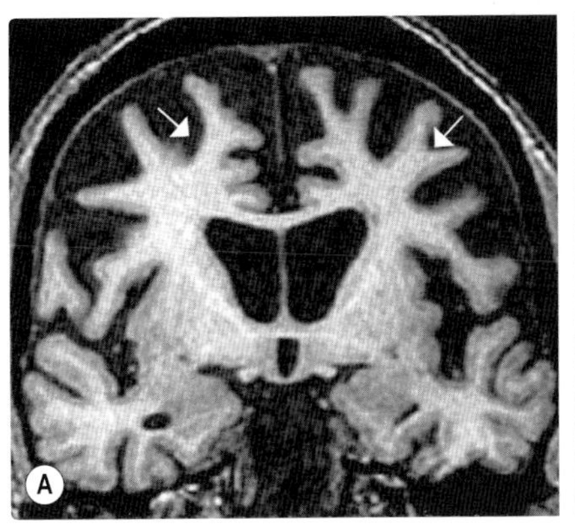

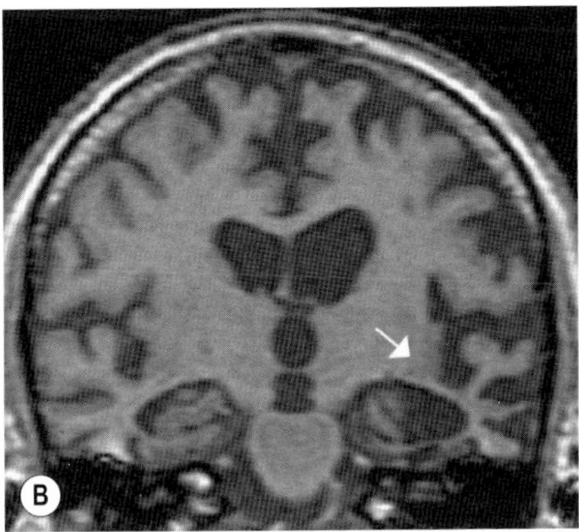

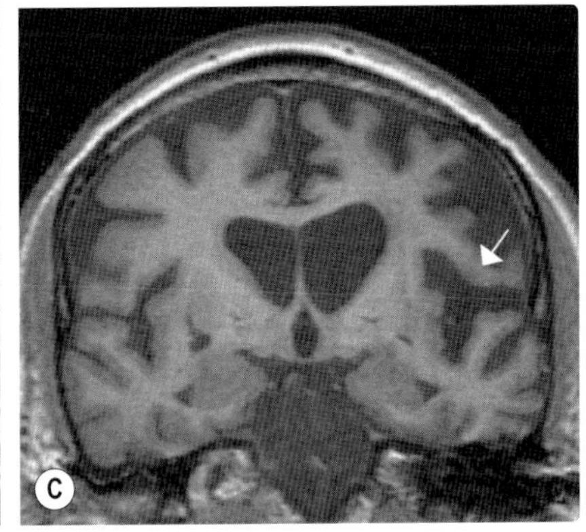

Fig. 12.22 **Neuroimaging findings in the three main variants of frontotemporal dementia (FTD). (A)** In the behavioural variant of FTD there is usually bilateral frontal lobe atrophy which is often worse on the non-dominant side; **(B)** In semantic dementia severe bilateral temporal lobe atrophy is typical; **(C)** Progressive non-fluent aphasia is characterized by dominant (usually left) hemisphere atrophy in the inferior frontal gyrus and perisylvian region, corresponding to the left-hemisphere language areas. [Coronal T1-weighted MRI scans. The arrows indicate the most severely affected areas.] From Schott, JM and Fox, NC: Structural imaging in the dementias. J Psychiat (Old Age Psychiatr) (2007, pp. 503–507) with permission.

Progressive non-fluent aphasia

Individuals with **progressive non-fluent aphasia** (**PNFA**) have marked expressive language difficulties (**aphasia**) with word substitutions and word-finding problems, together with errors in grammar, syntax and pronunciation. This tends to affect verbs, prepositions and function words more than nouns (cf. **Broca's dysphasia**; see Ch. 3). In some cases there is **progressive apraxia of speech**, which has more to do with motor control of the speech articulators. Neuroimaging in PNFA typically shows asymmetric brain atrophy which is most severe in the left inferior frontal lobe and 'perisylvian region', meaning the area surrounding the lateral sulcus, corresponding to the left-hemisphere language areas (Fig. 12.22C).

FTD and motor neuron disease

Up to 15% of patients with frontotemporal dementia also have features of **motor neuron disease** (**MND**). This is characterized by **progressive muscle weakness** and wasting, together with **increased muscle tone** and **reflexes**, due to loss of motor neurons in the cerebral cortex and spinal cord (see Ch. 4, Clinical Box 4.9). In these cases a diagnosis of **FTD-MND** is made. Conversely, at least 30% of patients with motor neuron disease develop cognitive decline which may be severe enough to meet the criteria for frontotemporal dementia. This reflects an overlap between the molecular pathology of FTD and MND (discussed below).

Pathological features

The range of pathological entities presenting clinically as frontotemporal dementia is referred to by pathologists as **frontotemporal lobar degeneration** (**FTLD**). It is important to emphasize that FTLD is a pathological description rather than a clinical term.

Diagnosis is based on the recognition of **pathological inclusions** (composed of disease-specific proteins) within neurons and glial cells, using immunohistochemistry (antibody labelling). However, the clinical features reflect the **anatomical distribution** of the degenerative changes rather than the particular protein present.

Molecular classification

In 50% of FTLD cases, the pathological inclusions are predominantly composed of the 43 KDa RNA processing protein **TAR DNA binding protein 43**. This protein, **TDP-43**, is also responsible for the majority of sporadic and familial motor neuron disease cases, which partially accounts for the link between frontotemporal dementia and MND. The pathological diagnosis in these cases is FTLD-TDP.

In another 40% of cases inclusions are composed of **tau**. FTLDs in this group are therefore classified as **tauopathies**. The pathological diagnosis in these cases is thus FTLD-tau.

In most of the remaining cases the inclusions are composed of another **RNA processing protein** called **FUS** (the name comes from its role in a type of soft tissue cancer, meaning 'fused in sarcoma'). This protein has also been shown to underlie a proportion of familial motor neuron disease. The pathological diagnosis in these cases is FTLD-FUS.

Genetic factors in FTD

Around 60% of frontotemporal dementia is sporadic. In the 40% of cases with a family history, the inheritance pattern is usually not straightforward. In 10% of cases (a quarter of those with a family history) there is clear **autosomal dominant inheritance** and a known mutation can often be identified in one of two genes on chromosome 17 or a locus on chromosome 9.

Key Points

- Frontotemporal dementia is a clinical term for a rare group of conditions (accounting for 5% of dementia cases) in which there is selective degeneration of the frontal and temporal lobes.
- The behavioural variant accounts for 50% of cases and is dominated by changes in personality and behaviour. Semantic dementia and progressive non-fluent aphasia are less common.
- Some patients with FTD also have features of motor neuron disease (MND), whilst a proportion of people with MND develop frontal dementia, due to an overlap in the molecular pathology.

Key Points

- Examination of the brain in patients with frontotemporal dementia shows variable frontal and temporal lobe atrophy: frontotemporal lobar degeneration (FTLD).
- In the majority of FTLD cases, pathological inclusions can be identified in neurons and glial cells. These are most often composed of TDP-43 (50%), tau (40%) or FUS (5%).
- Importantly, the clinical features depend on the anatomical distribution of the pathological changes and neuronal loss, rather than the particular protein involved.

Mutations in the **tau gene** (*MAPT*) on chromosome 17 cause frontotemporal lobar degeneration with tau-positive inclusions (FTLD-tau). In another group there are mutations in the **progranulin gene** (*PGRN*), which is close to the tau gene on chromosome 17. In these cases the inclusions are composed of TDP-43 rather than progranulin, therefore the molecular diagnosis is FTLD-TDP. The function of progranulin in the CNS is uncertain, but it appears to take part in brain inflammatory responses.

Many cases of frontotemporal dementia (as well as motor neuron disease and FTD-MND) are now known to be associated with a **hexanucleotide repeat expansion** in a gene on chromosome 9, known as ***C9ORF72***. The function of this gene and its transcribed protein are unknown, but it may be involved in RNA processing like TDP-43 and FUS.

Key Points

- Most cases of frontotemporal dementia are sporadic (60%). In the 40% of cases with a family history, the inheritance pattern is often not straightforward.
- In 10% of FTD cases (a quarter of those with a family history) there is clear autosomal dominant inheritance and a known mutation can usually be identified in: (i) the tau or progranulin genes (*MAPT* or *PGRN*) on chromosome 17; or (i) the *C9ORF72* gene on chromosome 9.
- A proportion of patients with frontotemporal dementia also have features of motor neuron disease (FTD-MND) due to an overlap in the underlying molecular pathology.

Chapter 13
Parkinson's disease

CHAPTER CONTENTS

Parkinson's disease is a progressive degenerative disorder of the basal ganglia that affects the initiation and execution of voluntary movements (and is usually associated with a tremor). It is the second most common neurodegenerative disorder after Alzheimer's disease. The lifetime risk is 0.1%, but the incidence increases with age and the prevalence is 1–2% in people over 65. The mean age at onset is 60 and it is more common in males. Although there is no cure, symptoms can usually be well controlled for several years with dopamine replacement therapy (discussed below).

Clinical features

Most cases of Parkinson's disease are idiopathic (meaning that the cause is not known). The main symptoms and signs of **idiopathic Parkinson's disease** (**IPD**) are illustrated in Figure 13.1. The central feature is **akinesia** or poverty of movement (Greek: a-, without; kinesis, movement) together with marked muscular **rigidity**. It is therefore classified as an **akinetic-rigid syndrome**. Another prominent component is **bradykinesia**, meaning that movements are slow and deliberate (Greek: bradys, slow). In most cases there is also a coarse tremor. Parkinson's disease is sometimes referred to as an **extrapyramidal movement disorder** since the pyramidal (primary motor) pathway is unaffected.

Akinesia

Parkinson's disease is characterized by **poverty of movement**. Voluntary actions are initiated with effort and performed slowly (e.g. turning in bed, rising from a chair). **Gait freezing** is common and may be associated with a frustrating sense of being stuck to the floor. All spontaneous movements are reduced, including facial expressions and blinking. This creates a mask-like appearance, referred to as **facial amimia** (the 'parkinsonian stare'). On examination, there is progressive reduction in the speed and amplitude of repetitive movements such as apposition of the thumb and index finger. The voice may be slow and quiet (**hypophonia**), the handwriting small and illegible (**micrographia**).

Muscular rigidity

Increased muscle tone (**rigidity**) may present as stiffness, muscle pain or fatigue. On examination, there is uniform resistance to joint flexion and extension which has been compared to bending a piece of lead pipe. In contrast to spasticity, **lead-pipe rigidity** is constant (not velocity-dependent) and may be due to over-activity in the long-latency component of the stretch reflex (see Ch. 4).

Abnormal posture and gait

Patients with Parkinson's disease have a characteristic **flexed posture**. A slow **shuffling gait** is combined with reduced or **absent arm swing** and the hands are held in front of the body. Crossing boundaries such as doorways may be difficult and turning is often slow and awkward. Excessive trunk flexion brings the centre of gravity forward and the walking pace tends to accelerate as the feet try to keep up, termed a **festinating gait** (Latin: festinare, to hurry). This increases the risk of falling, particularly since **impairment of postural reflexes** is another common feature.

Rest tremor

Tremor is a rhythmic 'back-and-forth' movement in the limbs, head or jaw and occurs in 75% of patients with Parkinson's disease. The parkinsonian tremor is usually **asymmetric** and often begins in one hand or arm. It is classified as a **rest tremor** because it is much more prominent between movements. It is of large amplitude and low frequency (4–6 Hz) and is not present during sleep. Some patients have a classical '**pill-rolling**' **tremor** (Fig. 13.2) which is strongly suggestive of idiopathic Parkinson's disease. The combination of lead-pipe rigidity and tremor creates a jerky or 'ratchet-like' sensation on examination. This is termed **cogwheeling** and is best appreciated at the wrist.

Other features

Non-motor symptoms in Parkinson's disease reflect: (i) the role of the basal ganglia in cognition, emotion and behaviour (see Ch. 3); and (ii) the presence of widespread pathological changes in the brain stem, limbic lobe and neocortex. **Anxiety**, **depression** or **apathy** occurs in 40% of patients. There may be **sleep disorders** including: nocturnal hallucinations, excessive daytime somnolence, vivid dreams, nightmares or sleepwalking. Subtle cognitive changes are common, such as **bradyphrenia** (generalized slowing of thought) or **executive dysfunction** (difficulty with organization, planning and decision-making). One in five patients will eventually be diagnosed with dementia (Clinical Box 13.1).

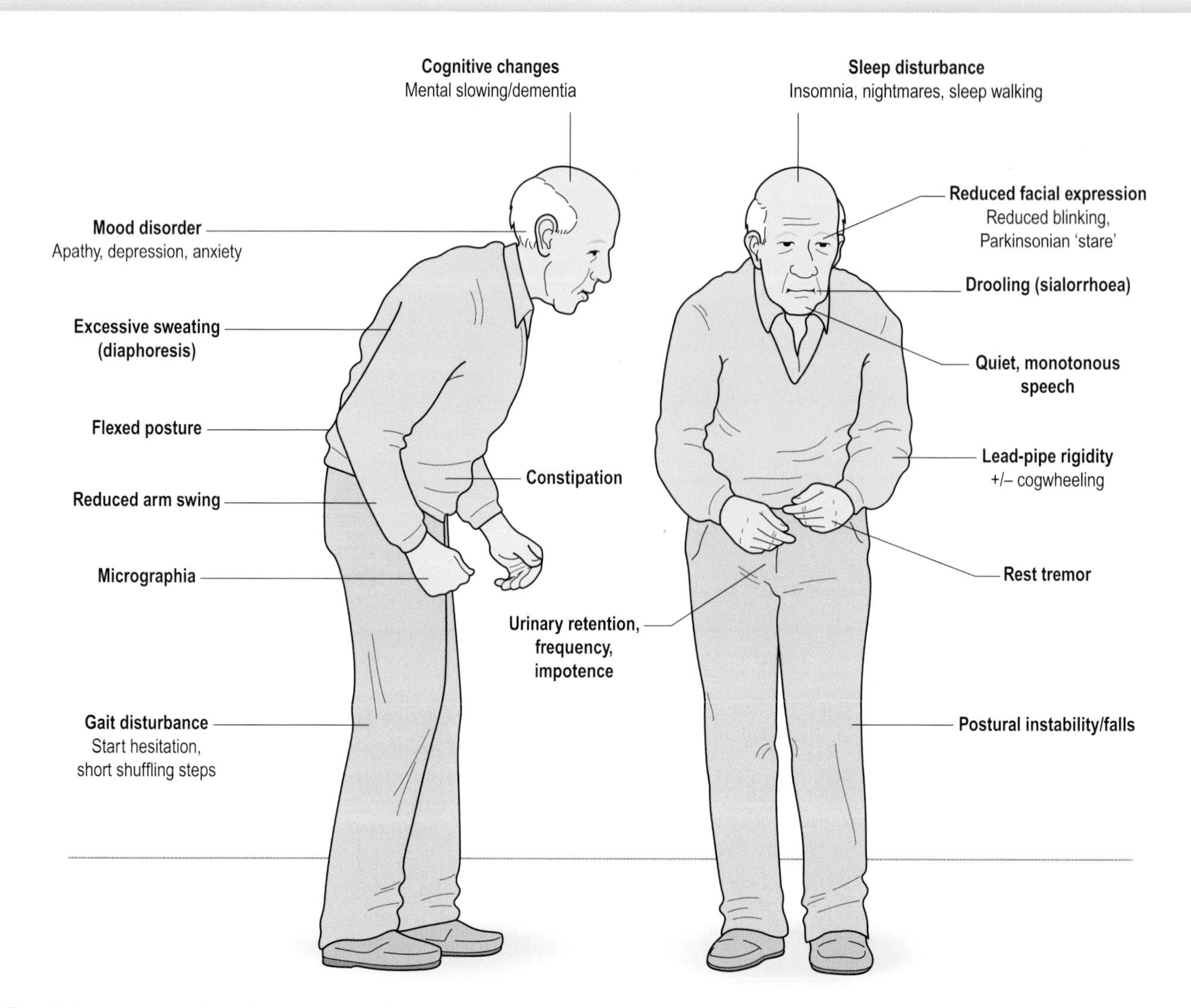

Fig. 13.1 **Features of idiopathic Parkinson's disease.** The combination of a flexed posture, slow shuffling gait, mask-like facial expression and unilateral tremor is highly characteristic.

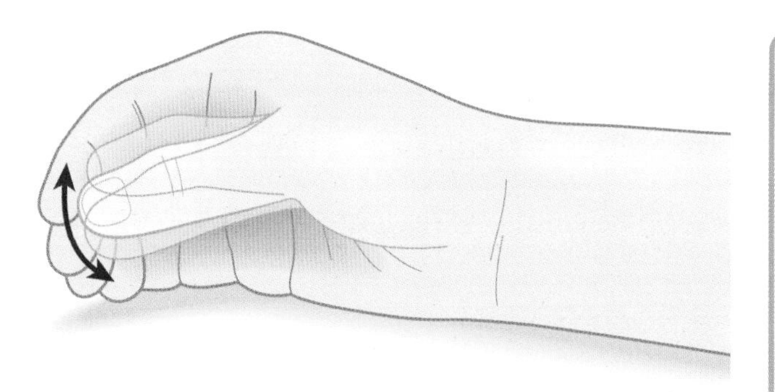

Fig. 13.2 **Tremor in Parkinson's disease.** The presence of a coarse, low-frequency 'pill-rolling' rest tremor (illustrated here) is virtually diagnostic of idiopathic Parkinson's disease. Tremor is often embarrassing for the patient and may be difficult to treat.

Diagnosis and course

The diagnosis of Parkinson's disease is primarily clinical. Routine MRI scans are often normal, but **dopamine deficiency** in the basal ganglia can be demonstrated using specialized tests (Fig. 13.3). Without treatment there is progressive decline over a 5–10-year period, with gradual deterioration of motor function, worsening postural instability, gait freezing and frequent falls. However, symptoms can usually be controlled for a number of years with **dopamine replacement therapy** and this is associated with a near-normal life expectancy.

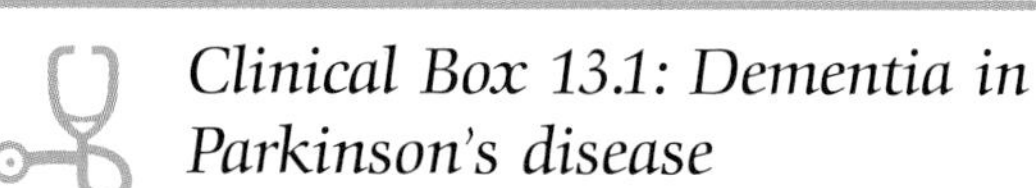

Clinical Box 13.1: Dementia in Parkinson's disease

Dementia occurs in at least 20% of patients with Parkinson's disease, usually after a number of years. If cognitive decline appears 12 months or more after the onset of parkinsonian features, then the term **Parkinson's disease with dementia** (**PDD**) is used. If cognitive decline occurs within a year of presentation (or at the same time as the motor features) then a diagnosis of **dementia with Lewy bodies** (**DLB**) may be made. Specific features of DLB, in addition to parkinsonism, include **fluctuations** in cognitive performance and **visual hallucinations**. It is important to note that the distinction between PDD and DLB is purely clinical, since the pathological changes are identical (see Ch. 12 for further discussion of dementia, including features that distinguish DLB from Alzheimer's disease).

Parkinsonism

Some patients presenting with an akinetic-rigid syndrome do not have idiopathic Parkinson's disease. This is referred to as **parkinsonism** and there are many underlying causes. Response to dopamine replacement tends to be poor, symptoms are typically more symmetric in distribution and there may be other **atypical features** such as gaze palsy,

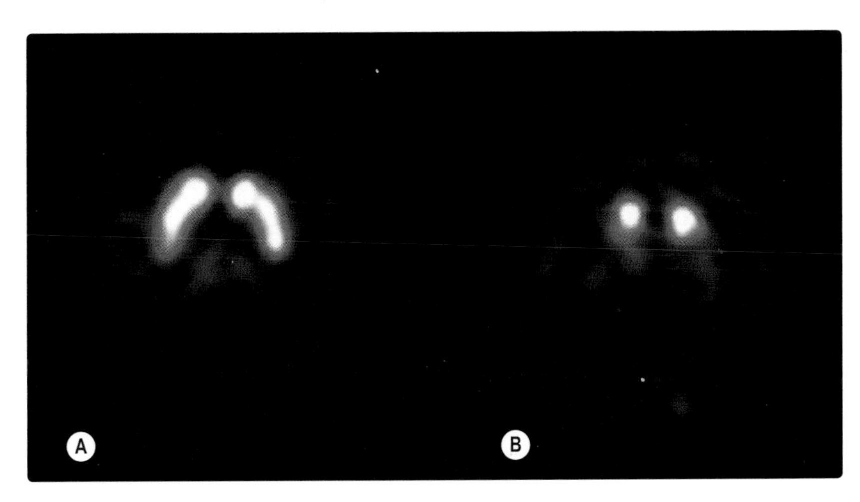

Fig. 13.3 **Functional imaging of dopamine transport in Parkinson's disease. (A)** Axial section through the basal ganglia showing the normal pattern of uptake in a healthy control. The characteristic 'comma' shape of the striatum (caudate nucleus and putamen) is seen; **(B)** In a patient with Parkinson's disease, there is markedly reduced signal in the putamen but not in the head of the caudate nucleus, creating a 'full stop' appearance. [Images obtained using single photon emission computed tomography (SPECT) with the radioactively labelled (^{123}I) beta-CIT.] From Seibyl, JP: Single-photon emission computed tomography and positron emission tomography evaluations of patients with central motor disorders. J Semin Nuclear Med (2008) with permission.

Key Points

- Idiopathic Parkinson's disease is the second most common neurodegenerative disorder after Alzheimer's disease, affecting 1–2% of people over the age of 65.
- The central feature is akinesia (poverty of movement). This is accompanied by bradykinesia (slow initiation and execution of movements), 'lead-pipe' rigidity and impaired postural reflexes.
- Tremor occurs in 75% of patients. It is not an invariable feature, but a classic 'pill-rolling' tremor is virtually diagnostic of idiopathic Parkinson's disease.
- Mood disorder occurs in about 40% of patients and subtle cognitive changes are common. One in five patients will eventually develop dementia, usually after a number of years.

Clinical Box 13.2: Corticobasal degeneration

This is a rare neurodegenerative disease of the cerebral cortex and basal ganglia that affects less than 1 in 100,000 people. Clinical features include **parkinsonism** (that responds poorly to dopamine replacement) together with limb **apraxia, pyramidal tract signs** and **frontotemporal dementia**. It often presents with a single clumsy or apraxic limb. Some patients experience autonomous hand or arm movements, referred to as an **alien limb.** CBD may also present as an isolated dementia syndrome without parkinsonian features.

axial rigidity, early falls or pyramidal tract signs. The most common forms are drug-induced, vascular and neurodegenerative.

Drug-induced parkinsonism

Administration of **antipsychotic** (**neuroleptic**) agents may cause 'extrapyramidal side effects' that mimic Parkinson's disease and this is the most common cause of parkinsonism. It occurs because neuroleptic drugs antagonize central dopamine receptors, including those within the basal ganglia.

Vascular pseudoparkinsonism

Patients with **cerebrovascular disease** may develop an akinetic-rigid syndrome. This is due to **microinfarcts** (small ischaemic strokes, see Ch. 10) in the basal ganglia or hemispheric white matter. In contrast to idiopathic Parkinson's disease, symptoms tend to be more severe in the lower limbs, response to dopamine replacement is poor and tremor is usually absent.

Neurodegenerative causes

A number of other neurodegenerative disorders may be confused with Parkinson's disease. The most important are **progressive supranuclear palsy** (**PSP**) and **multiple system atrophy** (**MSA**), each with a prevalence of approximately 1 in 20,000. An even rarer form is **corticobasal degeneration** (**CBD**), discussed in Clinical Box 13.2.

Progressive supranuclear palsy

This is the most common neurodegenerative mimic of Parkinson's disease, accounting for about 5% of people with a parkinsonian syndrome. In more than 50% of cases there is **axial rigidity**, a **hyperextended posture** and a characteristic **supranuclear gaze palsy** with failure in the cortical ('supranuclear') control of **vertical eye movements**. There may also be apathy, cognitive decline and outbursts of inappropriate laughter or tearfulness, termed **emotional incontinence**. This classical form of PSP is also referred to as **Richardson's syndrome**. In up to a third of cases the clinical features closely resemble idiopathic Parkinson's disease. In this subtype, referred to as **PSP-P**, the pathological changes are less severe and the clinical course is more favourable. Features of PSP and Parkinson's disease are compared in Figure 13.4.

Multiple system atrophy

Multiple system atrophy is characterized by **parkinsonism**, **cerebellar ataxia** and **autonomic dysfunction**. There are two patterns. **MSA-P** is dominated by rigidity, bradykinesia and postural instability and closely resembles idiopathic Parkinson's disease; whereas **MSA-C** combines features of cerebellar ataxia with corticospinal tract signs including increased muscle tone and reflexes (see Ch. 4).

Multiple system atrophy encompasses three entities that were previously regarded as separate diseases: **striatonigral degeneration** (corresponding to MSA-P), **olivopontocerebellar atrophy** or **OPCA** (corresponding to MSA-C) and the **Shy–Drager syndrome** (representing a form of primary autonomic failure). Autonomic features such as **postural hypotension** and **erectile dysfunction** may occur in both MSA-C and MSA-P and also in idiopathic Parkinson's disease.

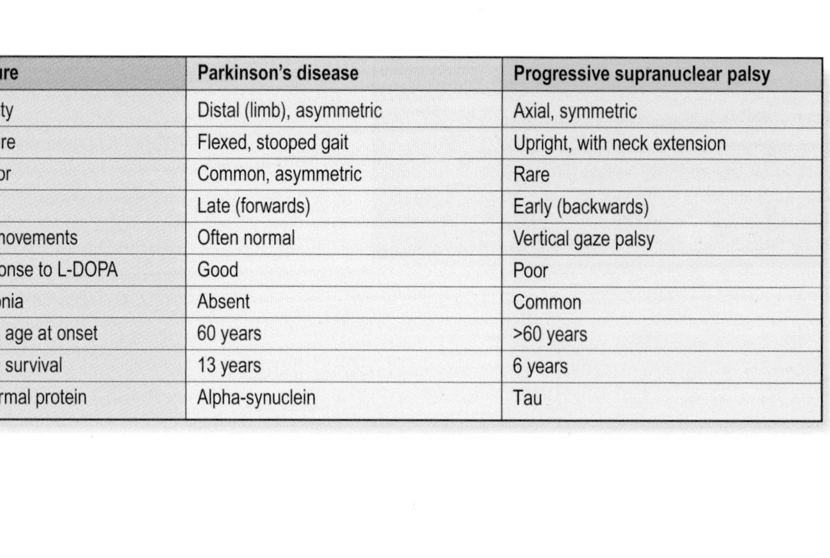

Feature	Parkinson's disease	Progressive supranuclear palsy
Rigidity	Distal (limb), asymmetric	Axial, symmetric
Posture	Flexed, stooped gait	Upright, with neck extension
Tremor	Common, asymmetric	Rare
Falls	Late (forwards)	Early (backwards)
Eye movements	Often normal	Vertical gaze palsy
Response to L-DOPA	Good	Poor
Dystonia	Absent	Common
Mean age at onset	60 years	>60 years
Mean survival	13 years	6 years
Abnormal protein	Alpha-synuclein	Tau

(A)

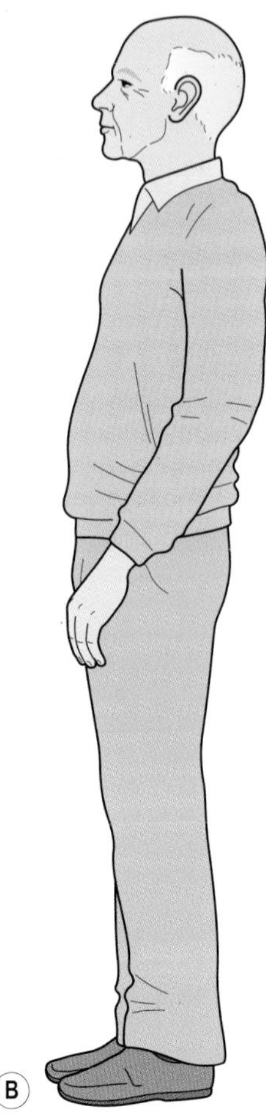

Fig. 13.4 **Comparison of idiopathic Parkinson's disease (IPD) and progressive supranuclear palsy (PSP).** The main clinical features including response to dopamine replacement therapy (L-DOPA) are compared in **(A)** and the characteristically erect posture seen in PSP is illustrated in **(B)**.

Key Points

- Akinetic-rigid syndromes other than idiopathic Parkinson's disease are referred to as parkinsonism. The main causes are drug-induced, vascular and neurodegenerative.
- The most common form of parkinsonism is seen in patients taking antipsychotic agents, which work by antagonizing central dopamine receptors ('extrapyramidal side effects').
- Vascular pseudoparkinsonism is due to small infarcts in the basal ganglia or their white matter connections.
- The most common neurodegenerative mimic of Parkinson's disease is progressive supranuclear palsy (PSP), characterized by axial rigidity, hyperextended posture and vertical gaze palsy.
- Others include multiple system atrophy (with parkinsonian and cerebellar subtypes: MSA-P and MSA-C) and the much less common corticobasal degeneration (CBD).

Pathology of Parkinson's disease

The key pathological change in Parkinson's disease is loss of dopaminergic neurons in the **substantia nigra** of the midbrain (Fig. 13.5). This is associated with degeneration of the **nigrostriatal tract**, leading to a profound reduction of dopamine in the basal ganglia (typically below 20% of normal at presentation). Surviving nigral neurons contain cytoplasmic inclusions called **Lewy bodies**, which can be identified by antibody labelling for the major component, **alpha-synuclein** protein. This reveals widespread pathological changes throughout the brain stem, limbic lobe and neocortex.

Neuronal loss

The substantia nigra is a large midbrain nucleus that can be divided into compact and reticular parts. The **pars compacta** contains the cell bodies of dopaminergic neurons contributing to the nigrostriatal tract, whereas the **pars reticulata** consists of GABAergic neurons and is analogous to the globus pallidus. The substantia nigra is almost black in the adult brain (Latin: nigra, black) due to the accumulation of **neuromelanin** as a by-product of **dopamine synthesis** (see Ch. 7). Loss of dopaminergic neurons in Parkinson's disease causes pallor of the substantia nigra which can be seen at post-mortem examination. The lateral part of the substantia nigra (which projects to the putamen or 'motor striatum') is more severely affected than the medial portion (which projects to the caudate nucleus).

Neuronal loss is also seen in other parts of the nervous system in patients with Parkinson's disease. These include the noradrenergic **locus coeruleus** of the pons (see Ch. 1). Post-mortem examination of the brain in Parkinson's disease may therefore show pallor of the loci coerulei as well as the substantia nigra. Despite normal age-related degeneration of the substantia nigra, most people have sufficient **reserve capacity** so that striatal dopamine levels never fall below 20% of normal.

Lewy bodies

The pathological hallmark of Parkinson's disease is the **Lewy body** (Fig. 13.6). This is a type of **pathological inclusion** (abnormal protein aggregate) found in the cytoplasm of surviving neurons. Lewy bodies are spherical structures,

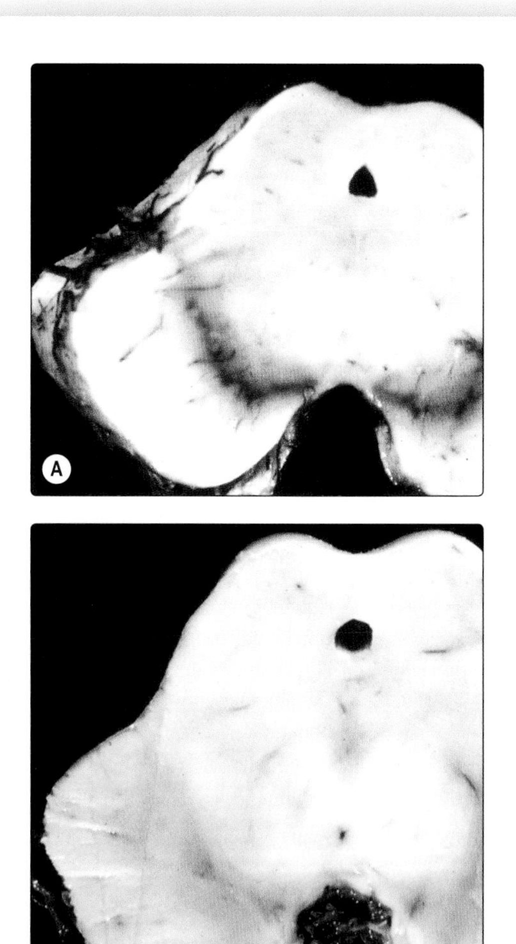

Fig. 13.5 **Degeneration of the substantia nigra in Parkinson's disease. (A)** Normal midbrain (in cross section) with a deeply pigmented substantia nigra; **(B)** Pallor of the substantia nigra in a case of Parkinson's disease. From Kumar et al: Robbins and Cotran's Pathologic Basis of Disease 7e (Saunders 2004) with permission.

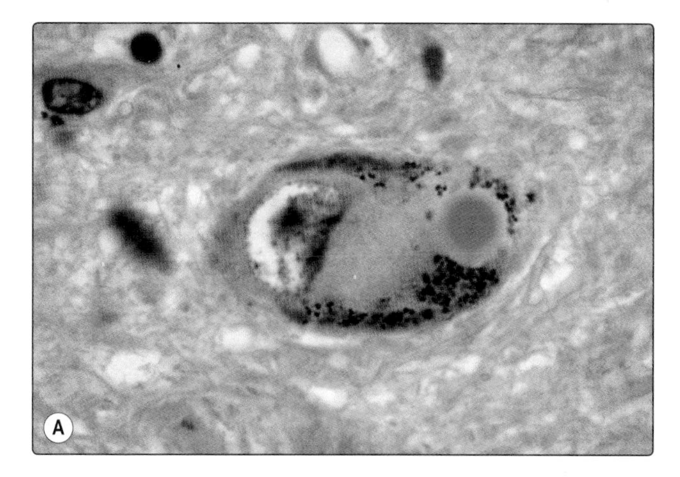

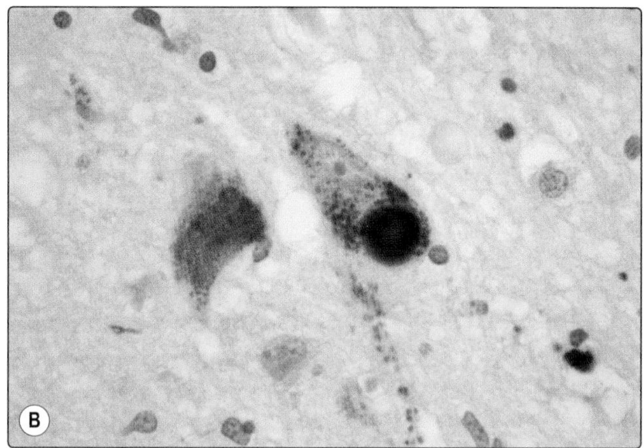

Fig. 13.6 **Lewy bodies. (A)** On routine haematoxylin and eosin (H&E)-stained sections Lewy bodies appear as bright pink structures in the neuronal cytoplasm, surrounded by a pale halo; **(B)** They can also be demonstrated by immunohistochemistry for alpha-synuclein protein, which is the main constituent. Courtesy of Professor Steve Gentleman.

measuring 5–30 μm in diameter. They are pink on standard histological preparations (because they take up the red tissue dye **eosin**) and are surrounded by a pale halo.

Progression of Lewy body pathology

Lewy body pathology begins in the medulla and olfactory bulbs, spreading progressively through six **Braak stages** to involve the pons, midbrain, limbic lobe, amygdala and neocortex (Fig. 13.7). **Cortical Lewy bodies** are similar to those encountered in the brain stem, but do not have a halo and are present even in cases without dementia. Pathological inclusions are also found in the **autonomic nervous system**, including the enteric nervous system in the gastrointestinal tract.

Spread of Lewy body pathology may reflect **selective vulnerability** of certain brain regions (so that they are affected earlier) or could be due to stepwise spread along anatomical pathways. Since the olfactory bulb is affected first, the possibility of a **pathogenic virus infection** gaining access to the brain via the nasal mucosa has been postulated.

Alpha-synuclein

The main constituent of Lewy bodies is **alpha-synuclein**. This is a synaptic protein that is present in **presynaptic terminals** in association with synaptic vesicles. It seems to be involved in neurotransmitter release and **synaptic plasticity** (which is critical for learning and memory; see Ch. 7). It may also take part in the regulation of dopamine storage and synaptic vesicle recycling.

The **synuclein gene** (***SNCA***, on chromosome 4) has six exons and encodes a natively unfolded 140-amino-acid protein. This has three domains, including a central hydrophobic region that is involved in protein aggregation. The most common familial forms of Parkinson's disease are caused by **duplications** or **triplications** of the synuclein gene. In other cases ***SNCA*** **point mutations** encourage alpha-synuclein aggregation and Lewy body formation.

Key Points

- The key pathological change in idiopathic Parkinson's disease is loss of dopaminergic neurons in the substantia nigra (pars compacta) of the midbrain, resulting in degeneration of the nigrostriatal tract.
- This leads to profound reduction in striatal dopamine (<20% of normal at presentation). The projection to the putamen ('motor striatum') is most severely affected, with less pronounced dopamine deficiency in the caudate nucleus.
- The pathological hallmark of Parkinson's disease is the Lewy body, a cytoplasmic neuronal inclusion composed predominantly of the synaptic protein alpha-synuclein.
- Lewy body pathology begins in the olfactory bulb and medulla, progressing through six Braak stages to involve the pons, midbrain, amygdala, limbic lobe and neocortex.

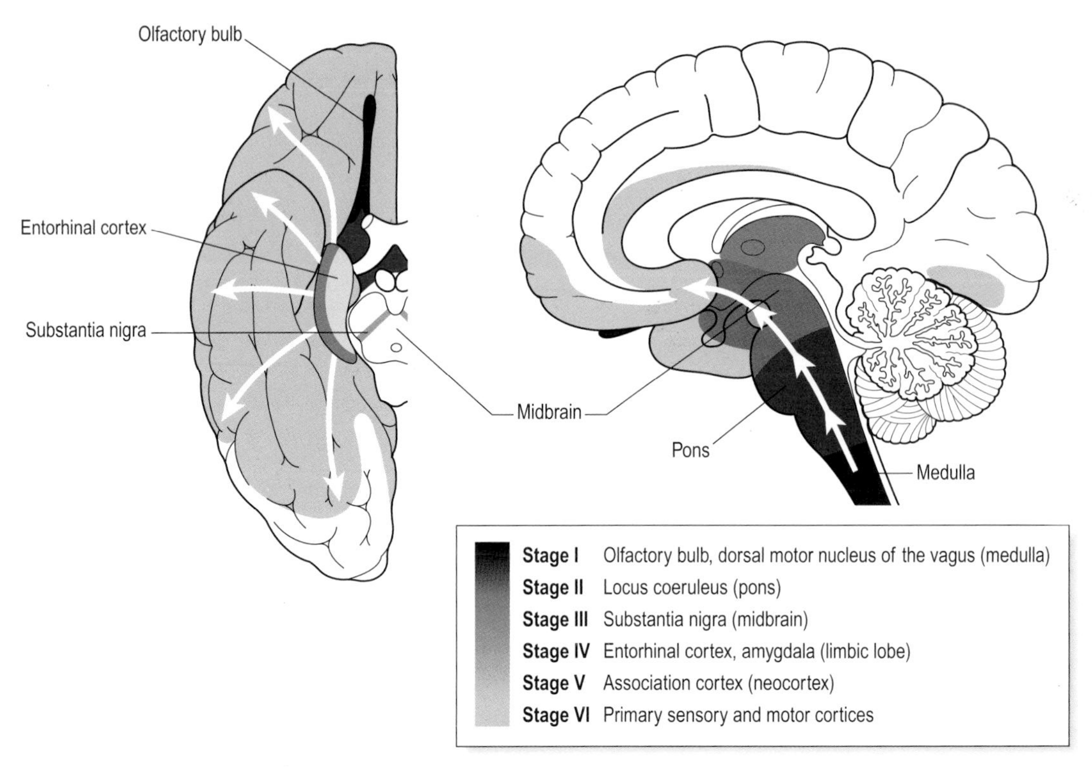

Fig. 13.7 **Progression of Lewy body pathology.** Lewy bodies first appear in the medulla and olfactory bulb and then progressively spread to the pons, midbrain, limbic lobe and neocortex. Key anatomical structures involved in each of the six Braak stages are indicated and disease progression is colour-coded on the inferior and midsagittal views of the cerebral hemisphere. Modified from Braak H et al: Neurobiology of Aging 24 (2003) with permission.

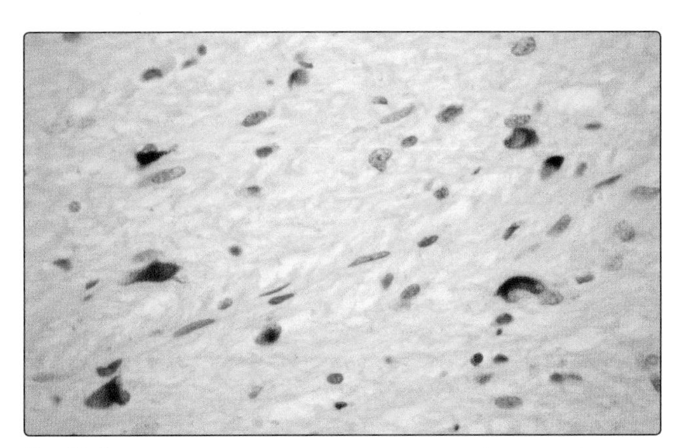

Fig. 13.8 **Synucleinopathies such as Parkinson's disease and multiple system atrophy (MSA) are characterized by pathological neuronal and glial inclusions composed of alpha-synuclein protein.** This microscopic image shows glial cytoplasmic inclusions (GCIs) within oligodendrocytes in a case of MSA, highlighted by immunohistochemistry (antibody labelling). Courtesy of Professor Steve Gentleman.

Accumulation of alpha-synuclein (within neurons and glia) occurs in several other parkinsonian syndromes including Parkinson's disease with dementia, dementia with Lewy bodies (DLB) and MSA (Fig. 13.8) which are all classified as **synucleinopathies.** In other forms of parkinsonism such as PSP and CBD there is accumulation of the microtubule-associated protein **tau** and these disorders are therefore classified as **tauopathies**. The molecular classification of neurodegenerative diseases is discussed in Ch. 8.

Familial Parkinson's disease

Five to ten percent of Parkinson's disease is familial. Around a dozen genes have been identified and the six best understood are shown in Figure 13.9. Some genes have one name connected with the protein encoded and another that is based on the order of discovery (*PARK1, PARK2,* etc.). The names can be confusing (for instance, it turns out that *PARK1* and *PARK4* are the same gene).

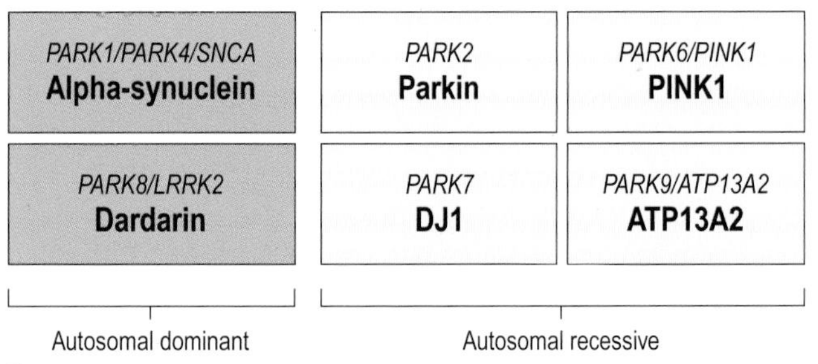

Fig. 13.9 **Genes involved in familial Parkinson's disease.** Around a dozen genes have been identified in association with familial Parkinson's disease, but the six best understood are illustrated. In each case the different names for the genes are shown above the protein encoded.

Autosomal dominant PD

The first Parkinson's disease gene to be identified was ***SNCA*** (also known as *PARK1/PARK4*), which encodes **alpha-synuclein.** This led to the discovery that alpha-synuclein is the main constituent of Lewy bodies. The gene was identified by genetic linkage analysis in a large Italian family known as the **Contursi kindred**. This family carries an alanine to threonine point mutation (**A53T**) in the alpha-synuclein gene on chromosome 4. Different point mutations (**A30P, E46K**) have been found in other families, all of which produce a severe, **autosomal dominant Parkinson's disease** with variable penetrance. The clinical and pathological features are similar to sporadic Parkinson's disease.

The most common form of autosomal dominant Parkinson's disease is caused by mutation of the **leucine-rich repeat kinase 2** gene (*LRRK2/PARK8*). This is a large gene composed of 51 exons which encodes a 2,527-amino-acid protein called **Dardarin** (Basque: dadara, tremor). The protein is part of an intracellular **second messenger cascade** which activates intracellular **kinases**. A number of pathogenic mutations have been identified. These produce a late-onset, **dopamine-responsive parkinsonian syndrome** that resembles idiopathic Parkinson's disease.

Autosomal recessive PD

Mutations in the genes that encode the proteins **Parkin, PINK1** and **DJ1** all cause a similar **dopamine-responsive parkinsonism** with **dystonia** (abnormal muscle tone and posture).

With Parkin gene (*PARK2*) mutations, disease onset is usually below the age of 40 years and these mutations account for 50% of **autosomal recessive juvenile parkinsonism** (**ARJP**). Parkin is a **ubiquitin-ligase** which is involved in ubiquitination and targeting of proteins for degradation by the **proteasome** (discussed below; see also Ch. 8). Most Parkin gene mutations reduce the ability to form protein aggregates and Lewy bodies are therefore absent.

PINK1 (**PTEN-induced kinase 1**) is a serine/threonine **protein kinase** that translocates to mitochondria and is thought to protect cells from stress-induced mitochondrial dysfunction. Mutations in the PINK1 gene (*PINK1/PARK6*) explain around 5% of autosomal recessive Parkinson's disease.

DJ1 is a **molecular chaperone protein** that prevents aggregation of synuclein and also seems to protect against oxidative stress. Mutations in the DJ1 gene (*PARK7*) account for a small proportion of autosomal recessive parkinsonism.

Mutations in the **ATPase Type 13A2** gene (*ATP13A2/PARK9*) are associated with **juvenile-onset autosomal recessive Parkinson's disease** which is accompanied by hallucinations, cognitive changes, gaze palsy and pyramidal tract signs. The gene encodes a **lysosomal ATPase** that is present at high concentration in the substantia nigra and may be involved in degradation of alpha-synuclein.

> *Key Points*
>
> - Five to ten percent of Parkinson's disease is familial and may be autosomal dominant or recessive.
> - The first gene to be identified was *SNCA* (the alpha-synuclein gene) which causes an autosomal dominant parkinsonism with features similar to idiopathic Parkinson's disease.
> - The other familial forms have variable clinical and pathological features, some with dystonia (abnormal muscle tone and posture).
> - Parkin gene (*PARK2*) mutations account for 50% of autosomal recessive juvenile parkinsonism (ARJP). These cases do not have Lewy bodies.

Treatment of Parkinson's disease

The core features of Parkinson's disease can be treated by replacing striatal dopamine, enhancing transmission at dopaminergic synapses or by stimulating dopamine receptors (see Fig. 13.10; and discussion in following sections).

Dopamine replacement

The mainstay of treatment for idiopathic Parkinson's disease is **levodopa** (or **L-dopa**), the amino acid precursor of dopamine. Levodopa (**L-3,4-dihydroxyphenylalanine**) is absorbed orally and, unlike dopamine, readily crosses the blood–brain barrier. It does so via the transport mechanism for **large neutral amino acids**. Levodopa is first taken up by dopaminergic neurons and astrocytes, then converted to dopamine by **dopa decarboxylase**. Dopamine can be stored by surviving nigral neurons and released at striatal synapses. It is also liberated directly into the interstitial fluid by astrocytes.

Levodopa is a **prodrug** because it has to be taken up by neurons and glia where it is converted to the active drug, dopamine. Peripheral activation would release dopamine into the bloodstream, causing **hypotension** and **nausea** (Clinical Box 13.3). Uptake by sympathetic neurons and conversion to noradrenaline would also interfere with autonomic control of the cardiovascular system. These side effects are avoided by co-administration of a **dopa-decarboxylase inhibitor** that is unable to cross the blood–brain barrier, increasing availability to the brain and significantly reducing the oral dose. Two commonly used peripheral decarboxylase inhibitors are **carbidopa** and **benserazide** (contained in combined preparations: co-careldopa and co-beneldopa).

Problems with levodopa therapy

Levodopa provides excellent symptomatic control in early Parkinson's disease, but in the later stages its efficacy gradually declines and a number of debilitating side effects emerge.

Reduction in efficacy

With time, single doses of levodopa wear off sooner, causing **end-of-dose fluctuations** in motor performance. There may be unpredictable shifts from a mobile ('on') state to an immobile ('off') state which can be very disabling.

Loss of effectiveness may be due to the natural progression of the disease. For instance, as nigral neurons continue to degenerate there is reduced capacity for neurotransmitter synthesis and storage, so that striatal dopamine levels are increasingly dependent on the **plasma concentration**. Competition for uptake into the brain via the transporter for large neutral amino acids may therefore become more important and striatal dopamine levels may fall after protein-rich meals.

Delivery of dopamine can be evened out by **modified-release preparations** or by continuous gastrointestinal delivery, via a tube inserted into the jejunum.

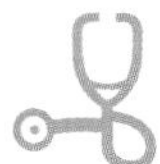

> *Clinical Box 13.3: Nausea in Parkinson's disease*
>
> Nausea is a common side effect of Parkinson's disease drugs, due to stimulation of dopamine receptors in the **emetic** (vomiting) centre of the medulla. It can be treated with **domperidone**, a dopamine receptor antagonist that does not cross the blood–brain barrier and cannot therefore interfere with central dopamine receptors. It acts directly at the **chemoreceptor trigger zone** of the emetic centre, which lies outside of the blood–brain barrier. Most anti-emetic agents are unsuitable as they block central dopamine receptors and exacerbate parkinsonism.

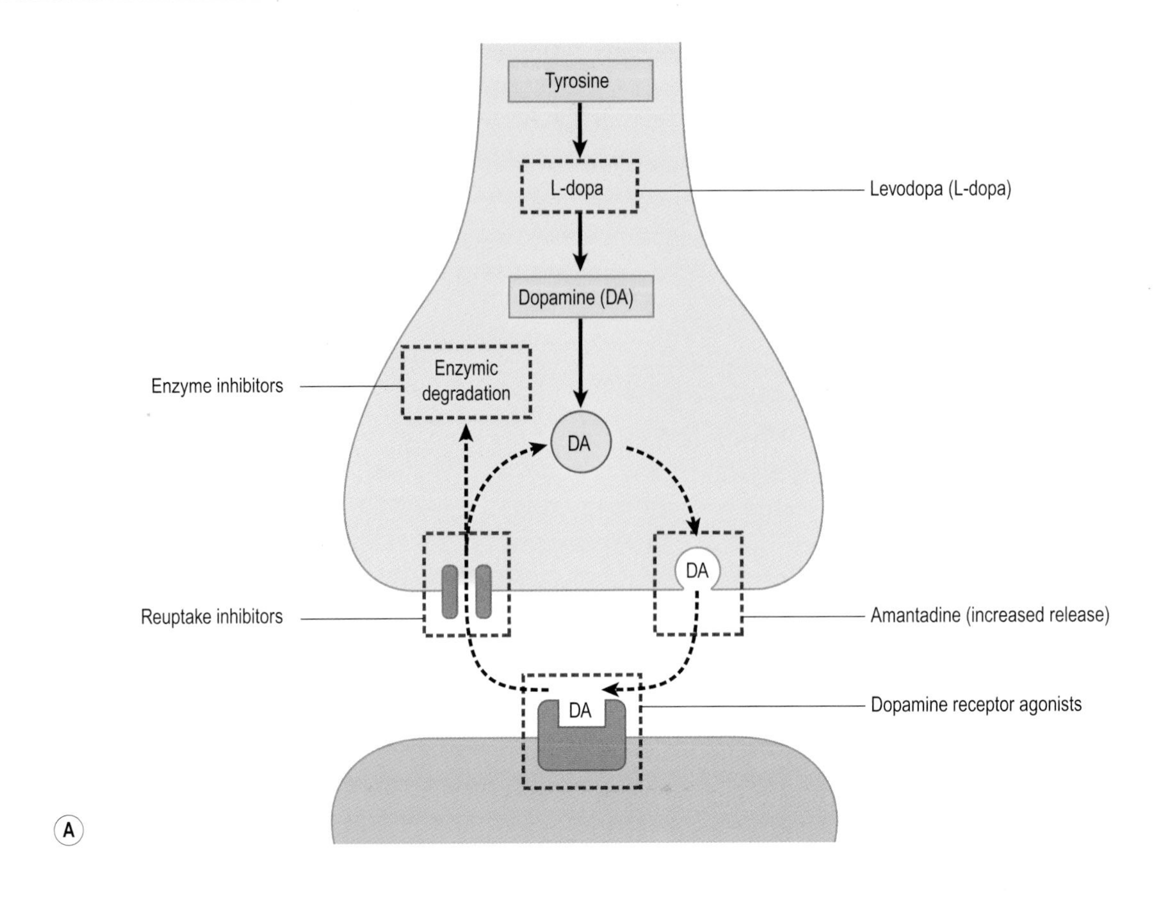

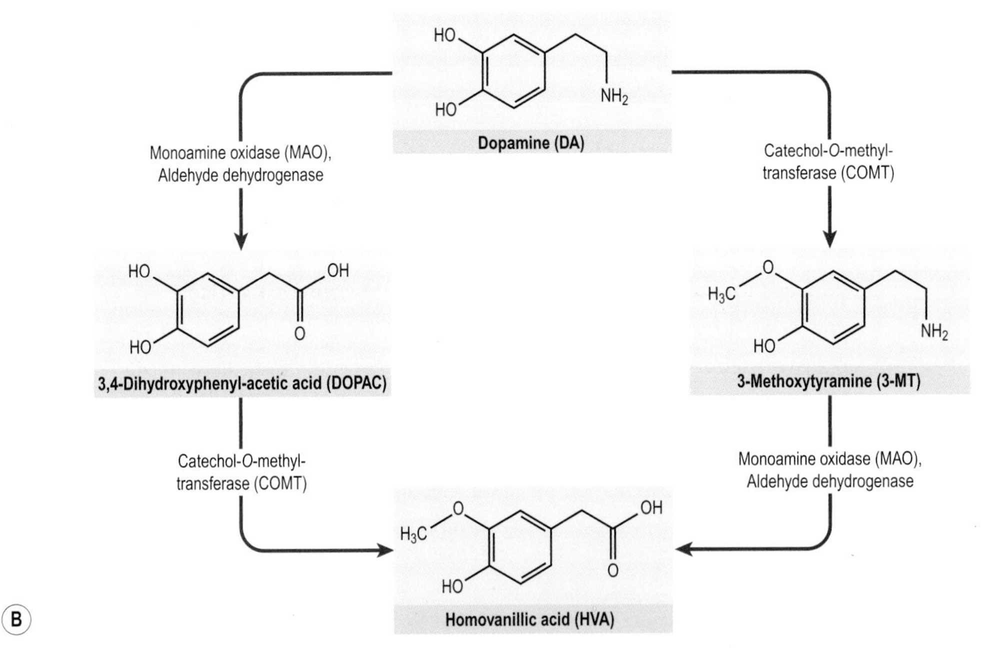

Fig. 13.10 **Treatment of Parkinson's disease. (A)** Several agents used in the symptomatic treatment of Parkinson's disease act at the dopaminergic synapse, affecting dopamine synthesis, release, reuptake or metabolism. A number of dopamine receptor agonists are also available which act directly at post-synaptic dopamine receptors in the striatum; **(B)** The two main pathways for enzymic degradation of dopamine are shown, via monoamine oxidase (MAO) and catechol-ortho-methyltransferase (COMT). MAO/COMT inhibitors are also used in Parkinson's disease to increase availability of dopamine.

Side-effects of levodopa

Patients on long-term levodopa therapy develop disabling **dyskinesias** (involuntary movements). This occurs at a rate of approximately 10% of patients per year. It does not happen in the natural history of Parkinson's disease and represents a specific side effect of dopamine replacement therapy.

Excessive dopaminergic stimulation may also cause **psychotic features** which may be difficult to manage as most **antipsychotic agents** block central dopamine receptors and therefore exacerbate parkinsonism. Some patients respond to 'atypical' neuroleptics (e.g. **clozapine**) which also antagonize serotonin receptors. Other side effects include confusion and behavioural changes (Clinical Box 13.4).

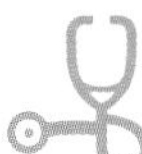

Clinical Box 13.4: Dopamine dysregulation syndrome

A small percentage of patients with Parkinson's disease become 'addicted' to their medication and use much higher doses than they need. This is associated with **impulse control** problems (e.g. hypersexuality, pathological gambling, over-eating, over-spending). Another feature is **punding**, the compulsive repetition of purposeless actions (e.g. lining up objects in rows). Dopamine dysregulation syndrome is thought to be caused by over-stimulation of dopamine receptors in the **ventral striatum**, part of the basal ganglia that is known to be involved in **reward-based learning** and addiction (see Ch. 3).

Other agents

Other drugs used to treat the symptoms of Parkinson's disease include dopamine receptor agonists, enzyme inhibitors (see Fig. 13.10) and anticholinergic agents.

Anticholinergics

Anticholinergics such as **benztropine** and **benzhexol** provide modest symptomatic benefit (by an uncertain mechanism) and are more effective in treating **tremor** than akinesia or rigidity. These agents may also offer some improvement in drooling and urinary frequency. Side effects include blurred vision, constipation, memory loss and confusion (which are more problematic in the elderly).

Amantadine

This was originally used as an **antiviral agent** to treat influenza, but provides mild symptomatic benefit in early Parkinson's disease. It can be used as a **dopamine-sparing agent**, delaying the onset of levodopa-associated side effects and loss of efficacy. Amantadine increases dopamine release and reduces its reuptake. It is also a weak antagonist at the NMDA glutamate receptor (see Ch. 7). The beneficial effect of amantadine is modest overall and tends to wear off after a few weeks. Side effects include ankle oedema, skin rash, confusion and hallucinations.

Enzyme inhibitors

Inhibitors of **catechol-O-methyltransferase** (**COMT**) such as **entacapone** and **tolcapone** block degradation of levodopa. This boosts the effective plasma half-life and increases the amount available to enter the brain. These agents are therefore similar to peripheral decarboxylase inhibitors. COMT inhibitors tend to cause **gastrointestinal side effects** including diarrhoea and liver toxicity.

Inhibitors of **monoamine oxidase** prevent degradation of dopamine and therefore prolong its action. Specific inhibitors of the central nervous system isoform (**MAO-B**) such as **selegiline** have been used in early Parkinson's disease to delay initiation of levodopa therapy. It has been suggested that selegiline might slow disease progression by blocking conversion of a putative environmental agent to its neurotoxic form, but this has not been proven.

Dopamine receptor agonists

Numerous dopamine receptor agonists are used in the treatment of Parkinson's disease, such as **pramipexole** and **ropinirole** (others include lisuride, bromocriptine and cabergoline). They are not as effective as levodopa, but may be less likely to cause dyskinesias and can be used to delay administration of levodopa or reduce the required dose.

The effectiveness of a dopamine agonist depends in part on its receptor specificity. An ideal drug would stimulate both main types of dopamine receptor (D1 and D2). **Apomorphine** is such an agent, but can only be administered by subcutaneous infusion via a syringe driver, which makes it more expensive and less practical.

Key Points

- The mainstay of Parkinson's disease treatment is levodopa, a prodrug which is able to cross the blood–brain barrier where it is taken up by neurons/glia and converted to dopamine.
- It is administered as a combined preparation together with a peripheral decarboxylase inhibitor (e.g. carbidopa or benserazide) to minimise unwanted systemic effects.
- Nausea is a common side effect of drugs used in the management of Parkinson's disease and can be treated with domperidone, a dopamine receptor antagonist that does not cross the blood–brain barrier.
- The efficacy of levodopa treatment gradually falls over time, so that: (i) single doses wear off sooner; (ii) there are unpredictable 'end-of-dose fluctuations' in motor performance; and (iii) the patient may experience abrupt shifts from a mobile 'on' state to an immobile 'off' state.
- In addition, patients on long-term levodopa therapy tend to develop disabling dyskinesias (involuntary movements). This occurs at a rate of approximately 10% of patients per year.
- Dopamine receptor agonists (e.g. pramipexole, ropinirole) are also used in the treatment of Parkinson's disease. They are not as effective, but less likely to cause drug-induced dyskinesias.
- Other agents include: anticholinergics (e.g. benztropine, benzhexol) which may be particularly helpful in tremor; amantadine (an antiviral agent that increases dopamine availability); and inhibitors of enzymes that degrade dopamine or levodopa (e.g. COMT, MAO).

Surgery in Parkinson's disease

Neurosurgery may be an option in longstanding Parkinson's disease that is no longer responsive to levodopa, particularly in patients with severe dyskinesias and no evidence of dementia. Destructive lesions in the thalamus or pallidum (**thalamotomy** and **pallidotomy**) can be effective and a small number of patients have received experimental transplants from the substantia nigra of fetuses (Clinical Box 13.5). However, the most successful surgical approach

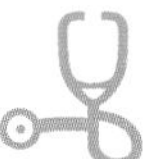

Clinical Box 13.5: Fetal nigral transplants

Some patients with Parkinson's disease have received **neuronal transplants** from the substantia nigra of fetuses (obtained following elective termination of pregnancy). **Fetal nigral cells** are grafted directly into the striatum where they have been shown to form synapses, synthesize dopamine and accumulate **neuromelanin**. Increased striatal dopamine has also been confirmed by **PET scanning**. However, the effect on parkinsonian symptoms in most patients has been disappointing and post-mortem studies in long-term survivors show that grafted cells also degenerate and eventually develop **Lewy bodies** (providing an important clue to the pathogenesis of Parkinson's disease).

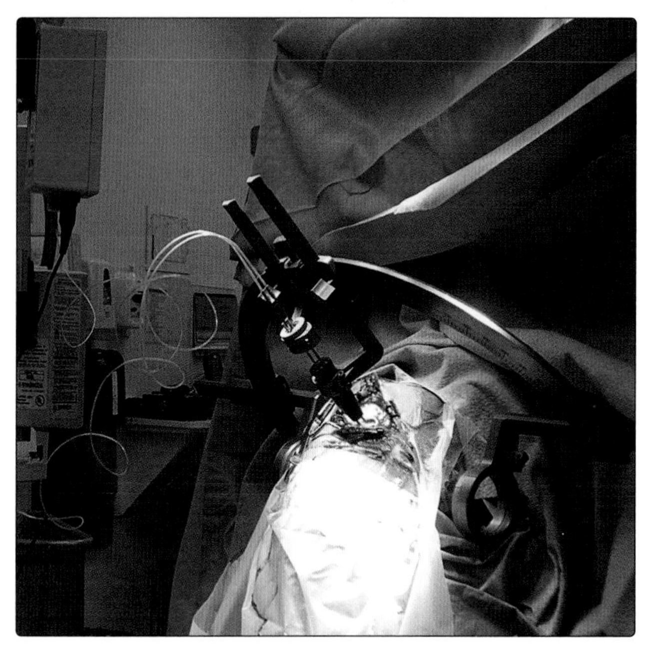

Fig. 13.11 **Surgery in Parkinson's disease.** Intraoperative photograph of a patient wearing a stereotactic frame undergoing functional neurosurgery for drug-resistant Parkinson's disease. From Larson, PS: Neurosurg Clin North Am 2010; 21(4): 691–698, with permission.

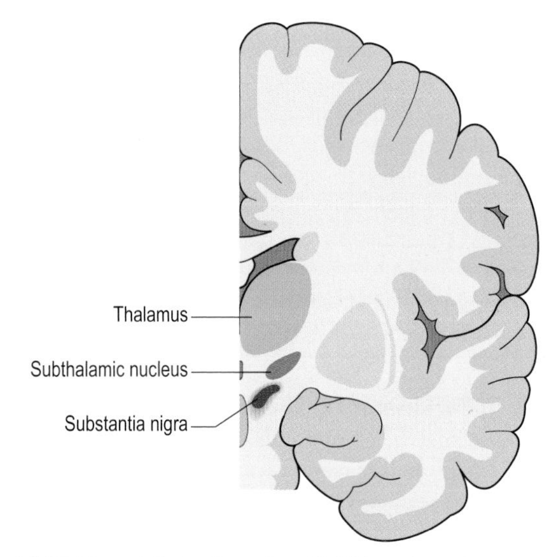

Fig. 13.12 **The subthalamic nucleus (STN) is an important target for deep brain stimulation in Parkinson's disease.** This small, lens-shaped nucleus belongs to the basal ganglia. It lies just below the thalamus, close to the substantia nigra and posterior limb of the internal capsule.

involves the placement of **deep brain electrodes** which are used to stimulate various parts of the basal ganglia.

Deep brain stimulation (DBS)

Using a **stereotactic frame** and MRI guidance (Fig. 13.11) it is possible to implant electrodes at precise subcortical targets, deep within the brain. Specific nuclei can then be stimulated via a subcutaneous pacemaker in the chest. The main surgical risks are intracerebral haemorrhage and infection, but serious complications occur in less than 2% of cases in specialist centres.

The most effective approach is bilateral stimulation of the **subthalamic nucleus** (Fig. 13.12) which provides excellent relief of akinesia and bradykinesia. It also allows the oral levodopa dose to be reduced and improves dopa-induced dyskinesias. Other DBS targets include the **thalamus** (particularly in people with severe, drug-resistant tremor) and, much less commonly, the **pedunculopontine nucleus** at the junction of the midbrain and pons (a small brain stem structure that is involved in gait initiation and is known to degenerate in Parkinson's disease).

The effect of deep brain stimulation on the target structure depends on **stimulation frequency**. Low-frequency stimulation (<80 Hz) appears to be excitatory, whereas stimulation at higher frequencies (>130 Hz) inhibits the target nucleus by an uncertain mechanism. This may be due to **depolarization blockade** (similar to the way that muscle-relaxant drugs work) or neurotransmitter depletion.

Key Points

- Neurosurgery may be an option in longstanding Parkinson's disease that is no longer responding to levodopa, particularly in patients with severe dyskinesias and no evidence of dementia.
- Destructive lesions in the thalamus and globus pallidus (thalamotomy and pallidotomy) have largely been replaced by deep brain stimulation (DBS).
- The most successful approach is bilateral stimulation of the subthalamic nucleus (STN) which provides excellent relief of both akinesia and bradykinesia. Surgery also permits a reduction in the oral levodopa dose, decreasing the risk of dopa-induced dyskinesias.
- Some patients with Parkinson's disease have received striatal transplants from the substantia nigra of fetuses, but clinical trials have been disappointing and post-mortem studies in long-term survivors show that grafted cells also degenerate and develop Lewy bodies.

Pathophysiology

The anatomy of the corpus striatum, its functional divisions and the concept of **basal ganglia loops** (including their non-motor roles in cognition, emotion and behaviour) have been introduced in Chapter 3. This section will explore the contribution of the basal ganglia to **voluntary movement** and how this is disturbed in Parkinson's disease.

The voluntary motor loop

Initiation of voluntary actions involves a basal ganglia loop that originates and terminates in the **supplementary motor area (SMA)** (Fig. 13.13; see also Ch. 3). Activity in the SMA and voluntary motor loop is facilitated by dopamine, which lowers the threshold for movement initiation. This helps to determine whether an **intention to act** is translated into an actual movement. Reduced activity in the SMA (due to striatal dopamine deficiency) is responsible for the **akinesia** (poverty of movement) in Parkinson's disease.

The SMA is involved in **self-initiated actions** (e.g. throwing a ball, rising from a chair) rather than movements that occur in response to an external stimulus or trigger (e.g. catching a ball, stepping over a piece of chalk). This has been exploited with the creation of **virtual reality glasses** that provide artificial **visual cues** for parkinsonian patients (projections of horizontal lines to 'step over'). This leads to improvement in gait initiation, stride length and pace, with fewer falls. In some cases, powerful emotions can overcome akinesia (Clinical Box 13.6).

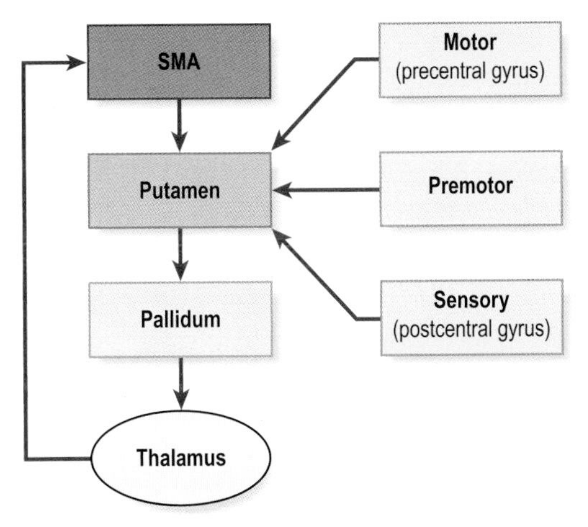

Fig. 13.13 **Voluntary motor loop of the basal ganglia.** The central, 'closed loop' component originates and terminates in the supplementary motor area (SMA) in the medial frontal lobe (see Ch. 3, Fig. 3.4b). Other sensory and motor areas form 'open-loop' components.

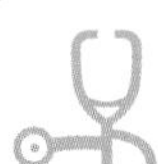

Clinical Box 13.6: Paradoxical kinesis

A strong **sense of urgency** or **fear** can sometimes overcome akinesia in patients with Parkinson's disease. The classic example is the profoundly akinetic patient who is suddenly able to run freely from a burning building, only to 'freeze' again once he reaches a place of safety. This is referred to as **paradoxical kinesis** and may be mediated by projections from the amygdala to the **ventral striatum** which is the 'limbic' (emotion-related) portion of the basal ganglia (see Ch. 3).

Key Points

- Initiation of voluntary movement is associated with increased activity in the supplementary motor area (SMA) and voluntary motor loop, which is facilitated by dopamine.
- The SMA is particularly involved in self-initiated (rather than externally triggered) actions and this type of movement is most affected in Parkinson's disease.
- In addition to the well-known (and best-understood) roles in motor control, the basal ganglia also contribute to numerous aspects of cognition, behaviour and mood.

Afferent and efferent connections

To understand how activity in the basal ganglia loops contributes to normal and **disordered voluntary motor control**, it is first necessary to review the general arrangement of the basal ganglia connections.

Projections into the basal ganglia

All basal ganglia loops arise and terminate in the frontal lobe. The frontal cortex projects to the **striatum** (caudate-putamen) which is therefore the afferent (or 'input') part of the basal ganglia. Cortical afferents terminate on **medium spiny neurons**, which make up 95% of basal ganglia cells. They are so-named because they have medium-sized cell bodies and numerous **dendritic spines** (Fig. 13.14). The **head** of each spine receives a single afferent projection from the frontal cortex, whereas the **shaft** receives a dopaminergic projection from the nigrostriatal pathway (which has a modulating effect). It is important to note that the vast majority of intrinsic basal ganglia cells are GABAergic and that the outflow of the basal ganglia is entirely **inhibitory**.

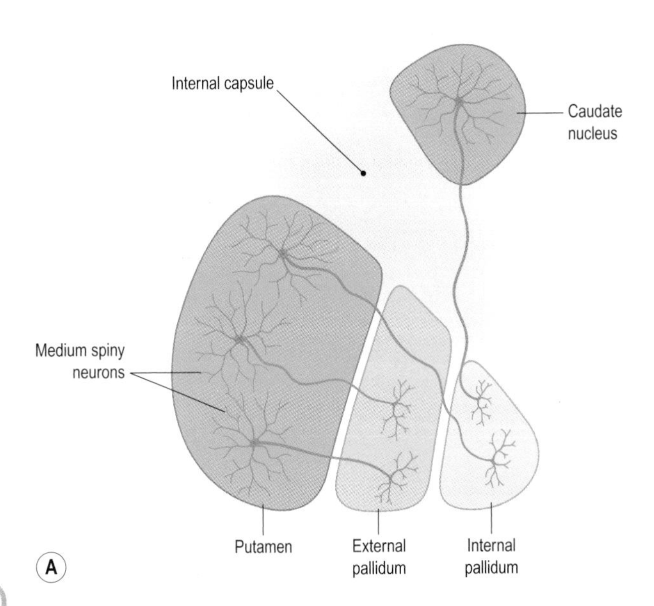

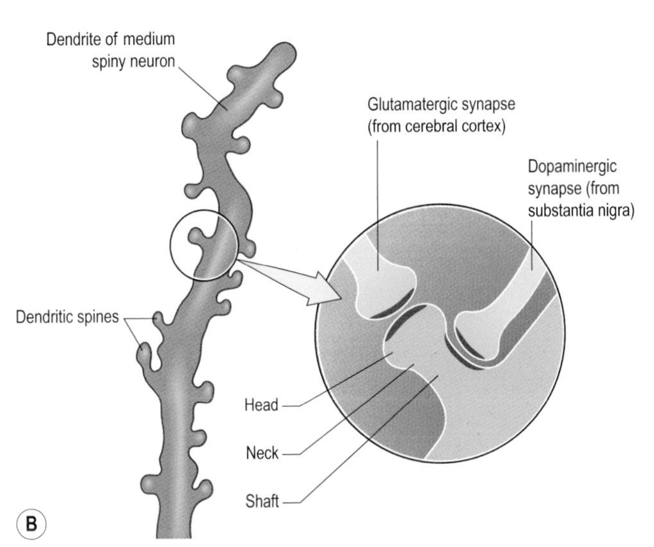

Fig. 13.14 **Medium spiny neurons in the striatum. (A)** Approximately 95% of basal ganglia neurons are classified as 'medium spiny' cells. Several medium spiny striatal neurons are illustrated in the figure: some projecting to the external pallidum, others projecting to the internal pallidum. These two types of neuron belong to the 'indirect' and 'direct' pathways, respectively [see text for further discussion]; **(B)** Medium spiny neurons in the striatum (caudate nucleus/putamen) receive excitatory projections from the frontal lobe. These excitatory cortico-striatal projections terminate on the heads of dendritic spines. In contrast, dopaminergic projections (from the substantia nigra) synapse on the shafts of dendritic spines, facilitating direct pathway neurons but inhibiting those belonging to the indirect pathway.

Outflow of the basal ganglia

The outflow of the basal ganglia arises from the **internal pallidum** (internal segment of the globus pallidus). The pars reticulata of the substantia nigra (SNpr) is functionally homologous and performs an equivalent role in an **oculomotor loop** that controls voluntary gaze. The internal pallidum/SNpr is therefore the efferent (or 'output') part of the basal ganglia and is entirely inhibitory.

By default, the internal pallidum inhibits **thalamocortical neurons** that take part in basal ganglia loops. The 'default action' of the basal ganglia is thus to prevent unwanted movements, thoughts and behaviours (Fig. 13.15). Although tonically active, the internal pallidum is also constantly stimulated by the **subthalamic nucleus**, which is excitatory and glutamatergic. This reinforces the 'default state' of pallidal

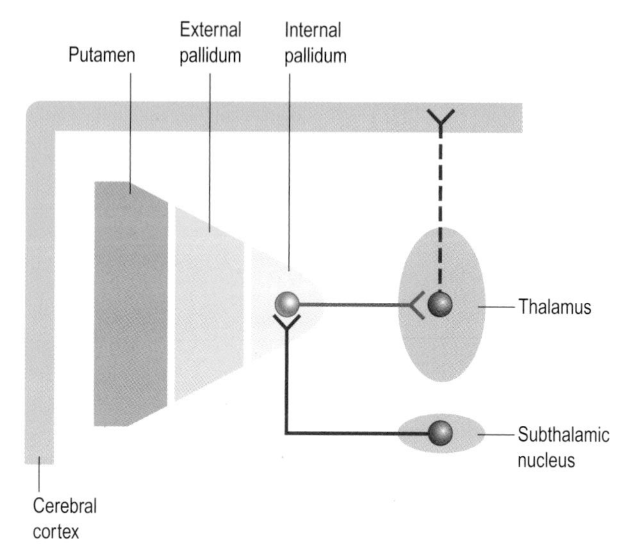

Fig. 13.15 **The output of the basal ganglia is inhibitory.** This simplified diagram illustrates the 'default' state of the basal ganglia. The internal pallidum is tonically active and powerfully inhibits nuclei in the ventral thalamus, blocking activity in thalamocortical projections that take part in basal ganglia loops. The subthalamic nucleus (which belongs to the basal ganglia) is constantly active and excites the internal pallidum, reinforcing its restraining action on the thalamus. (If the internal pallidum is a 'brake', then the subthalamic nucleus is a 'foot' on the brake pedal.)

Clinical Box 13.7: Hemiballismus

Hemiballismus is a rare condition characterized by violent flinging movements on one side of the body (Greek: hemi, half; ballismos, jumping). It is usually caused by a small stroke (Ch. 10) affecting the **subthalamic nucleus**, which normally helps to block unwanted movements by exciting the internal pallidum (which is the inhibitory outflow nucleus or 'brake' of the basal ganglia). In the absence of excitation from the subthalamic nucleus, the internal pallidum no longer suppresses unwanted movements. It is as though the 'foot' has been taken off the 'brake'.

inhibition and explains why destruction of the subthalamic nucleus causes involuntary movements (Clinical Box 13.7).

Key Points

- All basal ganglia loops arise and terminate in the frontal lobe. The frontal cortex projects to the striatum (caudate-putamen) which is the afferent or 'input' part of the basal ganglia.
- Cortico-striatal projections terminate on the dendritic spines of medium spiny neurons and the influence of the cortical afferent is facilitated or inhibited by the nigrostriatal dopamine projection (which terminates on the shafts of dendritic spines).
- The internal pallidum is the main 'outflow structure' of the basal ganglia and is entirely inhibitory. It exerts a powerful restraining influence on thalamocortical neurons. It is tonically active (helping to prevent unwanted thoughts and actions), and this is reinforced by constant excitatory drive from the subthalamic nucleus (which belongs to the basal ganglia).

Direct and indirect pathways

The striatum gives rise to two sets of basal ganglia connections: the **direct** and **indirect pathways**, which are both stimulated by afferent (corticostriatal) projections. Dopamine stimulates striatal neurons belonging to the

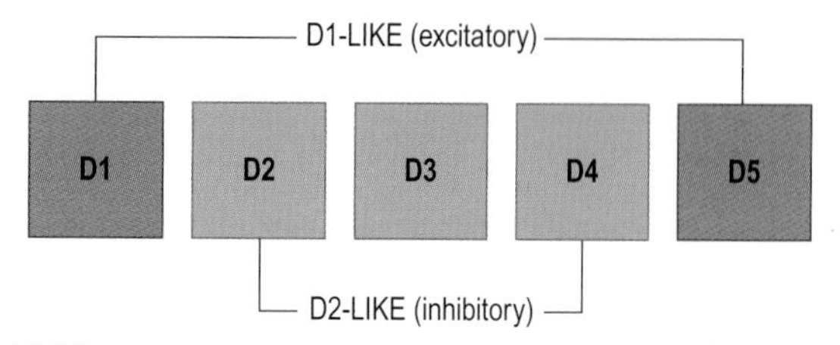

Fig. 13.16 **Dopamine receptor subtypes.** There are two major subtypes of dopamine receptor. D1-like receptors (D1, D5) are excitatory, whereas D2-like receptors (D2, D3, D4) are inhibitory.

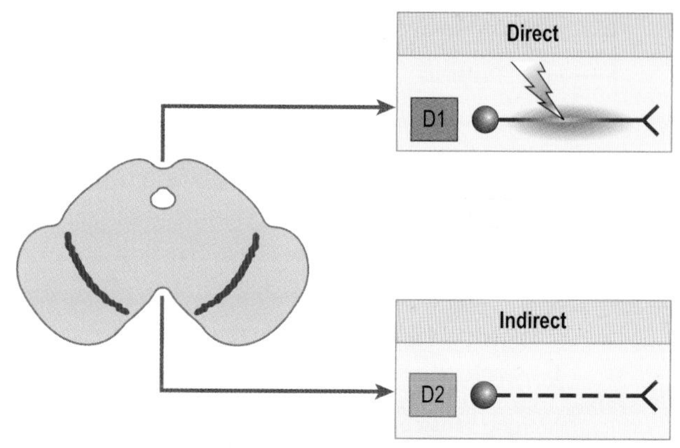

Fig. 13.17 **The effect of dopamine on a striatal medium spiny neuron depends on the type of dopamine receptor that it expresses.** Neurons that are part of the direct pathway express D1-like dopamine receptors and are excited by dopamine. Neurons that are part of the indirect pathway express D2-like dopamine receptors and are inhibited by dopamine. Dopamine therefore shifts the balance of activity in favour of the direct pathway.

direct pathway, but at the same time inhibits those of the **indirect pathway**. This is because the two types of neuron express different **dopamine receptors**. There are five main types of dopamine receptor, arranged in two groups: D1-like and D2-like (Fig. 13.16). Direct pathway neurons are excited by dopamine since they express D1-like receptors; indirect pathway neurons are inhibited by dopamine because they express D2-like receptors (Fig. 13.17). The action of dopamine is therefore to **shift the balance** in favour of the direct pathway and this leads to increased activity in the SMA/motor loop.

Direct pathway

The internal connections of the basal ganglia work by **disinhibition** (release of inhibition). This happens when two inhibitory neurons are arranged in series, so that the first one inhibits the braking action of the second (illustrated in Fig. 13.18).

The arrangement of connections in the **direct pathway** is shown in Figure 13.19A in the context of the voluntary motor loop. Striatal neurons belonging to the direct pathway project directly to the **internal pallidum** and inhibit it, thereby releasing thalamocortical neurons from their normal state of inhibition. This promotes activity in the motor loop and SMA, facilitating voluntary movement.

Indirect pathway

The indirect pathway is illustrated in Figure 13.19B. Striatal neurons belonging to the indirect pathway project to the **external pallidum**, where they inhibit a group of cells that would normally reduce the firing rate of the subthalamic nucleus. This means that the indirect pathway disinhibits the subthalamic nucleus and accentuates its excitation of the internal pallidum. The indirect pathway therefore reinforces the 'default' (inhibitory) outflow of the basal ganglia. Selective loss of indirect pathway neurons leads to involuntary movements in **Huntington's disease** (Clinical Box 13.8).

Key Points

- The internal connections of the basal ganglia are arranged as a set of direct and indirect pathways which are both stimulated by afferent (corticostriatal) projections.
- The connections of the basal ganglia work by disinhibition. Increased activity in the direct pathway disinhibits thalamocortical projection neurons by 'switching off' the restraining influence of the internal pallidum.
- In contrast, activity in the indirect pathway disinhibits the subthalamic nucleus, which increases activity of the internal pallidum and reinforces the 'default state' of inhibition.
- The effect of dopamine on striatal neurons depends upon the receptors that they bear. Dopamine stimulates direct pathway neurons (which have D1 receptors) but inhibits indirect pathway neurons (which have D2 receptors).
- The effect of dopamine on the striatum is therefore to shift the balance in favour of the direct pathway. In the voluntary motor loop, this facilitates movement.

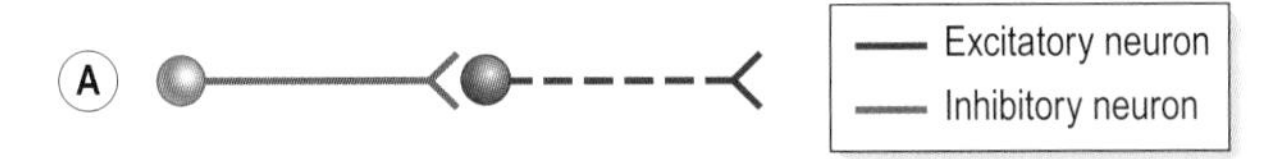

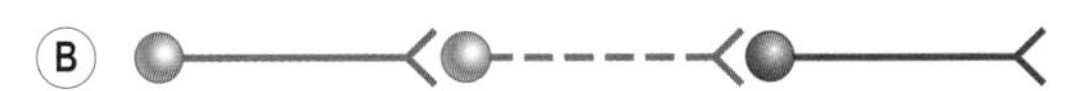

Fig. 13.18 **The connections of the basal ganglia work by inhibition and disinhibition. (A)** Simple illustration of an inhibitory interaction between two nerve cells. Activity in the excitatory neuron (red) is inhibited by an inhibitory interneuron (blue); **(B)** Disinhibition (release of inhibition) occurs when two inhibitory neurons occur in sequence. In this case the excitatory neuron (red) has been released from inhibition (or 'disinhibited') as the neuron that was previously restraining its action has itself been inhibited. In functional terms, disinhibition is equivalent to excitation.

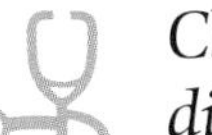

Clinical Box 13.8: Huntington's disease

This is an **autosomal dominant** disorder with variable penetrance caused by expansion of a **CAG (trinucleotide) repeat** within the **huntingtin gene** on chromosome 4. It is therefore classified as a trinucleotide repeat expansion disorder and the number of abnormal repeats determines disease severity and age at onset. Huntington's disease is characterized by involuntary movements with a 'jerky' or dance-like quality, termed **chorea** (Greek: khoreia, a choral dance). This is caused by selective loss of **indirect pathway** neurons which normally inhibit movement. Accompanying degeneration of the caudate nucleus and cerebral cortex is associated with **dementia** and **psychiatric features** (Fig. 13.20).

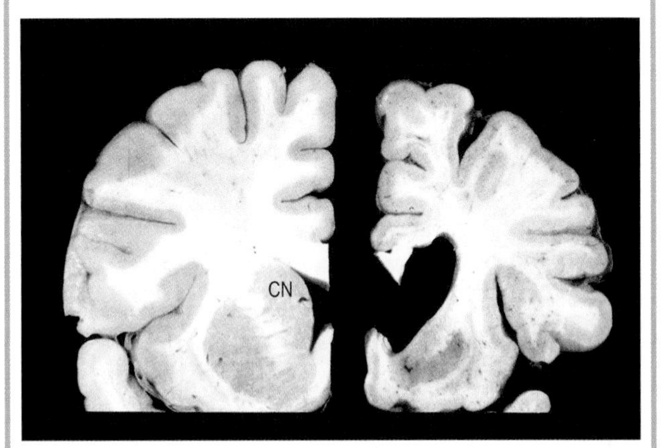

Fig. 13.20 **Huntington's disease.** Post-mortem examination of the brain in an individual with Huntington's disease [right] compared to a normal control brain [left] shows marked cortical thinning, extensive loss of subcortical white matter and dilation of the lateral ventricle. There is also striking atrophy of the caudate nucleus (labelled "CN" in the normal control brain) which takes part in basal ganglia loops passing through the prefrontal cortex that are concerned with cognition and behaviour. From Kumar et al.: Robbins and Cotran's Pathologic Basis of Disease 7e (Saunders 2004) with permission.

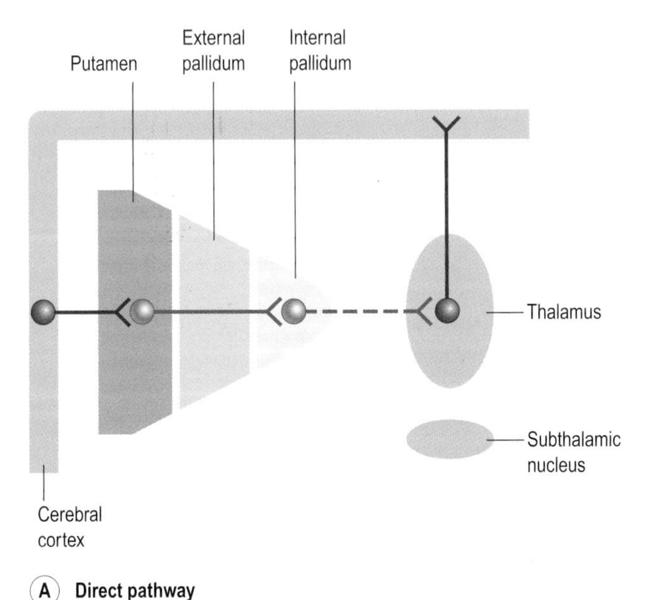

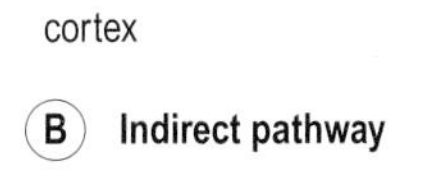

Fig. 13.19 **Direct and indirect pathways of the basal ganglia. (A)** Striatal neurons belonging to the direct pathway project directly to the internal pallidum and inhibit it, thereby releasing thalamocortical neurons from inhibition. In the voluntary motor loop, the direct pathway therefore facilitates movement; **(B)** Striatal neurons belonging to the indirect pathway project to the external pallidum, where they inhibit a group of neurons that would normally reduce the firing rate of the subthalamic nucleus. This means that the indirect pathway disinhibits the subthalamic nucleus and accentuates its excitation of the internal pallidum. The indirect pathway therefore reinforces the default (inhibitory) outflow of the basal ganglia and prevents unwanted movements.

Basal ganglia oscillations

Some of the results of stereotactic surgery do not fit well with the direct and indirect pathway model of the basal ganglia. For instance: (i) the model does not always correctly predict the effect of focal basal ganglia lesions; and (ii) a similar effect on movement can sometimes be obtained either by stimulating or by destroying a particular structure ('the paradox of stereotactic surgery').

These findings may be partly explained by recordings from **deep brain electrodes** in experimental animals (and patients with Parkinson's disease). These show that the basal ganglia engage in **rhythmic oscillations** consisting of synchronized discharges in which nuclei 'lock step' with one another at various frequencies:

- **Low frequency** (<10 Hz), associated with tremor and dystonia (abnormal muscle tone and posture).
- **Beta band** (13–30 Hz), typical of akinetic states or dopamine deficiency (e.g. in Parkinson's disease).
- **Gamma band** (>60 Hz), which occurs during voluntary movement and in response to dopamine replacement.

In Parkinson's disease there is **excessive beta activity**, which is normalized by dopamine replacement. The effect of surgical intervention (whether by stimulation or destruction) may be to interfere with **pathological oscillations**, which might enable other parts of the brain to compensate. This is summarized in the idea that 'silence is better than noise'.

> *Key Points*
>
> - Some of the results of stereotactic surgery do not fit well with the direct and indirect pathway model of the basal ganglia ('the paradox of stereotactic surgery').
> - This may be partially explained by recordings from deep brain electrodes in experimental animals and in patients with Parkinson's disease which show rhythmic oscillations.
> - Oscillations occur at characteristic frequencies, associated with: (i) tremor (<10 Hz); (ii) akinesia or dopamine deficiency (13–30 Hz); and (iii) voluntary activity or treated parkinsonism (>60 Hz).
> - Destruction or stimulation of various basal ganglia targets may be sufficient to disrupt pathological oscillations and allow functional compensation ('silence is better than noise').

Aetiology and pathogenesis

The precise cause of sporadic Parkinson's disease is not known, but appears to be due to an interaction between genetic and environmental factors.

Risk factors

The main risk factor for Parkinson's disease is advancing age. It is also more common in males and in people with a history of head injury. A possible link with industrialization, use of herbicides or pesticides and drinking well-water has also been described. Twin studies show a similar incidence of sporadic Parkinson's disease in identical and fraternal twin pairs and any genetic contribution to sporadic disease is thought to be mediated by multiple (unknown) **susceptibility genes**.

Environmental factors

There are several examples of **acquired akinetic-rigid syndromes** that have features in common with idiopathic Parkinson's disease. These are caused by various environmental, infectious or toxic agents (e.g. carbon monoxide, manganese and carbon disulphide). Parkinsonian syndromes have also been described following viral or bacterial infections (see Clinical Boxes 13.9 and 13.10).

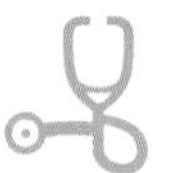

> *Clinical Box 13.9: Encephalitis lethargica*
>
> In the early 20th century a viral pandemic swept across central Europe. Features included fever, headache and marked somnolence or coma caused by inflammation of the brain: **encephalitis lethargica** (the 'sleepy sickness'). It affected children and young adults and carried a mortality of 40%. More than half of the survivors developed a syndrome of **post-encephalitic parkinsonism** and these individuals were among the first recipients of levodopa therapy in the 1960s. Post-mortem examination of the brain showed degeneration of the substantia nigra and accumulation of **neurofibrillary tangles** in surviving neurons, similar to those found in **Alzheimer's disease** (Ch. 12).

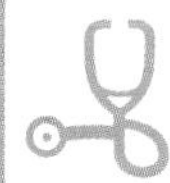

> *Clinical Box 13.10: Autoimmune basal ganglia damage*
>
> The extrapyramidal movement disorder **Sydenham's chorea** is characterized by 'jerky' involuntary limb movements ('St Vitus's dance'). It is now rare, but classically occurred a few weeks after recovery from **rheumatic fever** (caused by a streptococcal infection that affects the heart and joints). There is also a group of conditions referred to as **PANDAS** (paediatric autoimmune neuropsychiatric disorders associated with streptococcal infection). Affected children may develop **tics**, features of **obsessive-compulsive disorder** (see Ch. 3, Clinical Box 3.10) or **Tourette's syndrome**. The underlying cause in both disorders is autoimmune CNS damage due to 'cross-reaction' with a basal ganglia surface antigen that is similar to one present on the streptococcal bacterium. Interestingly, adults with OCD and related disorders are significantly more likely to show serological evidence of a previous streptococcal infection than controls.

Frozen addict syndrome

The most informative acquired parkinsonian syndrome occurred in a group of heroin addicts in California in 1982. These individuals developed an akinetic-rigid syndrome within days of injecting a synthetic heroin derivative, contaminated by the neurotoxin **MPTP** (1-methyl-4-phenyl-1,2,3,6-tetrahydropyridine). This had been inadvertently produced during the illegal manufacture of **MPPP** (1-methyl-4-phenyl-4-propionoxypiperidine), a heroin analogue related to the opiate analgesic **pethidine** (called **meperidine** in the USA). **MPTP-induced parkinsonism** is a reliable and reproducible model of Parkinson's disease and is now the primary non-human primate model of this condition. It also demonstrates conclusively that parkinsonism can be caused by an environmental agent.

MPTP in animal models

Administration of MPTP to non-human primates causes selective damage to the dopaminergic neurons of the substantia nigra and to the nigro-striatal pathway, with profound reduction of striatal dopamine. This leads to an akinetic-rigid syndrome similar to Parkinson's disease.

CH_3 N Monoamine oxidase CH_3 N^+

MPTP MPP+

(A)

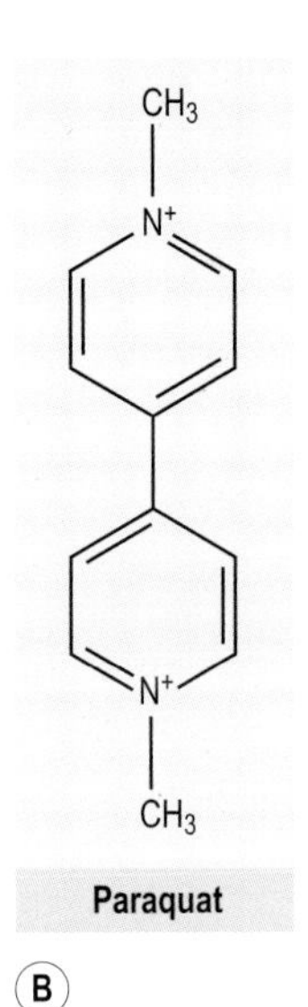

(B)

Fig. 13.21 **MPTP (1-methyl-4-phenyl-1,2,3,6-tetrahydropyridine). (A)** MPTP is converted to the neurotoxic agent MPP+ by monoamine oxidase B. MPP+ is then taken up by dopaminergic neurons; **(B)** MPP+ is structurally similar to the neurotoxic herbicide paraquat.

Mechanism of MPTP toxicity

MPTP crosses the blood–brain barrier where it is taken up by neurons and astrocytes and metabolized by **monoamine oxidase** (**MAO**) to form **MPP+** (**1-methyl-4-phenylpyridinium**) (Fig. 13.21A). This molecule is a highly reactive free radical species with an unpaired electron and is similar to the neurotoxic herbicide **paraquat** (Fig. 13.21B). MPP+ is taken up by dopaminergic neurons (via a specific monoamine transporter) where it binds to neuromelanin and becomes concentrated. MPP+ has been shown to inhibit **complex I** of the mitochondrial respiratory chain, leading to **oxidative stress** in dopaminergic neurons.

> *Key Points*
>
> - There are several examples of acquired akinetic-rigid disorders caused by an environmental agent (e.g. carbon monoxide, manganese, carbon disulphide) or a virus (e.g. post-encephalitic parkinsonism).
> - Autoimmune-mediated basal ganglia damage may also occur following infection with particular types of streptococcal bacteria (e.g. Sydenham's chorea and PANDAS).
> - The most informative acquired akinetic-rigid syndrome is frozen addict syndrome, caused by accidental exposure to the neurotoxin MPTP in a group of heroin addicts in the 1980s.

Mitochondria and oxidative stress

Inhibition of **complex I** of the **mitochondrial electron transport chain** (NADH dehydrogenase) is a key event in the pathogenesis of Parkinson's disease. This reduces ATP production and impairs energy-dependent cellular processes. It also leads to the generation of **free radicals**, causing additional **oxidative stress** and lowering the threshold for **apoptosis** (programmed cell death; see Ch. 8).

Animal models using toxins such as **MPTP** or **paraquat** (or the pesticide **rotenone**, another complex I inhibitor) cause selective nigral degeneration and parkinsonism but lack pathological inclusions. However, Lewy bodies are produced in chronic, low-grade toxicity models, mimicking the core features of idiopathic Parkinson's disease.

There is evidence of reduced complex I function (in brain tissue, muscle and platelets) in patients with Parkinson's disease. Markers of oxidative stress have also been found in post-mortem studies, such as increased **lipid peroxidation** of cell membranes. The role of mitochondrial dysfunction and complex I inhibition is further supported by the existence of autosomal recessive forms of familial Parkinson's disease caused by loss-of-function mutations affecting proteins that protect against oxidative stress or mitochondrial dysfunction (e.g. **DJ1**, **PINK1**).

Protein aggregation

A pathological hallmark of Parkinson's disease is **aggregation of alpha-synuclein** protein to form Lewy bodies. Excessive production of alpha-synuclein is known to be a factor in some familial forms of Parkinson's disease (e.g. with duplication or triplication of the synuclein gene) and this presumably overloads protein disposal mechanisms.

Neurotoxicity of alpha-synuclein

It is not clear whether or not Lewy bodies are neurotoxic and it may be that an intermediate **oligomeric species** (formed during their synthesis) is responsible for damaging the cell. It has been shown that monomers of alpha-synuclein associate with cell membranes and form ring-like **oligomeric assemblies** with a central pore that can perforate the cell membrane. This is similar to the **membrane attack complex** of the complement cascade and enables **free calcium** to enter the cell (a final common pathway in neuronal cell death; see Ch. 8). A similar mechanism has been postulated for amyloid beta toxicity in Alzheimer's disease (Ch. 12).

Inclusion bodies may also trigger **free radical stress**, either in response to the aggregated insoluble protein or as a result

> *Key Points*
>
> - Inhibition of complex I of the mitochondrial respiratory chain is a key event in the pathogenesis of Parkinson's disease and underlies MPTP-induced parkinsonism.
> - Administration of MPTP to non-human primates selectively damages dopaminergic neurons of the substantia nigra and causes an akinetic-rigid syndrome similar to Parkinson's disease.
> - MPTP crosses the blood–brain barrier and is metabolized by monoamine oxidase to MPP+. This is a highly reactive free radical species that resembles the neurotoxic herbicide paraquat and is taken up by dopaminergic neurons, leading to mitochondrial dysfunction.
> - Mitochondrial dysfunction impairs energy-dependent cellular processes and leads to generation of free radicals, creating oxidative stress.

of mitochondrial dysfunction. Protein aggregation may reduce activity in the **ubiquitin-proteasome system**, either by overloading/blocking it or as a secondary consequence of oxidative stress or mitochondrial dysfunction (since it is an active, energy-dependent process; see below).

Abnormal phosphorylation

Abnormal protein phosphorylation may also be a factor in the pathogenesis of Parkinson's disease (analogous to hyperphosphorylation of tau in Alzheimer's disease). This is in line with some inherited forms of Parkinson's disease in which **kinase dysfunction** is implicated (e.g. mutations of *PINK1* or *LRRK2*). In particular, it has been shown that **post-translational modification of serine residue 129** in the alpha-synuclein protein promotes fibril formation (native alpha-synuclein is not phosphorylated).

Dysfunction of the ubiquitin-proteasome system

The ubiquitin-proteasome system (UPS) is an important cellular mechanism for the disposal of abnormal or misfolded proteins, particularly when attempts to deal with them have failed (e.g. the **unfolded protein response** or upregulation of **molecular chaperones**, see Ch. 8).

Evidence implicating UPS dysfunction in Parkinson's disease includes the recognition that **Parkin** is an **E3 ubiquitin ligase** that is involved in tagging abnormal proteins for proteasomal destruction. Similarly, mutations of the gene encoding **UCH-L1** (**ubiquitin C-terminal hydrolase L1**), an enzyme involved in ubiquitin recycling, are responsible for some forms of familial Parkinson's disease.

Importantly, proteasome dysfunction may interact with both protein aggregation and mitochondrial stress since: (i) excessive quantities of abnormal protein overwhelm cellular disposal mechanisms; and (ii) mitochondrial dysfunction leads to reduced cellular ATP, which has a negative impact on the proteasome (since it requires ATP to function).

Interaction of pathogenetic mechanisms

Sporadic Parkinson's disease is thought to be caused by a combination of environmental and constitutional factors. There are three main elements (illustrated in Figure 13.22):

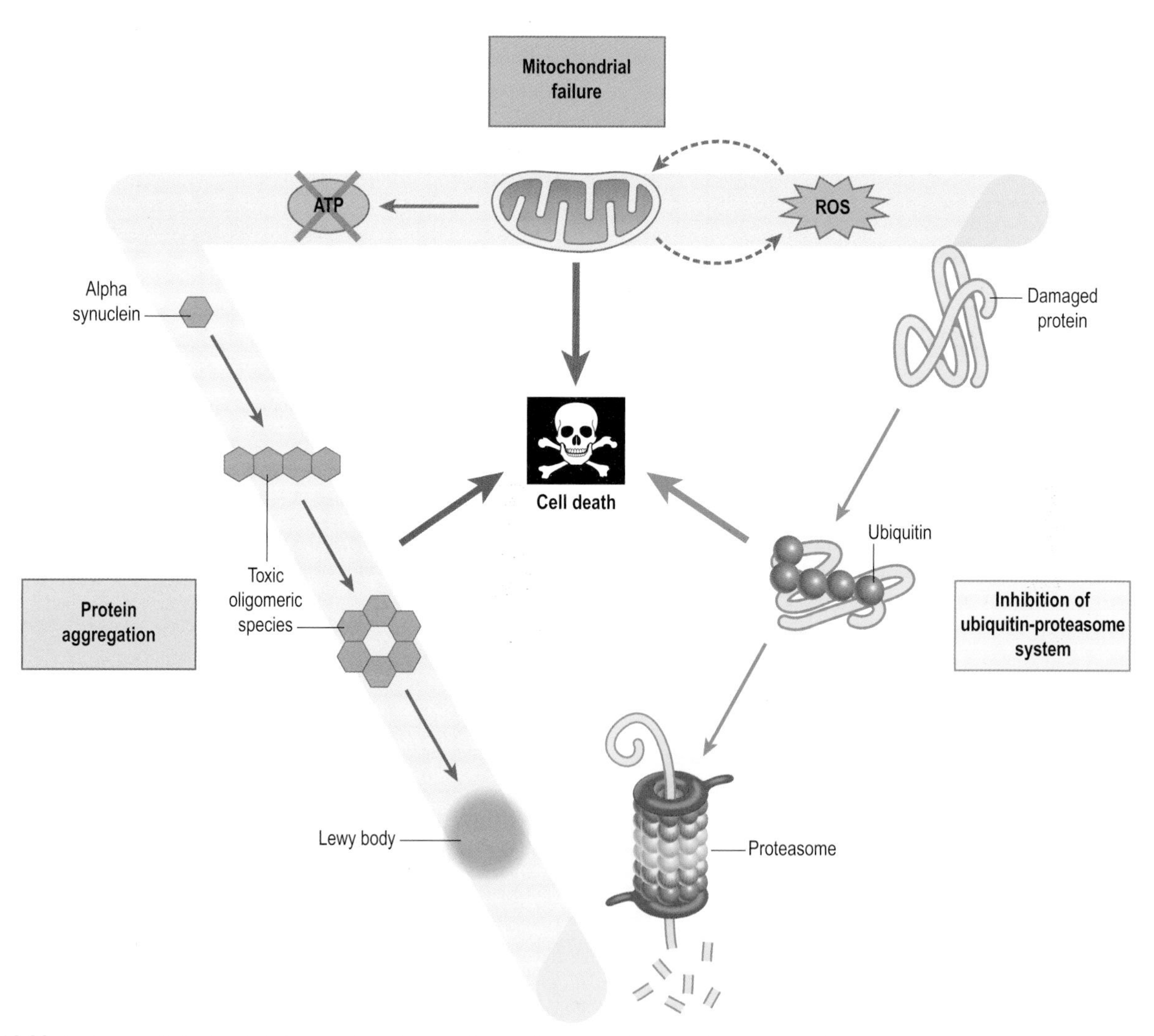

Fig. 13.22 **Pathogenetic factors in idiopathic Parkinson's disease.** Interaction between the three main factors creates a vicious cycle in dopaminergic neurons (ROS = reactive oxygen species).

- **Mitochondrial compromise**, with complex I inhibition, reduced cellular ATP production, increased oxidative stress and lowered threshold for programmed cell death.
- **Protein aggregation**, with generation of toxic oligomeric species, increased oxidative stress, secondary mitochondrial dysfunction and overload of protein disposal mechanisms.
- **Ubiquitin-proteasome dysfunction**, with accumulation of misfolded proteins leading to Lewy body formation, exacerbated by reduced mitochondrial function and ATP depletion.

Exposure to a relevant environmental or toxic factor in a genetically predisposed individual (e.g. with reduced capacity to deal with **oxidative stress**, **mitochondrial dysfunction** or to handle **misfolded proteins**) is thought to trigger a set of events that culminates in a **vicious cycle** incorporating these three key pathogenetic elements. This occurs on a background of variable nigral **reserve capacity** and normal age-related degeneration (in some cases with additional contributory factors, such as head injury).

Key Points

- A hallmark of Parkinson's disease is aggregation of alpha-synuclein (in the form of Lewy bodies) in the brain stem, cerebral hemispheres and autonomic nervous system.
- It is not certain if Lewy bodies are themselves neurotoxic, but oligomers of alpha-synuclein can form pores that are able to perforate the neuronal membrane.
- Pathological aggregates of insoluble protein are also likely to cause free radical stress which may in turn impair the function of mitochondria and the ubiquitin-proteasome system.
- UPS-dysfunction has been demonstrated in a number of neurodegenerative diseases, including two forms of autosomal recessive parkinsonism (caused by mutations affecting Parkin and UCH-L1 proteins). Importantly, this may interact with both mitochondrial stress and protein aggregation.

Chapter 14
Multiple sclerosis

CHAPTER CONTENTS

Multiple sclerosis is an inflammatory demyelinating disease of the central nervous system, with a lifetime prevalence of approximately 1 in 800. It typically presents between the ages of 20 and 40 and two-thirds of patients are female. Although the course is highly variable, MS is a progressive and incurable disease. It is responsible for a considerable burden of long-term neurological disability and is the most common chronic neurological disorder in young adults.

Demyelination

Axonal myelination is discussed in Chapter 5. The term **demyelination** refers to the loss of normally formed myelin and can be classified as primary or secondary:

- **Primary demyelination** is selective loss of myelin with relative preservation of axons. Multiple sclerosis is the most common and important cause.
- **Secondary demyelination** is degeneration of the myelin sheath following axonal loss.

It is important to distinguish demyelination (loss of structurally normal myelin) from **dysmyelination** in which the myelin sheath is not normally formed in the first place. Conditions characterized by dysmyelination are usually due to a metabolic abnormality or enzyme deficiency and are often inherited (Clinical Box 14.1).

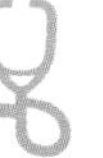

Clinical Box 14.1: Leukodystrophies

The leukodystrophies are a large group of cerebral white matter diseases (Greek: leukos, white) caused by **abnormal myelin formation** in the brain and spinal cord. These conditions usually present in infancy or childhood with **developmental delay** or progressive neurological deterioration and there may be gradual regression of cognitive, language or motor abilities in a previously normal child. Neuroimaging confirms abnormal cerebral white matter. Most of the leukodystrophies are genetic in origin and may show a recessive, dominant or X-linked pattern of inheritance.

Key Points

- Multiple sclerosis (MS) is the most common inflammatory demyelinating disease of the CNS. It typically presents between the ages of 20 and 40 and two-thirds of patients are female.
- MS is the most common and important cause of primary demyelination, which is characterized by loss of structurally normal myelin with relative preservation of axons.
- Secondary demyelination is degeneration of the myelin sheath as a result of axonal loss. In dysmyelination (e.g. in the leukodystrophies) myelin formation is abnormal.

Clinical features of MS

Multiple sclerosis is usually a relapsing-remitting disorder. Each clinical episode (or relapse) is caused by a focus of demyelination in the brain or spinal cord, which is referred to as a **plaque**. When a relapse occurs, symptoms typically develop over a few days and gradually resolve over a number of weeks, as the inflammation subsides and the plaques **remyelinate** to a greater or lesser degree.

Common symptoms

Although plaques can occur anywhere in the brain or spinal cord, including the central visual pathways, some sites are more likely to be affected than others. This means that certain symptoms and signs are more common (Fig. 14.1). The most frequently encountered presenting features are **weakness** in one or more limbs (40% of cases) and **optic neuritis** (up to 25% of cases; discussed below).

Loss of vision

Inflammatory demyelination of the optic nerve (termed **optic neuritis**) is common in MS. This causes blurred vision in one eye, with reduced light and colour perception, combined with **retrobulbar pain** (discomfort behind the affected eye, exacerbated by movement). In some cases there is a blind spot or **scotoma** (Greek: scotos, darkness). Symptoms usually resolve completely within a few weeks, but there may be a persistent **afferent pupillary defect** (Clinical Box 14.2). Optic neuritis can occur as an isolated phenomenon, but 75% of affected individuals will eventually develop multiple sclerosis. Another common visual problem in MS is discussed in Clinical Box 14.3.

Pain and fatigue

Up to 90% of people with MS suffer from **chronic fatigue**, which is characterized by overwhelming mental and physical exhaustion (regarded by many patients as one of the most disabling features). Painful symptoms may include

neuropathic-type burning and gnawing pains in the extremities (e.g. the hands and feet). Some patients experience **trigeminal neuralgia**, characterized by stabbing facial pains in the territory of the trigeminal nerve. This is extremely unpleasant and is sometimes called 'the suicide disease'. Chronic pain may also result from muscle spasms and contractures.

Paroxysmal symptoms

Paroxysmal sensory and motor symptoms are common in MS, such as temporary episodes of slurred speech, incoordination, muscle spasms or painful stabbing sensations. These may be due to abnormal electrical impulses in acutely demyelinating lesions. Another characteristic feature is **Lhermitte's phenomenon**. This is a sudden shooting pain elicited by neck flexion that may be described as an electric shock passing down the spine and radiating to the legs. It is caused by cervical cord demyelination and is virtually diagnostic of multiple sclerosis.

Cognitive and emotional changes

Cognitive, emotional and behavioural changes occur in at least 40% of patients with MS. There may be subtle disturbances in **frontal executive function** (e.g. attention, working memory, decision-making; see Ch. 3) and a small proportion of patients develop more severe cognitive decline or even **dementia** (Ch. 12). **Euphoria** is often described, but **depression** is more common (seen in up to 50% of patients) and the risk of suicide is also increased. **Psychotic features** (delusions and hallucinations) are rare.

Bladder, bowel and sexual dysfunction

Bladder problems such as **urinary retention** and **frequency** are common in multiple sclerosis, but faecal incontinence is rare. Sexual function may be compromised in longstanding disease and up to 40% of male patients experience some degree of **erectile dysfunction**. These are important (and potentially embarrassing) problems which can have a major impact on quality of life.

Cerebellar features

Involvement of the cerebellum or its connections with the brain stem may cause **dysarthria** (slurred speech), **ataxia** (incoordination) or **nystagmus** (a rhythmic abnormality of gaze fixation, with a frequency of 1–4 Hz, consisting of a slow drift phase and a brisk corrective 'snap'). There may also be a cerebellar **intention tremor**. This is worse towards the end of deliberate or precise movements

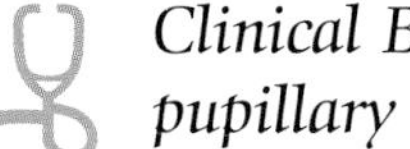

Clinical Box 14.2: Relative afferent pupillary defect

The pupillary light reflexes (see Ch. 3, Clinical Box 3.11) are often abnormal in patients with MS. Loss of myelin in the optic nerve may reduce the afferent drive to constrict the pupils when light is shone into the affected eye, causing a **relative afferent pupillary defect** (**RAPD**). This is demonstrated using the **swinging light test**. A pen torch shone into the normal eye causes strong constriction of both pupils. Quickly swinging the light across to the abnormal eye generates a weaker afferent drive to the pupil constrictor muscles (*relative* to the good eye) and both pupils paradoxically dilate slightly in response to the torch beam.

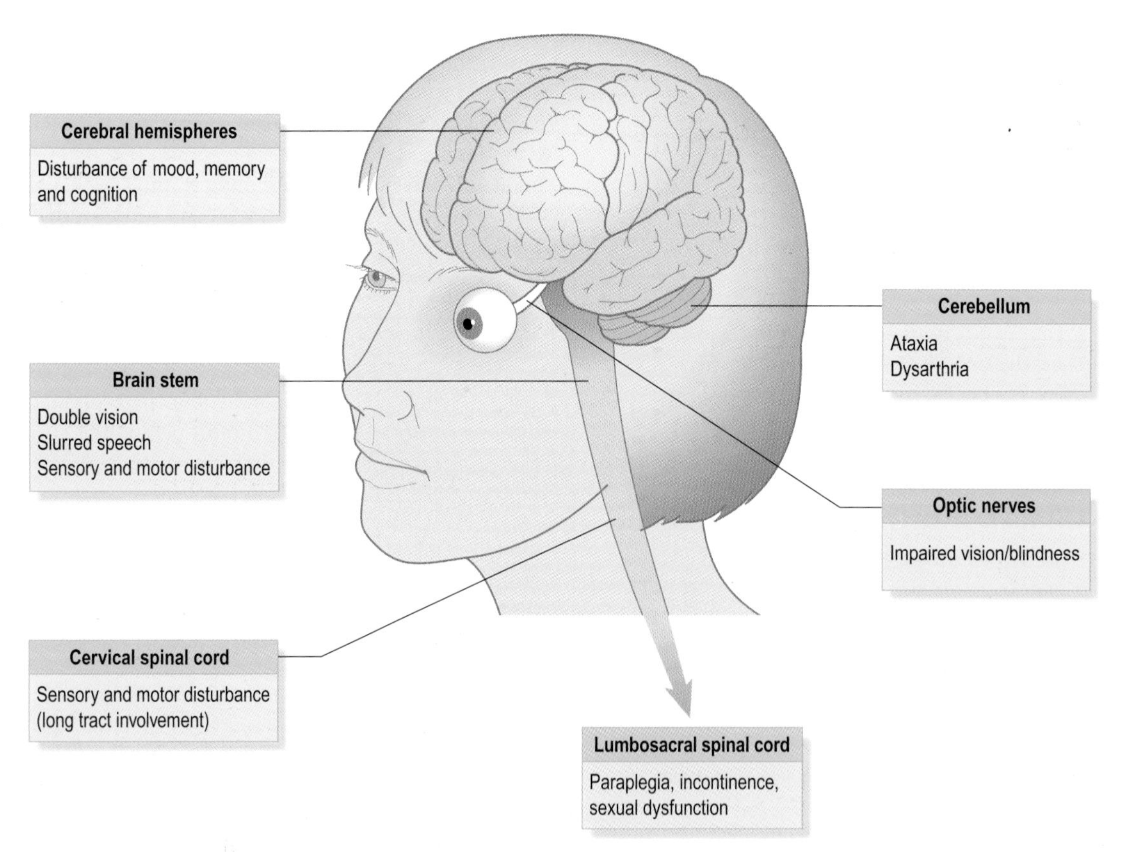

Fig. 14.1 **Common symptoms in multiple sclerosis.**

Clinical Box 14.3: Internuclear ophthalmoplegia

This is an eye movement abnormality that is caused by a small brain stem lesion that interrupts the connection between the **lateral gaze centre** (close to the abducens nucleus, CN VI, in the pons) and the **oculomotor nucleus** (CN III, in the midbrain). Interruption of the **medial longitudinal fasciculus** (**MLF**) causes failure of adduction in the affected eye on attempted contralateral gaze, illustrated in Fig. 14.2. It is important to note that the figure is a schematic representation and that in reality the two fasciculi lie close to each other on either side of the midline. This means that it is possible for a single lesion to interrupt both sides at once, leading to failure of adduction in both eyes (on attempted left and right lateral gaze).

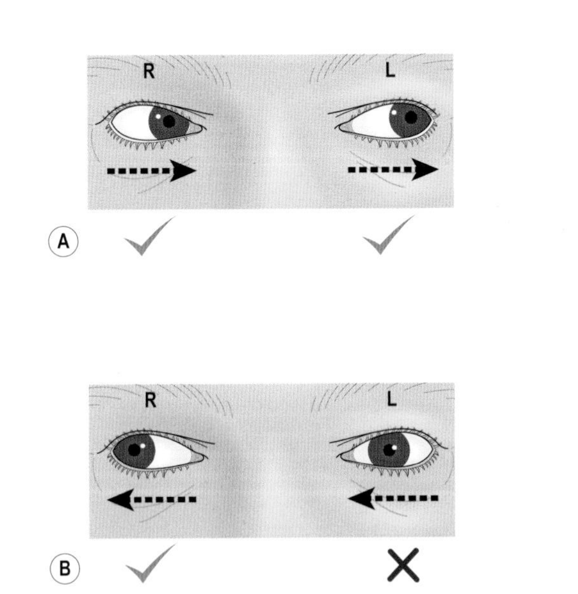

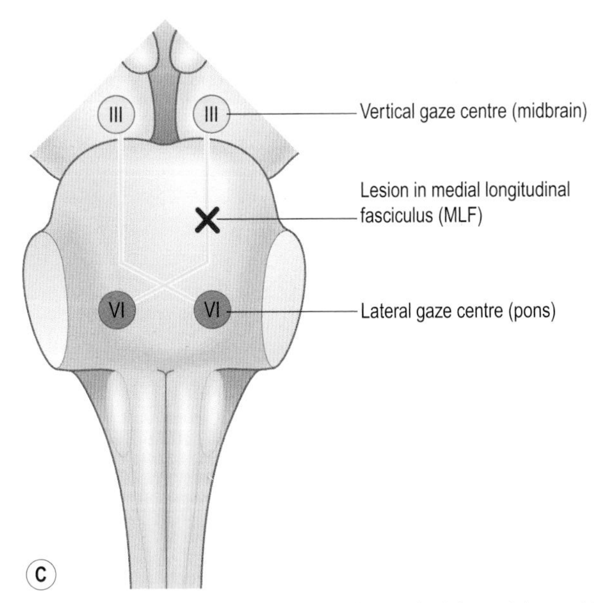

Fig. 14.2 **Internuclear ophthalmoplegia.** In this person left lateral gaze is normal **(A)** but on attempted right lateral gaze, the left eye fails to adduct **(B).** This is due to a lesion in the left MLF **(C)** which prevents the right lateral gaze centre from communicating with the opposite oculomotor nucleus (which it needs to do to recruit the medial rectus muscle).

(in contrast to the 'rest tremor' of **Parkinson's disease**; see Ch. 13).

Temperature sensitivity

Some MS symptoms are exacerbated (or clinically silent lesions unmasked) by an increase in body temperature. This can occur in a number of situations (e.g. a fever, hot bath or vigorous exercise) and is known as **Uhthoff's phenomenon**. It is thought that increased temperature prolongs inactivation of **voltage-gated sodium channels** (see Ch. 6) and therefore increases the chance of conduction failure in partially myelinated or incompletely remyelinated axons.

Key Points

- MS is usually a relapsing-remitting disorder and each clinical episode is caused by a focus of demyelination (or plaque) within the brain, spinal cord or central visual pathways.
- Common features include: optic neuritis, pain and fatigue, problems with bowel, bladder and sexual function and various paroxysmal symptoms (e.g. dysarthria, ataxia, Lhermitte's phenomenon).
- Nine out of ten people with MS suffer from chronic fatigue, which is one of the most disabling symptoms. Psychological features including anxiety and depression are also very common.
- Symptoms are often exacerbated by an increase in temperature (Uhthoff's phenomenon) which is thought to prolong sodium channel inactivation, leading to axonal conduction failure.

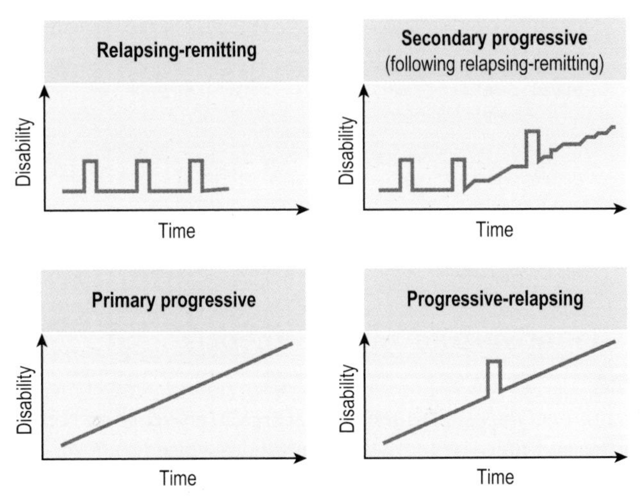

Fig. 14.3 **Clinical patterns of multiple sclerosis.**

Course and progression

The course of MS is highly variable and difficult to predict in a particular individual. The main clinical patterns are illustrated in Figure 14.3 and discussed further below.

Relapsing-remitting MS

Multiple sclerosis most often follows a **relapsing-remitting** course (85% of cases) and this is sometimes referred to as the **Charcot variant**. In this classic form of the disease, long periods of stability (**remissions**) are punctuated by discrete episodes of neurological dysfunction (**relapses**) followed by partial or complete recovery. A relapse is defined by new neurological symptoms or signs that are present for at least 24 hours and are not associated with a fever. One in five patients will experience this form of the disease for at least 20 years (**benign MS**) but most will eventually convert to a phase of gradual functional decline.

Secondary progressive MS

Individuals with relapsing-remitting MS who convert to a state of progressive decline are said to have **secondary progressive disease**. This is characterized by gradual accumulation of permanent neurological deficits. In addition to the steady functional decline, acute exacerbations or 'flare ups' may also continue. This is referred to as **progressive-relapsing MS**. The proportion of patients converting from relapsing-remitting to secondary progressive disease is around 50% at 10 years and more than 90% at 30 years.

Primary progressive MS

In **primary progressive MS** (which occurs in 10–15% of patients) there is steady functional decline from the start of the illness, with gradual accumulation of irreversible neurological deficits. Males and females are equally affected and age at onset is about ten years later than in relapsing-remitting disease, which coincides with the typical age of conversion from relapsing to secondary progressive MS. The most severe subtype is **acute multiple sclerosis**, also known as the **Marburg variant**. This is a rare, hyperacute form of MS that usually leads to death within six months (sometimes after only a few weeks).

Key Points

- The course of MS is highly variable, but a classical relapsing-remitting pattern (Charcot variant) is seen in 85% of cases and this lasts for more than two decades in 20% of people (benign MS).
- Most patients eventually convert to a state of steady functional decline (secondary progressive MS). This occurs in 50% of people within 10 years and 90% at 30 years.
- In primary progressive MS (seen in 10–15% of patients) there is steady functional decline from the start of the illness.

Diagnosis and management

Diagnosis of MS requires the demonstration of demyelinating central nervous system lesions that are disseminated in both space and time (i.e. more than one clinical episode, affecting at least two regions of the brain, spinal cord or visual pathways). There is no cure at present but a number of **disease-modifying agents** are available that may reduce relapse frequency and severity (see below).

Diagnosis

The diagnosis of multiple sclerosis is primarily clinical, but is confirmed and supported by neuroimaging, serological testing and electrophysiology.

Neuroimaging

The most sensitive method for demonstrating MS lesions is **magnetic resonance imaging** (**MRI**), which shows ten times more plaques than clinical episodes (since most lesions are clinically silent).

Demyelinating lesions are well-demonstrated on **T2-weighted MRI scans**, which highlight increased water content or decreased myelin (fat) content. However, since MS plaques tend to be periventricular, the T2 hyperintensity of normal CSF may make them more difficult to see. This is overcome using a **fluid attenuation inversion recovery** (**FLAIR**) sequence, which is similar to T2 but with a suppressed CSF signal (Fig. 14.4).

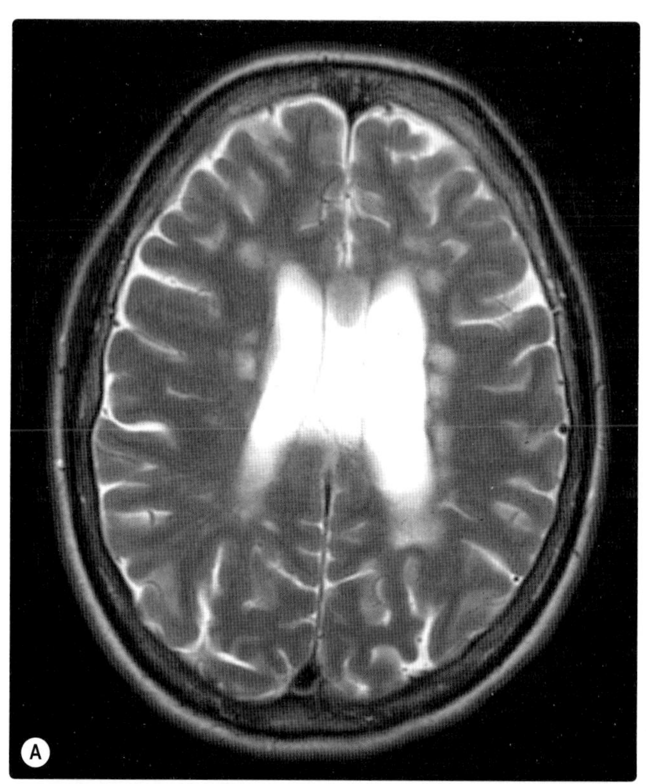

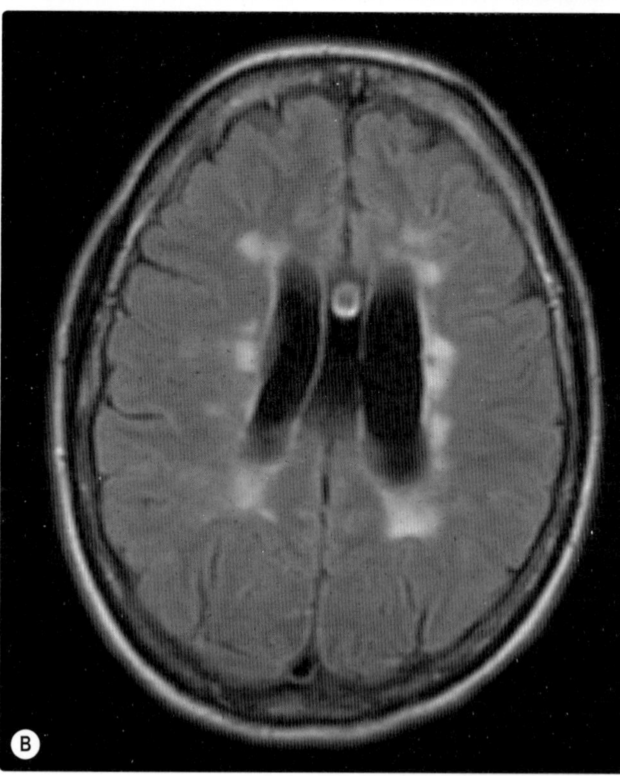

Fig. 14.4 **An axial, T2-weighted MRI scan (A) and a fluid attenuation inversion recovery (FLAIR) sequence (B) in a patient with multiple sclerosis.** There are numerous plaque-like lesions in the periventricular white matter, best seen on the FLAIR sequence [see text for explanation]. Courtesy of Dr Andrew MacKinnon.

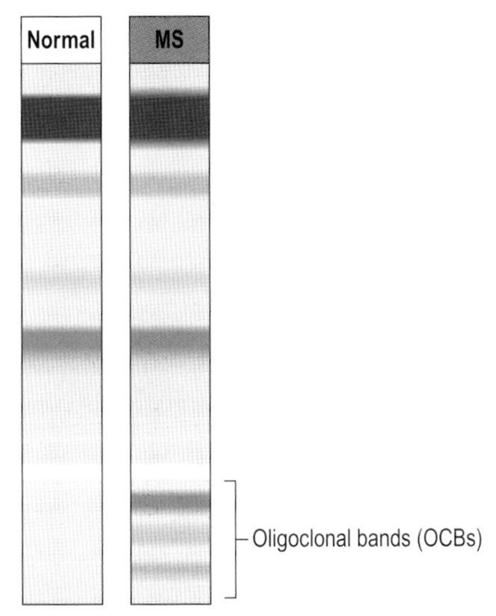

Fig. 14.5 **Oligoclonal bands in MS.** The presence of oligoclonal bands of immunoglobulin G (IgG) in the CSF that are not present in the peripheral blood provides evidence of CNS inflammation.

In patients with clinically definite multiple sclerosis, MRI shows multifocal white matter abnormalities in 95% of cases. Administration of the MRI contrast agent **gadolinium** is useful for demonstrating acute (active) lesions. This correlates with breakdown of the **blood–brain barrier** (see Ch. 5) in areas of active inflammation and demyelination.

Oligoclonal bands

The CNS inflammatory response in multiple sclerosis is associated with synthesis of antibodies (**immunoglobulins**) in the brain and spinal cord. It is therefore possible to detect antibodies in the CSF that are not present in peripheral blood. A sample of CSF is obtained by **lumbar puncture** (see Ch. 1, Clinical Box 1.3) and a specimen of venous blood is taken at the same time, for comparison. The two specimens are run on an **electrophoretic gel** to look for bands indicating the presence of **type G immunoglobulins** (**IgG**) that are only present in the CSF (which is indicative of CNS inflammation). These are known as **oligoclonal bands** (**OCBs**) and are found in 90% of people with MS (Fig. 14.5).

Visual evoked potentials

Decreased conduction speed in the central visual pathways can be demonstrated in the majority of patients with MS by obtaining **visual evoked potentials** (**VEPs**). Scalp electrodes record electrical activity in the occipital cortex in response to a changing visual stimulus such as an alternating chequerboard pattern. The stimulus-response sequence is repeated many times and averaged (to increase the signal-to-noise ratio). This reveals a characteristic **positive wave** in the visual cortex at 100 milliseconds (the **P100 wave**) which is delayed by 30–40 milliseconds in 95% of people with MS (Fig. 14.6).

Management

There is no cure for MS and the treatment is mainly supportive. Acute relapses are usually managed with a 3–5-day course of high-dose **intravenous corticosteroids** (e.g. **methylprednisolone**) or sometimes **oral prednisolone**. This has an immunosuppressive effect that shortens relapses and provides symptomatic relief, but does not improve long-term outcome.

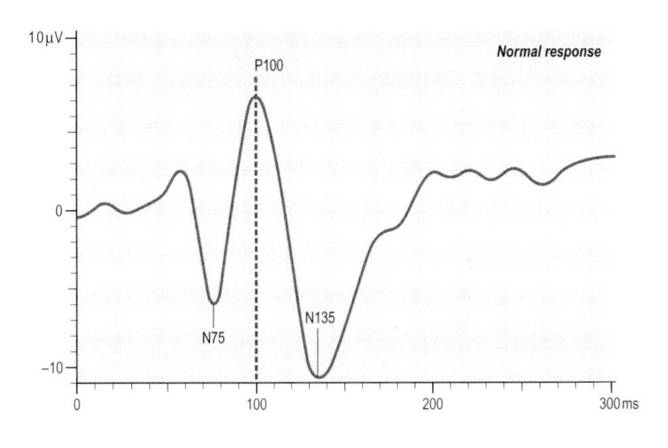

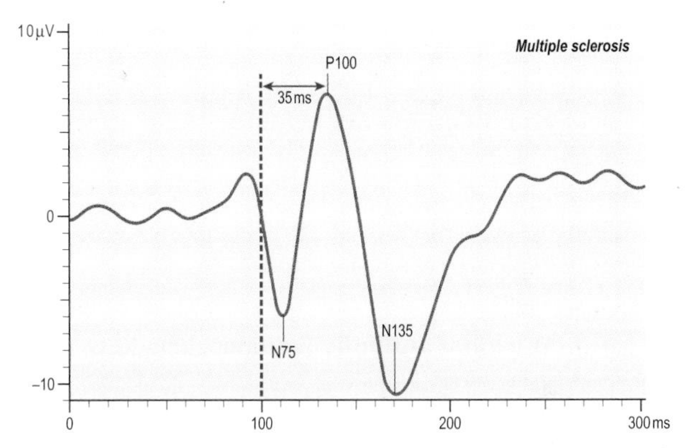

Fig. 14.6 **Delayed visual evoked potentials (VEPs) in MS.**

> ### *Key Points*
>
> - Diagnosis of MS is primarily clinical and requires demonstration of CNS demyelinating lesions that are disseminated in both space and time (confirmed by neuroimaging, serological testing and electrophysiology).
> - MRI (using a T2 FLAIR sequence) is the most sensitive method for demonstrating MS lesions (showing 10× more plaques than clinical episodes, since most lesions are clinically silent). The presence of gadolinium enhancement suggests there is breakdown of the blood–brain barrier.
> - Other findings in support of the diagnosis include oligoclonal bands (present in 90% of people with MS) and delay in the P100 wave on visual evoked potentials (in 95% of patients).

Disease-modifying drugs (DMDs)

Several **disease-modifying agents** are licensed for use in MS, but are mainly suitable for relapsing-remitting disease, with little effect once the patient has entered the progressive phase. Although disease-modifying agents are not curative, they do reduce relapse frequency and severity by up to two thirds. First-line treatment in MS includes (i) **interferon beta** and (ii) **glatiramer acetate**.

Interferon beta

Interferons are **cytokines** (inflammatory mediators) that influence immune responses and interfere with viral replication. The mechanism of action in MS is not certain, but interferons are known to have **immune modulating** and **anti-inflammatory properties**. Neuroimaging studies show that they reduce the number of inflammatory CNS lesions by more than 50%.

Two forms of interferon beta are used in the treatment of MS: **Interferon beta-1a** (administered by intramuscular or subcutaneous injection) and **interferon beta-1b** (administered subcutaneously). Side effects include **flu-like symptoms** (muscle aches, fever, chills and malaise) for 24–48 hours after injection. In the longer term, there is a risk of **liver function abnormalities** and **immunosuppression** (reduced white blood cell count). Interferons are not recommended for children or for women who are pregnant or breast feeding.

Glatiramer acetate

This is a synthetic mixture of polypeptides (a **copolymer**), containing four amino acids that are present in **myelin basic protein** (glutamic acid, alanine, tyrosine and lysine). It is administered by daily subcutaneous injection. The original rationale for its use was to compete with (or mimic) myelin basic protein but its actual mechanism of action is not certain. It appears to reduce antigen presentation and to promote secretion of **anti-inflammatory cytokines** from activated immune cells. There are usually no major side effects, in contrast to interferon beta, but this drug is also not recommended for children or for women who are pregnant or breast feeding.

Natalizumab

This is a **monoclonal antibody** (immunoglobulin G, IgG) which is given by intravenous injection every 28 days. Clinical trials show that it reduces the number of relapses by about two-thirds. Natalizumab recognizes an adhesion molecule called **α4 integrin** which binds to a **vascular cell adhesion molecule (VCAM-1)** on endothelial cells. This is designed to prevent leukocytes from binding to blood vessels, reducing the number of chronic inflammatory cells entering the CNS from the bloodstream. Side effects include headache, nausea, vomiting and skin rash. In rare cases it has been associated with an acute white matter disorder: **progressive multifocal leukoencephalopathy (PML)** (Clinical Box 14.4).

Fingolimod

This is the first **oral agent** that has been licensed for the treatment of MS. It has been shown in clinical trials to reduce the number of relapses by around 50%. It works by inhibition of **sphingosine 1-phosphate receptors** which blocks lymphocyte migration from lymph nodes. However, a number of potentially serious side effects have been described. These include **bradycardia**, **immunosuppression**, **liver toxicity** and **allergic reactions**. This drug is therefore only used in patients with severe relapsing-remitting MS, particularly people who are not responding to first-line treatments.

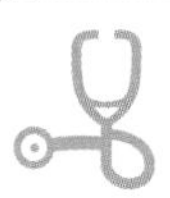

Clinical Box 14.4: Progressive multifocal leukoencephalopathy (PML)

This is a white matter disease associated with immune deficiency, often **HIV/AIDS**. It is an opportunistic infection caused by reactivation of a **papovavirus** that infects oligodendrocytes. The infectious agent is called **JC virus** (John Cunningham virus, named after a patient with PML). The pathological features include demyelination, chronic inflammation and reactive gliosis. Two key cellular elements are: (i) '**bizarre**' **astrocytes** with large irregular nuclei; and (ii) **transformed oligodendrocytes** with large nuclei that stain bluish-purple with routine stains (reflecting alterations in the nuclear DNA). The mortality rate is high and survivors are generally left with severe neurological disabilities.

Unlicensed drugs

Other drugs that may be useful in the management of MS are the immunosuppressive agent **azathioprine** and the chemotherapy drug **mitoxantrone**, but neither of these is licensed in the UK.

Mitoxantrone, in particular, may be beneficial in patients with secondary progressive MS and might also delay the transition from relapsing-remitting to progressive disease. It appears to work by suppressing activity in **lymphocytes** and **macrophages**, which are responsible for the immune-mediated attack on myelin (discussed below). In keeping with other anti-cancer drugs, side effects include **nausea**, **vomiting** and **hair loss**; more serious adverse effects sometimes occur, such as **cardiotoxicity** and **bone marrow suppression** (carrying a significant infection risk).

Intravenous immunoglobulin (IVIG) is pooled human **immunoglobulin G** that may be used in patients who are unable to tolerate standard disease-modifying treatments. The mechanism of action in MS is complex and incompletely understood, but is presumed to be immunomodulatory. It can be given to women who are unable to take their normal disease-modifying agents due to pregnancy or breast feeding. This is important, since one in three women experience a relapse in the post-partum period.

Long-term supportive care

Much of the long-term treatment for multiple sclerosis is supportive and aims to manage chronic symptoms such as fatigue, pain, muscle spasms and problems with bladder, bowel or sexual function:

- **Neuropathic pain** can be very troublesome and is managed with a number of agents including the anti-epileptic drugs **gabapentin** and **carbamazepine** (see Ch. 11).
- **Extreme tiredness** often responds to the Parkinson's disease drug **amantadine** (the stimulant effect is mediated by increased dopamine release at central synapses) (see Ch. 13).
- **Mood disorder** is common in patients with multiple sclerosis and can be treated with **antidepressants** or **anxiolytics**, in combination with counselling or cognitive-behavioural therapy.
- **Muscle spasms**, **musculoskeletal pain** and **spasticity** may be improved by physiotherapy or a muscle relaxant such as **baclofen**, **gabapentin**, **dantrolene** or a **benzodiazepine** (see Ch. 7).
- **Bladder problems** such as detrusor hyperactivity can be treated with antimuscarinic agents such as **oxybutynin** or **tolterodine** which relax smooth muscle of the urinary bladder; nocturia (increased urination during the night) may be treated by **desmopressin** (antidiuretic hormone).
- **Constipation** can usually be managed with **dietary measures** such as increased consumption of fruit and fibre. In some cases **aperients** (laxatives) or **stool softeners** may be appropriate.
- **Epilepsy** is also more common in patients with MS and this can be managed with **anti-epileptic drugs** if necessary (Ch. 11).

Careful attention to these long-term problems may have a considerable impact on **quality of life** and co-operation between the neurologist, family doctor and specialist team members (including nurses, physiotherapists and occupational therapists) is highly beneficial.

Key Points

- Acute MS relapses are treated with intravenous methylprednisolone (or oral prednisolone). This shortens relapses and provides symptomatic relief, but does not improve long-term outcome.
- First-line disease-modifying treatment for MS includes: (i) interferon beta (an inflammatory mediator that has immune-modulating and anti-inflammatory properties); and (ii) glatiramer acetate (a polypeptide copolymer mixture with an uncertain mechanism of action).
- Other disease-modifying agents include natalizumab and fingolimod (which prevent leukocyte migration into the brain) and immunomodulating or immunosuppressive agents such as mitoxantrone (a chemotherapy drug) and intravenous immunoglobulin (IVIG).
- Long-term supportive care aims to address chronic pain, fatigue, mood disorder, muscle spasms and problems with bowel, bladder or sexual function.

Pathological features

Post-mortem examination of the brain in a person with longstanding multiple sclerosis mainly shows **chronic (old) plaques**, but **acute lesions** are occasionally encountered.

MS plaques

In fresh post-mortem brain tissue, **chronic plaques** appear as sharply demarcated areas that lack normal myelin, giving them a salmon-pink appearance (Fig. 14.7). This is in contrast to **acute plaques** which have a yellowish colour due to the high lipid content. The presence of **gliosis** ('glial scarring'; see Ch. 8) gives plaques a firm or **sclerotic** consistency, from which the name multiple sclerosis is derived (Greek: sklerōs, hard). After the brain has been preserved, plaques have a greyish appearance (Fig. 14.8).

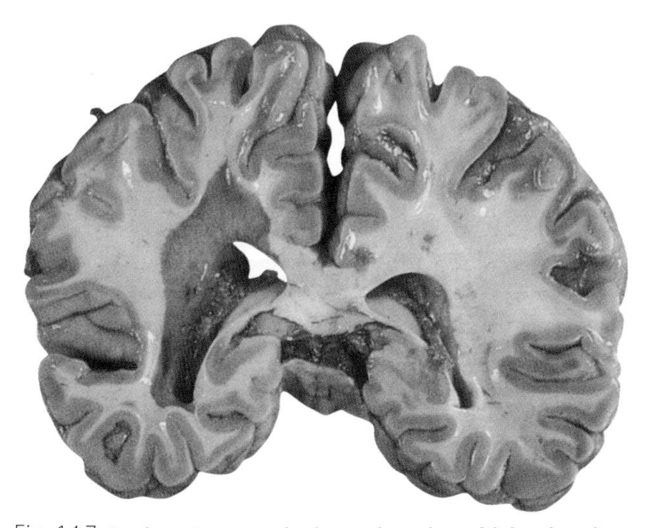

Fig. 14.7 **Fresh post-mortem brain specimen in multiple sclerosis showing salmon pink plaques in the periventricular white matter.** From Stevens and Lowe: Pathology 2e (Mosby 2000) with permission.

Plaque distribution

Plaques can occur anywhere in the brain or spinal cord, but they are most often found in the **periventricular white matter**. They are typically between 2–10 mm in diameter and have a well-defined margin (Fig. 14.9). Plaques also frequently occur at grey–white matter junctions (especially at the border between the cerebral cortex and subcortical white matter) and within the cortex itself, which also contains myelinated axons. In advanced cases extensive white matter loss may be associated with marked compensatory dilation of the ventricles, termed **hydrocephalus ex vacuo**. In a subset of patients, plaques are found only in the optic pathways and cervical spinal cord (Clinical Box 14.5).

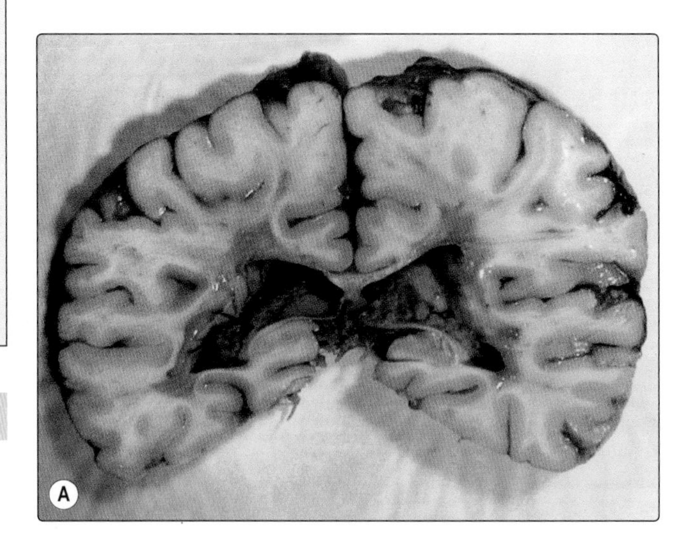

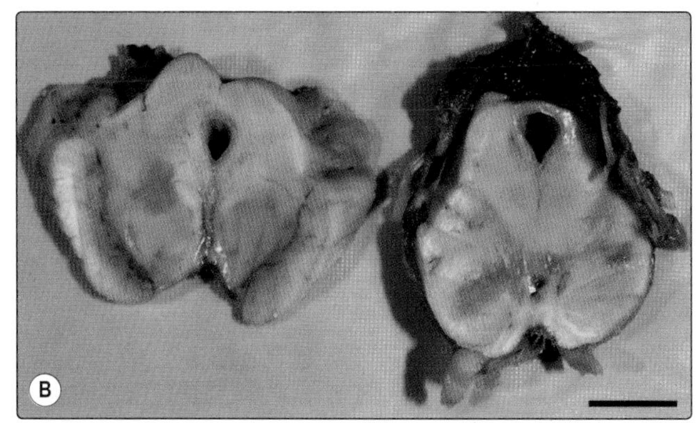

Fig. 14.8 **Sharply defined plaques of demyelination in (A) the periventricular white matter and (B) the brain stem.** In this case the brain has been preserved in formaldehyde prior to slicing. From Prayson, R: Neuropathology (Chuchill Livingstone 2005) with permission.

Acute and chronic plaques

The microscopic appearance of MS plaques depends on whether they are acute or chronic. **Acute plaques** are cellular, with sheets of **foamy macrophages** containing lipid-rich myelin debris and perivascular cuffs of **lymphocytes**. Importantly, there is relative **preservation of axons**.

Chronic plaques may be active or inactive. **Chronic active plaques** have a cell-poor centre which is gliotic (with numerous astrocytic processes) but shows little inflammation. This is surrounded by a peripheral margin of activity at the interface with healthy myelin. The rim of active demyelination contains macrophages and lymphocytes. **Chronic inactive plaques** are similar, but lack the

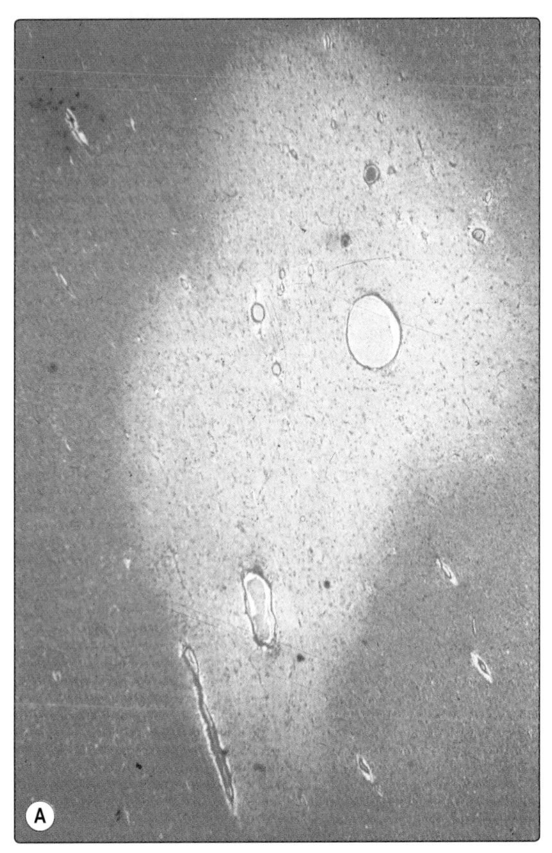

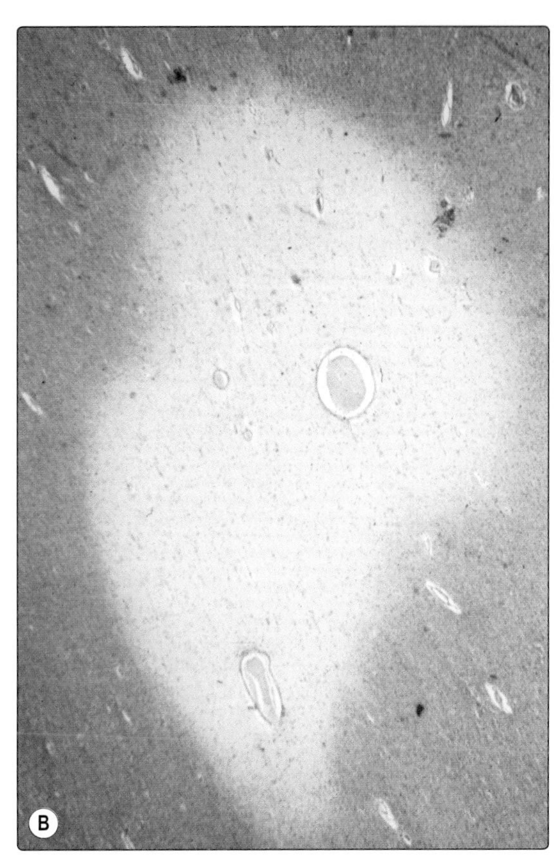

Fig. 14.9 **Appearances of a typical MS plaque with (A) a routine, haematoxylin and eosin or H&E stain and (B) with the myelin stain Luxol fast blue (LFB).** Note the sharp peripheral margin with the surrounding normal white matter. From Stevens, A, Lowe, JS and Young: Wheater's Basic Histopathology 4e (Churchill Livingstone 2002) with permission.

Clinical Box 14.5: Devic's disease

Devic's disease or **neuromyelitis optica** is an inflammatory demyelinating disorder that affects the cervical spinal cord (causing **tetraplegia**) and optic nerves (leading to **impaired vision** or blindness). It can be monophasic, recurrent or relapsing-remitting and may be regarded as a variant of **multiple sclerosis** or as a separate disease. In a proportion of cases there is an antibody-mediated autoimmune response to the membrane water channel **aquaporin-4**. Devic's disease can be managed with immunosuppressive agents including corticosteroids, but cannot be cured.

peripheral rim of demyelination. Some histological patterns are associated with a particular MS variant (Clinical Box 14.6).

Remyelination

After the inflammation has subsided, approximately 20% of MS plaques remyelinate to form a '**shadow plaque**' (Fig. 14.11). However, remyelination is often partial or inadequate, with thinner than normal myelin sheaths and shortened internodal segments.

Remyelination relies on recruitment from a pool of **oligodendrocyte precursor cells (OPCs)**. These cells migrate towards regions of demyelination before proliferating and differentiating into **mature oligodendrocytes** that are able to invest the denuded axons with a new myelin sheath.

Remyelination is more common in early MS lesions and is less likely in old (chronic) lesions. Inadequate remyelination may contribute to the gradual development of permanent neurological deficits in progressive disease, but the reason for myelination failure is not fully understood.

Failure of remyelination

Remyelination may be prevented by **on-going inflammation** and continued demyelination. In older plaques, the presence of **glial scarring** (see Ch. 8) may also be a factor. This is characterized by a dense meshwork of **astrocytic processes** at the centre of the lesion which may physically prevent inward migration of oligodendrocyte precursor cells.

Remyelination failure might also reflect **OPC depletion**, although successful recruitment and proliferation of progenitor cells has been demonstrated in some animal models, in which failure of **OPC differentiation** appears to be the most important factor.

Expression of certain cell-surface molecules on demyelinated axons may actively inhibit remyelination. These include the polysialylated form of **neural cell adhesion molecule (NCAM)**. Other inhibitory molecules are present in the extracellular matrix and in association with astrocytic processes (in areas of glial scarring).

Oligodendrocyte precursor cells express **Notch receptors** at the cell surface. These are stimulated by extracellular ligands such as the protein **jagged** (which is known to be

Clinical Box 14.6: Balo's concentric sclerosis

Balo's concentric sclerosis is a histological variant of MS which used to be regarded as a distinct form of the disease. Histological examination of the brain shows sharply defined **concentric rings of demyelination** alternating with bands of unaffected myelin, giving an 'onion-skin' appearance (Fig. 14.10). This was previously only diagnosed at **post-mortem examination** and was thought to be associated with an invariably aggressive (usually fatal) clinical course. However, it is now possible to identify Balo's disease in life using modern neuroimaging methods, which suggests that this pattern of demyelination is much more common and not necessarily aggressive.

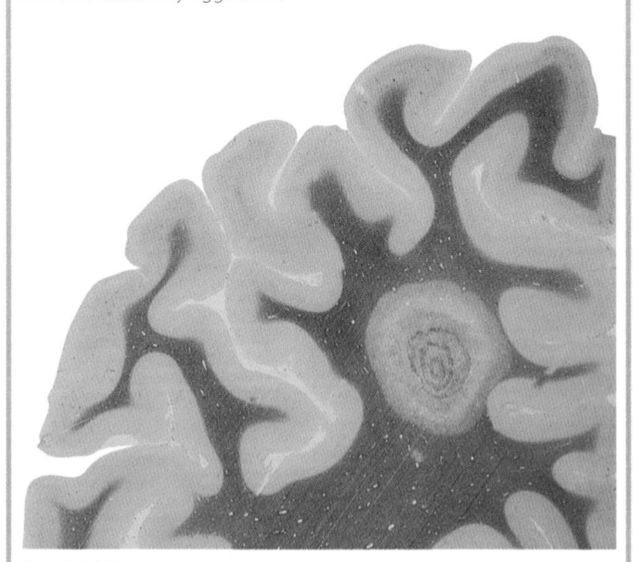

Fig. 14.10 **Balo's concentric sclerosis.** The presence of multiple concentric rings of demyelinated and myelinated axons creates an 'onion skin' appearance [section of cerebral hemisphere; Loyez stain], in which myelin appears black. From Ellison, D and Love, S: Neuropathology 2e (Mosby 2003) with permission.

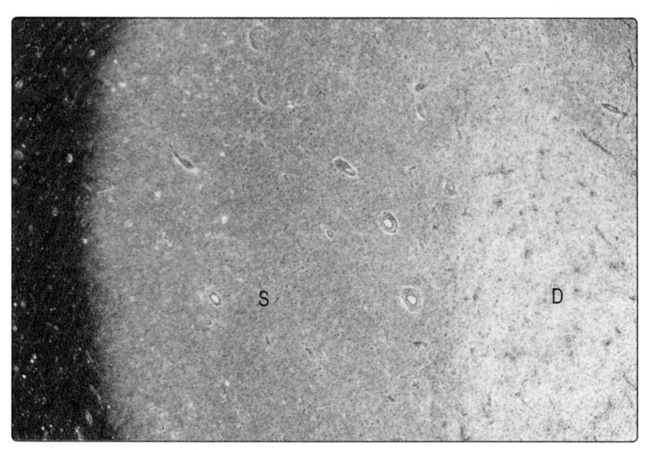

Fig. 14.11 **Shadow plaques represent areas of remyelination (or partial remyelination) in multiple sclerosis.** This section shows a shadow plaque (S) next to an area of active demyelination (D). Normal myelin (stained blue) can be seen at the far left-hand side of the image. From Ellison, D and Love, S: Neuropathology 2e (Mosby 2003) with permission.

present in MS plaques). The notch-jagged interaction inhibits differentiation of OPCs to mature oligodendrocytes and contributes to remyelination failure. **Notch inhibitors** are therefore potential disease-modifying agents in MS.

Key Points

- Pathological examination of the brain in MS shows acute, chronic active and chronic inactive plaques, which are 2–10 mm in diameter and often occur in the periventricular white matter.
- After the inflammation has subsided, approximately 20% of plaques remyelinate (particularly in the earlier stages of MS) to produce a partially remyelinated shadow plaque.
- Remyelination depends on the recruitment, proliferation and differentiation of oligodendrocyte precursor cells (OPCs).
- Failure of remyelination may be due to ongoing inflammation, the presence of an astroglial scar or failure of OPC differentiation. In the CNS, remyelination appears to be actively inhibited.

Aetiology

The cause of multiple sclerosis is not known, but it is widely believed to result from an interaction between genetic and environmental factors and may be triggered by exposure to a **virus infection**.

Genetic and immunologic factors

MS cannot be inherited in a simple Mendelian fashion and there are no familial forms. Nevertheless, concordance is around 25% in identical twins, compared to around 5% for fraternal twins and siblings – and the risk is up to 20 times higher in first-degree relatives of people with MS.

Familial clustering is likely to be due to a number of unknown **susceptibility genes**, but candidates have been difficult to identify. This is probably because the genetic effects are small and involve multiple genes, each making a modest contribution to overall risk.

Robust associations have only been found with certain **human leukocyte-associated antigen** (**HLA**) genes, particularly within the class II region of the **major histocompatibility complex** (**MHC**) of antigens on chromosome 6. The most consistently implicated subtype in Caucasians (the population at greatest risk) is **HLA-DRB1*15** (HLA-DR15 haplotype). In other populations, different HLA types may be more important and the estimated contribution to overall genetic susceptibility varies from 20–50%.

Environmental factors

The prevalence of multiple sclerosis varies with **distance from the equator** (Fig. 14.12). Equatorial regions tend to have comparatively low prevalence rates, whereas more temperate areas to the north and south have a progressively greater incidence. Some of the highest recorded rates of MS have been identified in the northern part of Scotland and in North America.

Migration studies

Geographic risk in MS relates to **location before puberty** (under the age of 15) and individuals who migrate after this age carry the risk of their original location. This may reflect exposure to an **environmental agent** (such as a **virus**) during a critical time-window prior to puberty. The time frame coincides with maximal development and involution of the **thymus gland**. This is the site of T-cell (thymus cell) maturation and the deletion of potentially auto-aggressive cells by apoptosis (see Ch. 8).

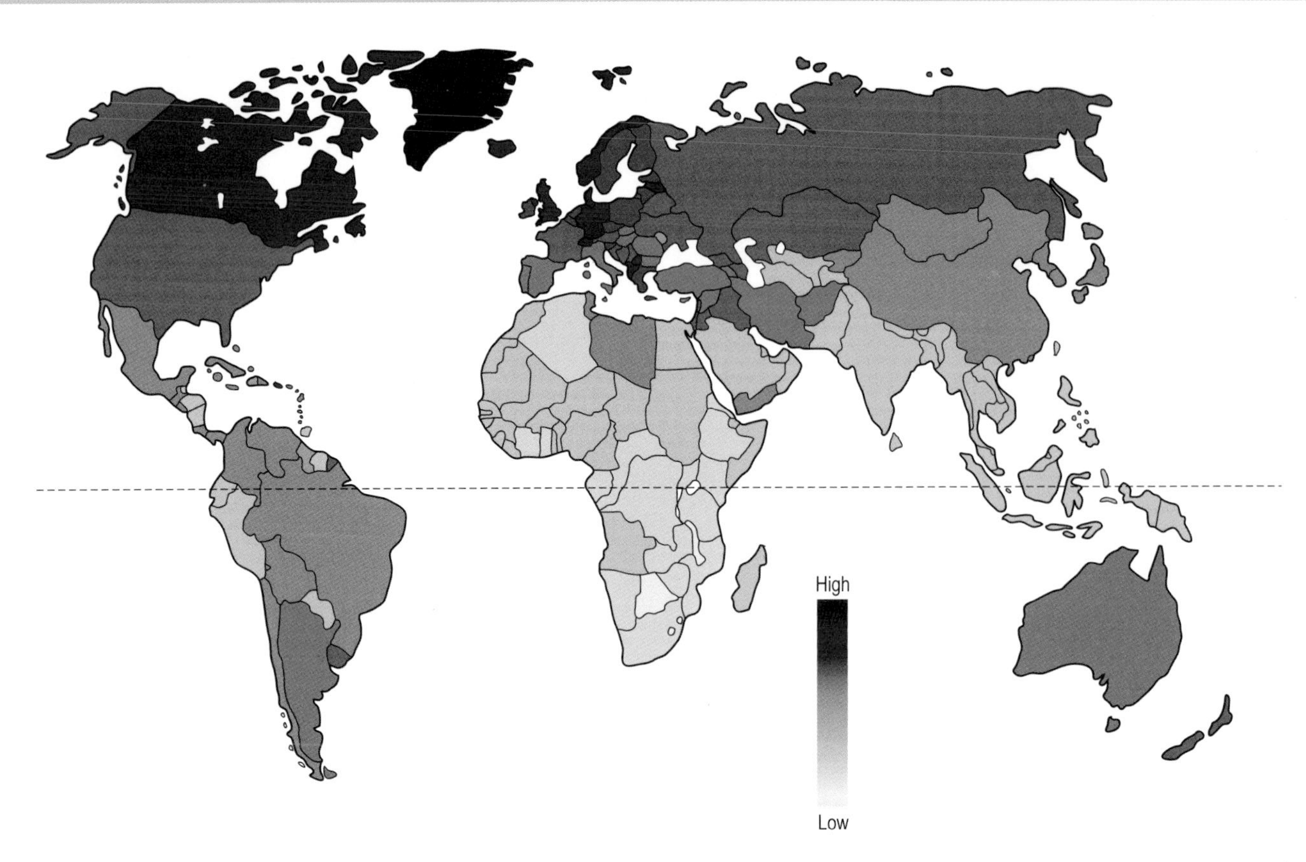

Fig. 14.12 **Geographical distribution of multiple sclerosis risk.** Individuals who are closer to the equator below the age of 15 years are at a lower risk of MS in adulthood, regardless of subsequent migration.

Sunlight and vitamin D

Proximity to the equator may reduce MS risk as a result of increased **sunlight exposure**. This could reflect a lower chance of encountering a particular **pathogenic virus** (since viruses are destroyed by ultraviolet radiation in sunlight) or higher levels of **vitamin D** (in keeping with research showing that supplementation may reduce relapse frequency). There is also a **month of birth effect**: in the Northern Hemisphere more people with MS are born in the spring than the autumn. This phenomenon may be related to maternal sunlight exposure or vitamin D status.

Viral and other infections

A number of infectious agents have been proposed as the cause of multiple sclerosis, including **Epstein–Barr virus** (**EBV**), **human herpes virus 6** (**HHV-6**) and many of the immunological features of MS are suggestive of a virally mediated process.

The bacterial agent *Chlamydia pneumoniae* has also been implicated – and bacterial infection is known to be associated with some cases of demyelination in the peripheral nervous system (Clinical Box 14.7). Nevertheless, no causative agent has been unequivocally implicated and no microorganisms have been isolated from human tissues.

Animal models of MS

A number of experimental models of CNS demyelination have been developed (which resemble multiple sclerosis to a greater or lesser degree) and have contributed to our understanding of its pathogenesis. Animal models fall into four major categories:

- Autoimmune.
- Virus-mediated.
- Chemically-induced.
- Genetic.

Key Points

- The cause of MS is not known, but it is widely believed to result from an interaction between genetic and environmental factors and may be triggered by a virus infection.
- MS cannot be inherited in a simple Mendelian fashion, but concordance rates are 5x higher in identical twins and risk is up to 20x higher in first-degree relatives of people with MS.
- The most robust association is with human leukocyte-associated antigen (HLA) subtypes and the most consistently implicated subtype in Caucasians (who are at greatest risk) is HLA-DR15.
- Prevalence of MS is higher with increasing distance from the equator and migration studies show that location prior to puberty determines adult risk. This may reflect increased risk of encountering a particular virus, but other factors have been implicated including sunlight exposure and vitamin D status.

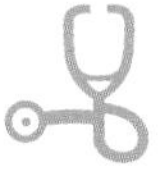

Clinical Box 14.7: Guillain–Barré syndrome

This is a peripheral neuropathy, also known as **acute inflammatory demyelinating polyneuropathy** (**AIDP**) that is characterized clinically by **ascending weakness**. This means that the lower part of the body is affected first, progressively spreading to involve more proximal muscle groups in the trunk and upper limbs. It can be life-threatening if paralysis reaches the respiratory muscles. In many cases the cause is not known but it is sometimes triggered by an infection and 30% of cases are preceded by an episode of **campylobacter enteritis** (caused by the bacterium *Campylobacter jejuni*). The pathogenesis is thought to involve **molecular mimicry**, in which a cell-surface antigen on the infectious organism is similar to a surface antigen in peripheral myelin, creating an **autoimmune inflammatory demyelination**. Unlike MS, it is restricted to the peripheral nervous system.

Autoimmune models

The most widely used model of central nervous system demyelination is **experimental autoimmune encephalomyelitis** (EAE). This system is used to evaluate potential disease-modifying therapies. The experimental animal is injected with homogenates derived from CNS tissue or protein extracts containing **myelin basic protein** (MBP) or **proteolipid protein** (PLP).

This induces a **T-cell-mediated** immune response (often in a rat or mouse, but sometimes in other species including non-human primates). This leads to brain and spinal cord inflammation with blood–brain barrier dysfunction, usually accompanied by demyelination. In particular, the immune response is mediated by **helper T-cells**, which is the same type of immune response seen in MS. This is accompanied by clinical signs and axonal changes, including conduction block. A criticism of this model is that since it produces a monophasic, post-vaccinial demyelinating disease, it has more in common with **acute disseminated encephalomyelitis** (Clinical Box 14.8).

> ## *Clinical Box 14.8: Acute disseminated encephalomyelitis*
>
> This is a self-limiting CNS disorder of childhood that presents with **meningism** (headache, fever, neck stiffness) and usually occurs 2–10 days after a virus infection or vaccine. Imaging shows bilateral hemispheric white matter changes corresponding to perivenous demyelination and oedema (Fig. 14.13). The clinical course is usually benign, with complete recovery. It is almost always monophasic. A hyperacute variant termed **acute haemorrhagic leukoencephalopathy** (**AHL**) or **Hurst disease** is characterized by widespread haemorrhagic lesions with brisk inflammatory infiltrates and marked brain oedema. This subtype is much more aggressive and usually fatal.
>
> 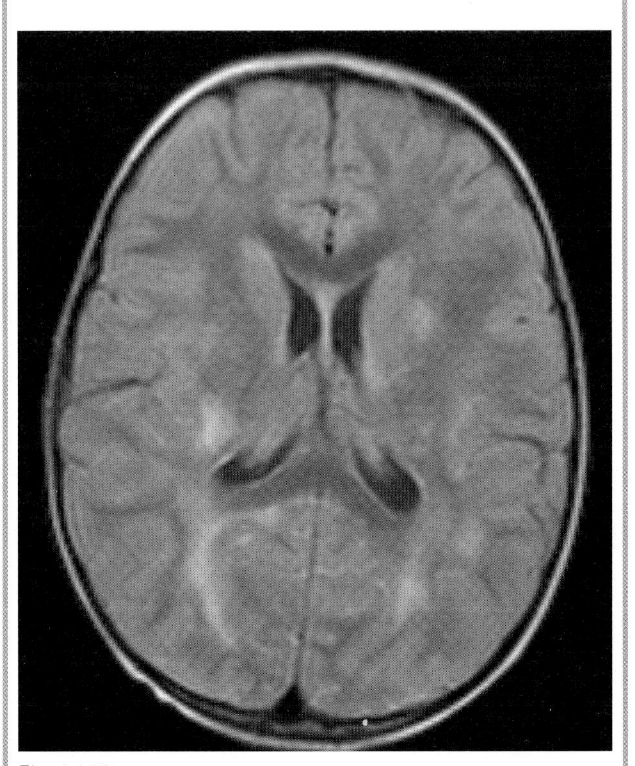
>
> Fig. 14.13 **Axial MRI FLAIR images in a boy age 2 years 8 months with acute disseminated encephalomyelitis (ADEM).** There are patchy signal changes widely distributed in the cerebral white matter bilaterally, including diffuse involvement of the internal capsules. Courtesy of Dr Andrew MacKinnon.

Viral models

A number of CNS viruses are known to cause demyelination in humans (such as JC virus in PML; see Clinical Box 14.4). Several animal models have been developed that exploit this phenomenon. Many of the viruses used in these models infect oligodendrocytes and are either directly cytotoxic or induce a **cell-mediated** immune response against oligodendrocytes.

Chemically-induced models

It is also possible to induce demyelination in experimental animals by systemic or targeted administration of substances that are toxic to oligodendrocytes. Examples include:
(i) **cuprizone**, a copper chelating agent that causes oligodendrocyte death following oral administration; and
(ii) **ethidium bromide**, a DNA-binding agent which can be injected into white matter pathways such as the dorsal columns or cerebellar peduncles.

Chemically-induced demyelination is monophasic and is usually followed by complete remyelination within a few weeks. These systems therefore enable systematic study of the processes involved in demyelination, clearance of myelin debris and remyelination, including OPC recruitment.

Genetic models

A number of models are available in which the experimental animal (usually a rodent) has a myelin gene mutation. These include animals with mutations in genes for **myelin basic protein** (e.g. Shiverer) and **proteolipid protein** (e.g. Rumpshaker and Jimpy). Gene knockout animals for myelin components also exist. However, animals with myelin gene mutations typically exhibit abnormal primary myelination (**dysmyelination**) and are thus more comparable to human **leukodystrophies** (see Clinical Box 14.1).

> ## *Key Points*
>
> - Animal models of CNS demyelination are useful to investigate the pathogenesis of MS and to test potential disease-modifying therapies. The main types are autoimmune, virus-mediated, chemically-induced and genetic.
> - The most common animal model of MS is experimental autoimmune encephalomyelitis (EAE) in which the experimental animal is injected with myelin extracts to trigger an immune reaction.

Pathogenesis

Our understanding of disease pathogenesis in MS is derived from a combination of findings in animal models and observations in human disease. Gadolinium-enhanced MRI scans in patients with MS suggest that disruption of the **blood–brain barrier** (see Ch. 5) may be an early event in acute lesions. Pathological studies confirm increased permeability of cerebral vessels, associated with immune activation of endothelial cells and passage of leukocytes from the bloodstream into the brain tissue.

Endothelial cells are activated by **pro-inflammatory cytokines** including **interferon-gamma**. This leads to upregulation of **MHC class II** molecules and alterations of cell-surface proteins involved in leukocyte–endothelial interactions, promoting cell adhesion and extravasation of

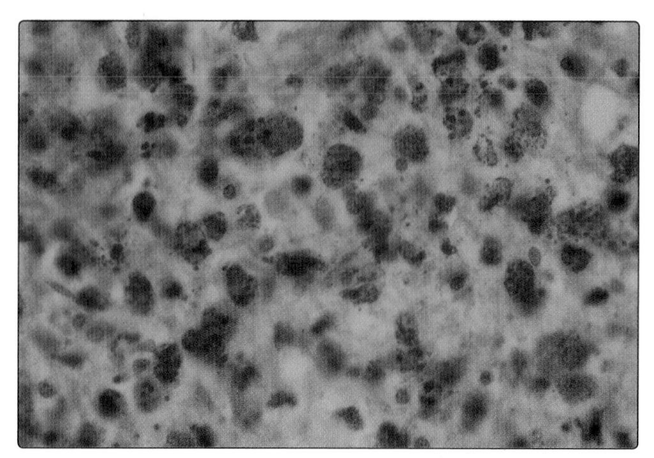

Fig. 14.14 **Foamy macrophages in an active MS plaque.** Stained with oil red-O which highlights lipid. From Ellison, D and Love, S: Neuropathology 2e (Mosby 2003) with permission.

white blood cells. Changes to **tight junctions** between endothelial cells lead to increased vascular permeability and movement of fluid and immune cells into the brain tissue, causing local **oedema** (swelling).

Inflammatory cells

Following endothelial cell activation and breakdown of the blood–brain barrier, a mixed inflammatory infiltrate enters the brain that is predominantly composed of **macrophages** and **lymphocytes**.

Macrophages

Macrophages (and **activated microglia**, which are of similar lineage) are the principal cellular mediators of demyelination. These cells actively strip axons of their myelin sheaths and digest its lipid and protein constituents. **Myelin debris** accumulates within activated macrophages to give a 'foamy' appearance (Fig. 14.14).

The number of macrophages is related to **lesion activity**. As myelin debris is cleared and inflammation subsides, macrophages gradually disappear from the centre of acute plaques, but remain prominent at the peripheral (active) margins of the lesion where there is continued expansion into the surrounding white matter.

T-lymphocytes

Active multiple sclerosis lesions are rich in **T-lymphocytes**. These can be divided into: (i) **helper T-cells** which express the cell-surface molecule CD4; and (ii) **cytotoxic T-cells** which express CD8. The CD4 and CD8 molecules help T-lymphocytes to recognize myelin constituents that have been processed and 'presented' to them by **antigen-presenting cells (APCs)** including activated microglia and macrophages (Fig. 14.15).

$CD4^+$ helper T-cells produce cytokines including **interleukin-1** and **2** (**IL-1** and **IL-2**), **tumour necrosis factor** (**TNF**) and **interferon-gamma** that are key inflammatory mediators. These molecules play a number of roles including upregulation of **cell-adhesion molecules** (facilitating leukocyte recruitment) and activation of microglia and macrophages.

$CD8^+$ cytotoxic ('killer') T-cells are also numerous in acute multiple sclerosis lesions and probably have a more direct role in damaging CNS tissues.

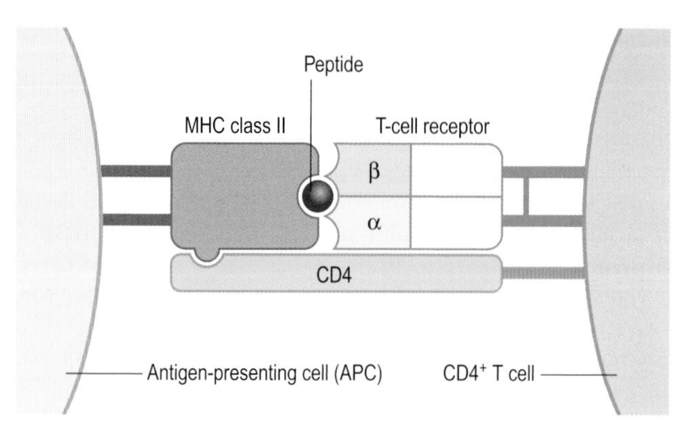

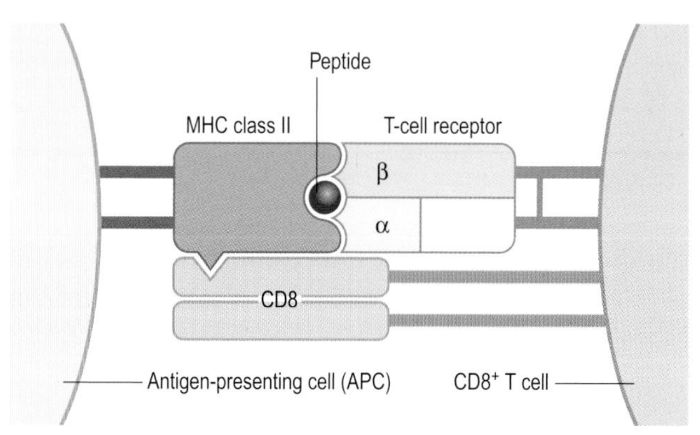

Fig. 14.15 **Antigen recognition by $CD4^+$ (helper) and $CD8^+$ (cytotoxic) T-lymphocytes.** The antigenic peptide (e.g. a myelin constituent) is first processed and presented by antigen-presenting cells.

B-lymphocytes

The role of **B-lymphocytes** (and antibody-producing **plasma cells** which derive from them) is demonstrated by the presence of IgG oligoclonal bands in the CSF of patients with multiple sclerosis.

Binding of myelin-specific autoantibodies disrupts the myelin sheath and triggers activation of the **complement cascade**, leading to attachment of proteins called **opsonins** that attract macrophages and microglia. Macrophages recognize and bind the opsonized myelin via complement receptors on the macrophage plasma membrane, leading to **receptor-mediated endocytosis**. Disrupted myelin fragments are thereby internalized by the macrophages and digested.

Key Points

- Gadolinium-enhanced MRI scans in patients with multiple sclerosis suggest that disruption of the blood–brain barrier is an early event in acute MS plaques.
- Endothelial cell activation (e.g. by pro-inflammatory cytokines such as interferon-gamma) is following by a chronic inflammatory infiltrate dominated by macrophages and lymphocytes.
- Macrophages (and activated microglia) are the principal mediators of demyelination and are involved in actively stripping and digesting the myelin sheath and its components.
- T-lymphocytes ($CD4^+$ helper T-cells and $CD8^+$ cytotoxic T-cells) are involved in cell-mediated myelin damage whereas B-cells (and plasma cells) produce myelin-specific autoantibodies.

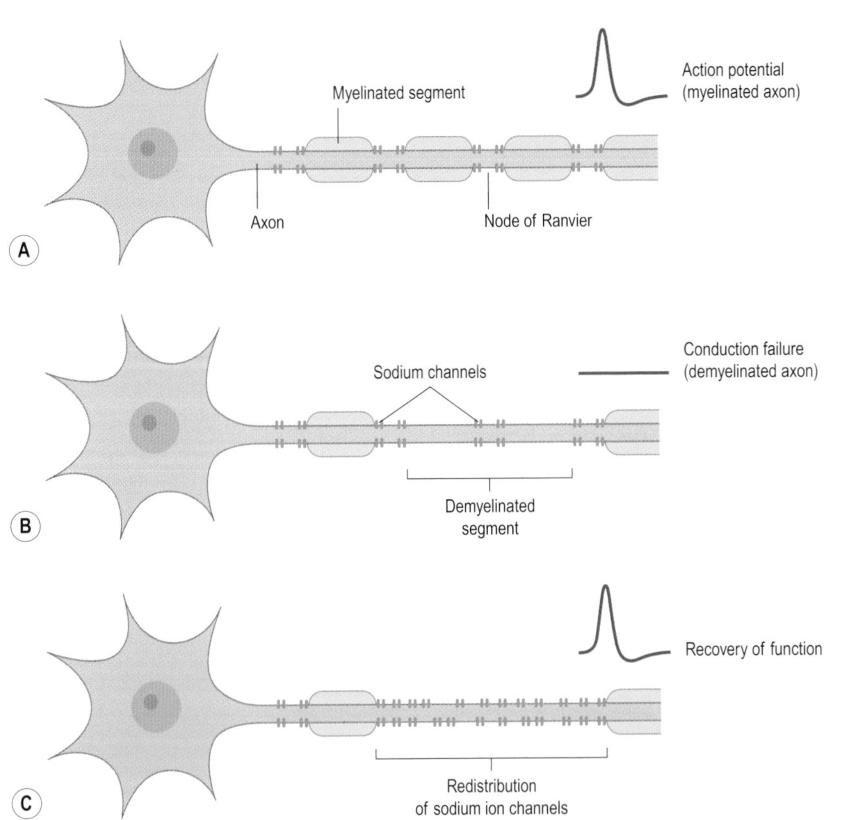

Fig. 14.16 **Conduction block and recovery of function in demyelinated axons.** See text for explanation.

Impact on axonal conduction

In myelinated fibres, voltage-gated ion channels are concentrated at the **nodes of Ranvier** (Fig. 14.16A). This means that following demyelination, the denuded portion of the axon is unable to transmit action potentials, leading to **conduction block** (Fig. 14.16B). Partial recovery of function may be possible due to redistribution or insertion of new voltage-gated sodium channels along the internodal region (Fig. 14.16C). However, this permits only continuous (rather than saltatory) conduction, which is considerably slower and much less energy-efficient (see Ch. 6).

Changes in the excitability and ion channel expression profile within the demyelinated axon can also generate **ectopic action potentials**. This may lead to 'positive' phenomena such as painful sensations or tingling (**paraesthesiae**). The hyperexcitable axonal segments may also be sensitive to mechanical deformation, which might explain Lhermitte's phenomenon (discussed above).

Types of active plaque

Studies of post-mortem brain tissue (and diagnostic brain biopsies in living patients) have provided evidence of **four distinct patterns** in early (active) MS plaques, each with a different pathophysiological mechanism (Fig. 14.17). In a particular patient, all plaques are of the same type.

The basic mechanism in multiple sclerosis (**pattern I**) is characterized by a **T-cell-mediated immune response** with macrophage-associated demyelination. This accounts for around 20% of MS cases. In many patients, the basic T-cell response is supplemented by a specific **antibody** and **complement-mediated** assault on CNS myelin (**pattern II**). This appears to be the most common type overall, accounting for more than 50% of cases. It is typified by **Devic's disease** and in this particular case the antibodies are raised against the water channel **aquaporin-4** (discussed above; see Clinical Box 14.5).

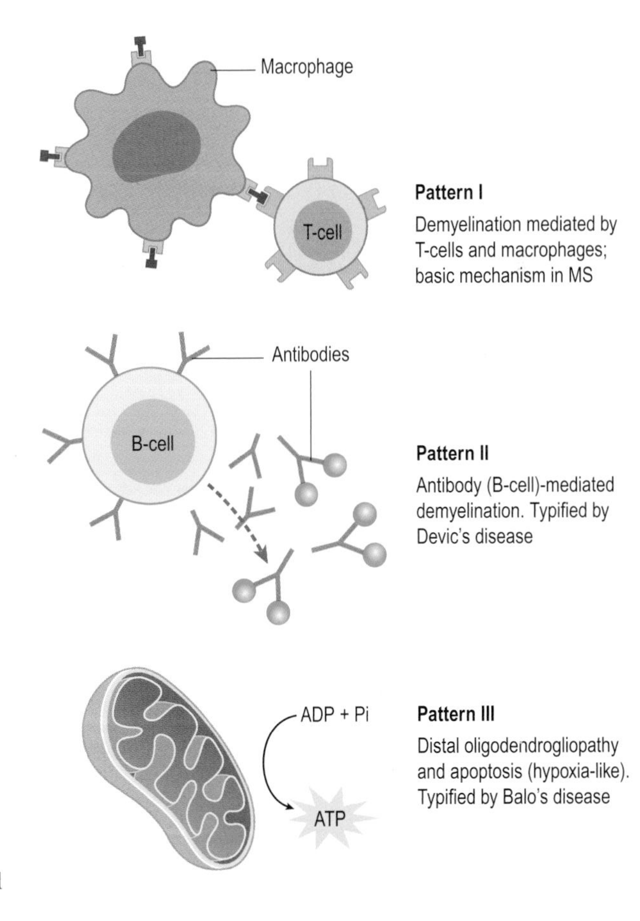

Fig. 14.17 **Subtypes of active plaque in multiple sclerosis.**

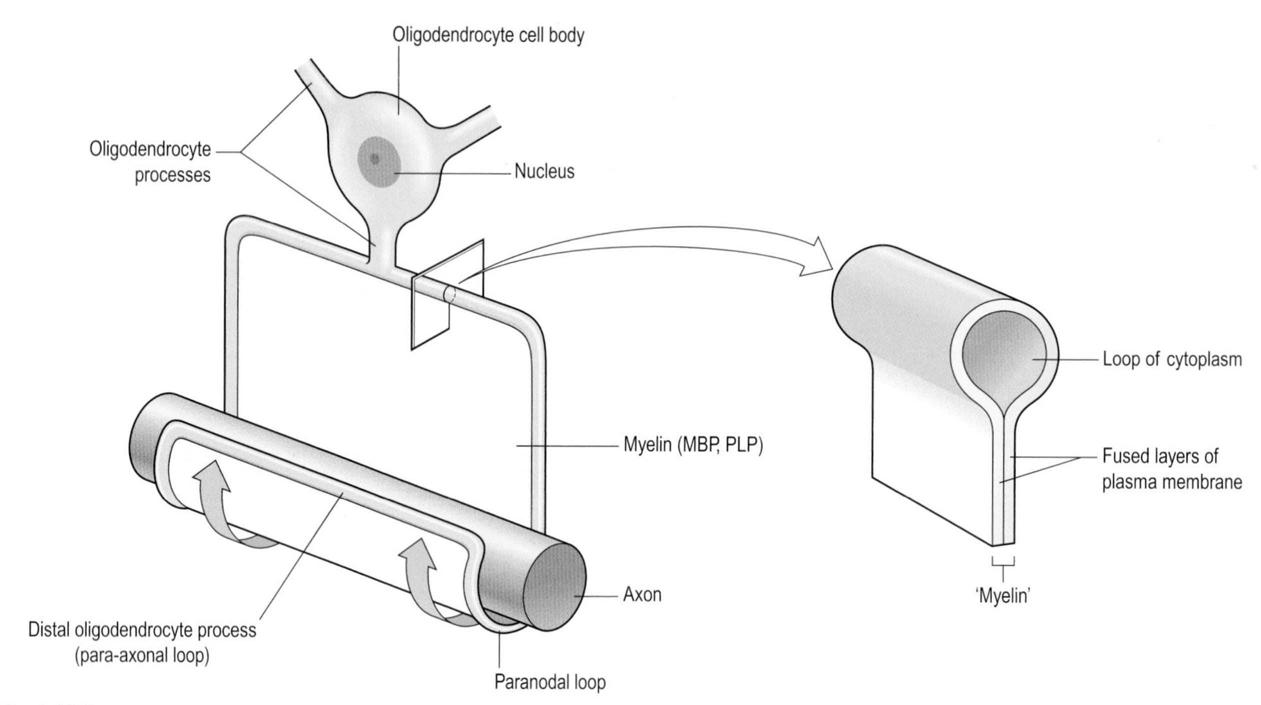

Fig. 14.18 **An oligodendrocyte process investing part of an axon.** The distal oligodendrocyte process (or para-axonal loop) is indicated. This is the target in 'dying-back' oligodendrogliopathy, the characteristic finding in pattern III multiple sclerosis plaques.

Pattern III is referred to as a **distal oligodendrogliopathy** because the target is the distal (para-axonal) loop of myelin that lies in intimate contact with the axon (see Fig. 14.18); the oligodendrocyte cell body remains intact, but there is a 'dying back' of its processes, with consequent demyelination. There is also evidence of **mitochondrial dysfunction** in this type of plaque, which has features in common with **hypoxic** or **ischaemic cell death** (see Ch. 10). Pattern III is typified by **Balo's disease** in which multiple waves of hypoxic-type damage create an onion skin appearance (see Clinical Box 14.6) and accounts for approximately 25% of lesions overall.

Rarely (in less than 5% of cases) there is a **genetic predisposition** leading to primary oligodendrocyte degeneration, followed by secondary demyelination (**pattern IV**).

Key Points

- Studies of post-mortem brain tissue and diagnostic brain biopsies in living patients have provided evidence that there are four different types (or patterns) of MS plaque.
- The basic mechanism in MS (pattern I) is characterized by a T-cell-mediated immune response (20%) supplemented by an antibody-mediated attack (pattern II) in a further 50% of cases.
- Pattern III (25% of cases) is referred to as a distal (dying-back) oligodendrogliopathy in which the distal oligodendrocyte processes are lost, with relative preservation of the cell body. Pattern IV is rare (<5% of cases) and is associated with a mutation that promotes oligodendrocyte apoptosis.
- In each of the four patterns, demyelination leads to: (i) conduction failure, associated with 'negative' neurological symptoms such as weakness and numbness; and (ii) ectopic action potentials, which leads to 'positive' symptoms including pain and paraesthesiae.

Neurodegeneration in MS

In the progressive phase of MS, there is gradual white matter atrophy, with ventricular dilatation and thinning of the cerebral cortex (Fig. 14.19). This is associated with accumulation of permanent neurological disability and is thought to be due to axonal damage and loss of cortical neurons.

Axonal damage

Axonal disruption and transection occurs in **acute MS plaques** and at the peripheral margins of **chronic active plaques**. In general, the degree of axonal damage correlates with the intensity of inflammation, but axon loss is also present in **normal-appearing white matter** (**NAWM**).

Disrupted axons (**axon swellings**) can be demonstrated using silver stains or by immunohistochemistry for axonal proteins such as neurofilament protein. Immunolabelling for **beta amyloid precursor protein** (**β-APP**) is a sensitive method for demonstrating axonal disruption, which is also used in traumatic head injury (see Ch. 9).

In recent years **progressive axonal loss** has become an increasing focus of research interest and is now regarded as an important cause of long-term neurological disability. Axonal and neuronal damage is likely to be responsible for the cumulative deficits that appear as the patient makes the transition to secondary progressive disease.

Mechanism of axonal injury

The precise cause of axonal loss in MS plaques is not known, but may reflect 'bystander' damage to neurons and axons. This refers to injury mediated by **cytotoxic molecules** including pro-inflammatory cytokines, nitric oxide and other toxic substances released by activated macrophages, lymphocytes and astrocytes during the inflammatory response.

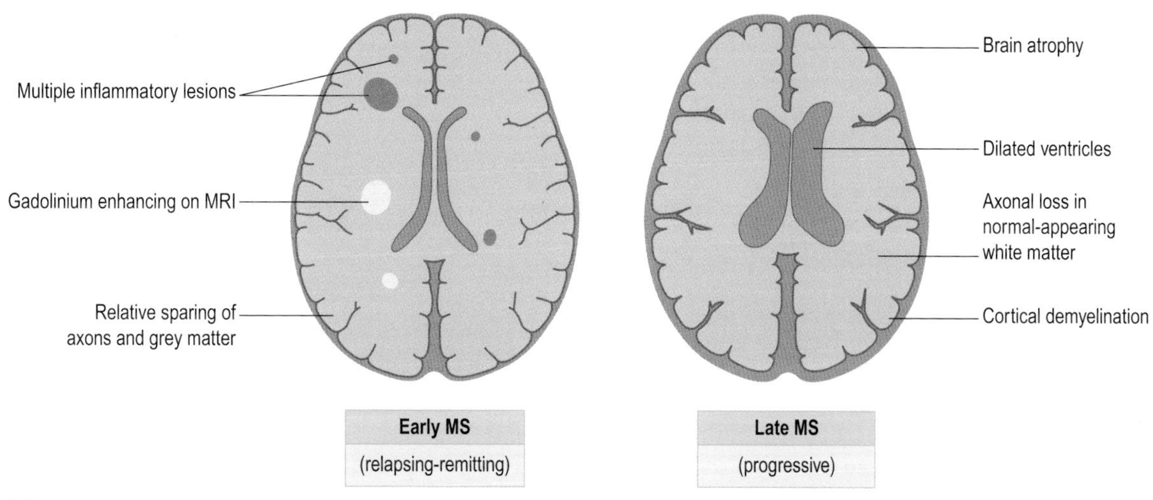

Fig. 14.19 **Neurodegeneration in multiple sclerosis.** In most patients, the early stages of MS are characterized by a relatively benign relapsing-remitting course with episodes of acute inflammatory demyelination and discrete clinical relapses, often with very good functional recovery. Most patients convert to a progressive phase of neurological decline, characterized by axonal loss (even in the normal-appearing white matter), together with plaques and neuronal loss in the cerebral cortex. The degenerative phase of MS is associated with brain atrophy and dilation of the ventricles.

Glutamate-mediated **excitotoxicity** (see Ch. 8) has also been implicated, with axonal calcium overload as a final common pathway. In experimental models of inflammation, axonal degeneration can be triggered by **nitric oxide** (which is known to be present in MS plaques and is generated in response to excess glutamatergic stimulation). In addition, the presence of **antineuronal antibodies** in the CSF of patients with MS raises the possibility of more direct, immune-mediated axonal damage.

Loss of demyelinated axons

In some cases demyelinated axons survive the acute inflammatory response but subsequently degenerate. One reason for loss of chronically demyelinated axons is lack of their normal **trophic support** from oligodendrocytes. This includes soluble mediators and trophic molecules that are required for continued neuronal survival.

Metabolically active demyelinated axons appear to be most at risk and **energy depletion** is considered to be an important factor. This may be due in part to redistribution of **sodium channels** along the internodal segments as a result of demyelination (see Fig. 14.16). This permits impulse conduction across the denuded axonal segments, but makes axonal conduction less efficient and increases axonal energy demands.

If there is inadequate ATP generation (to cope with the increased metabolic demands) then reduced activity of the ATP-dependent sodium–potassium pump may lead to the accumulation of sodium ions within the axon. This leads to impairment of the **sodium–calcium exchange pump** (which relies on the sodium gradient) with a consequent rise in the axonal free calcium concentration, triggering cell death pathways. Drugs that inhibit voltage-gated sodium or calcium channels may therefore be useful as potential neuroprotective agents in multiple sclerosis.

Cortical demyelination

The cerebral cortex also contains myelinated axons and **cortical plaques** are present in the majority of patients with MS (Fig. 14.20). Pathological studies in longstanding MS show that more than 25% of the cortex may contain plaques, which are of three types:

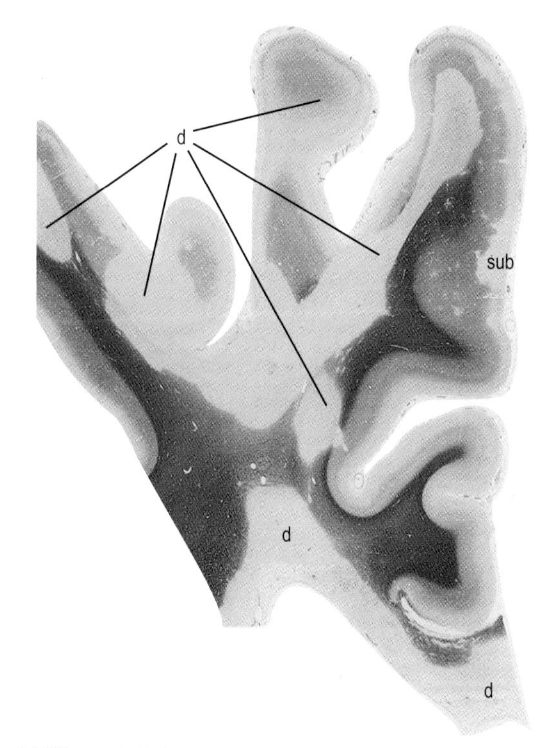

Fig. 14.20 **Cortical demyelination in multiple sclerosis.** This image shows numerous plaques of demyelination (labelled "d") at the cortical–subcortical junction, within the cerebral cortex and in the subcortical white matter. A prominent area of subpial demyelination (labelled "sub") is also indicated. [Micrograph of the cerebral hemisphere; the tissue has been stained with Luxol fast blue, which is used to demonstrate myelin]. From Ellison, D and Love, S: Neuropathology 2e (Mosby 2003) with permission.

- **Type I lesions** affect the lower half of the cerebral cortex and span the cortical–subcortical junction, therefore affecting both grey and white matter.
- **Type II lesions** are small foci of cortical demyelination that surround small blood vessels. They are the least

common and probably make a relatively minor contribution to cortical pathology.

- **Type III lesions** consist of large, confluent areas of subpial demyelination that affect the superficial half of the cortex, often spanning several adjacent gyri.

Cortical plaques are not associated with chronic inflammation, which makes them less obvious in pathological preparations. They are also difficult to identify using clinical imaging because there is no associated compromise of the blood–brain barrier (so they do not appear on T2-weighted MRI scans or with gadolinium contrast enhancement).

Pathological studies of cortical plaques show associated **axonal degeneration**, reduction in dendritic density and **neuronal apoptosis**, contributing to a greater than 20% reduction in cortical neuronal density in patients with progressive MS. Although chronic inflammatory infiltrates are not seen in association with cortical demyelination, there is prominent **microglial activation** and these cells (or cytotoxic inflammatory mediators released by them) may be responsible for the neuronal injury.

Key Points

- In the progressive phase of MS there is gradual white matter atrophy, with ventricular dilatation and thinning of the cerebral cortex, due to loss of axons and neurons.
- This degenerative element of the disease is less associated with inflammatory-demyelination and may be caused by excitotoxicity, cytopathic inflammatory mediators, antineuronal antibodies and (in the case of chronically demyelinated axons) loss of trophic support from oligodendrocytes.
- In addition to white matter lesions, there is also cortical demyelination in MS, affecting up to 25% of the cortical ribbon in late disease. This is associated with microglial activation and cytokine release rather than inflammation and is not visible with standard neuroimaging.

Appendix
Anatomical language

In anatomical descriptions, the human body is imagined to be in a standard position (Fig. A.1) so that relationships between body parts remain constant. For instance, the eyes are always 'superior to' the nose (meaning 'above' the nose in anatomical language) even when a person is lying down.

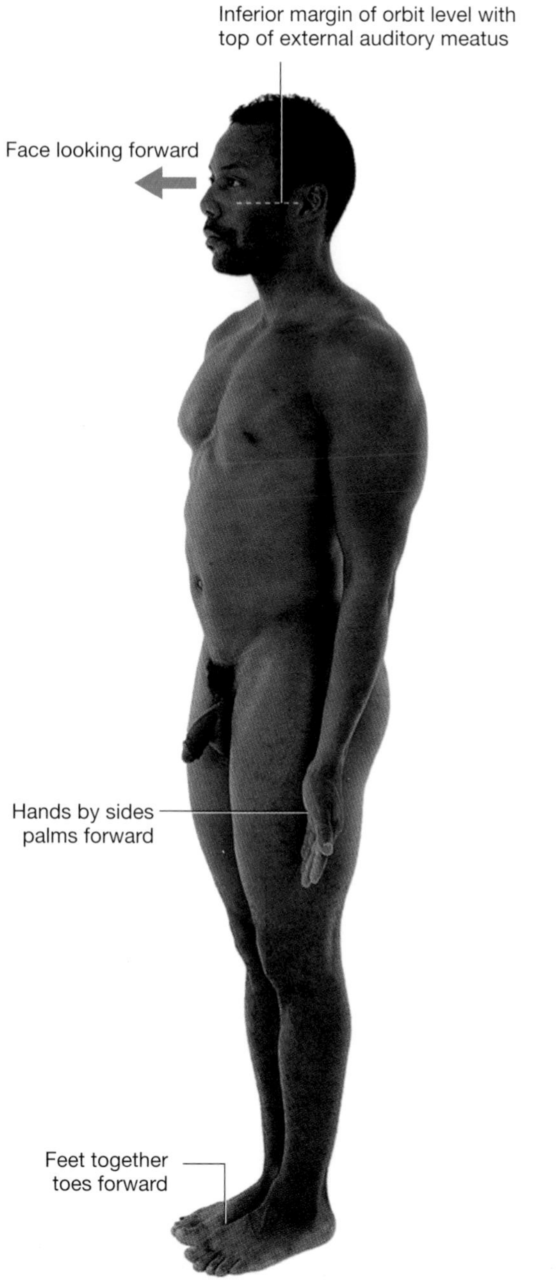

Inferior margin of orbit level with top of external auditory meatus
Face looking forward
Hands by sides palms forward
Feet together toes forward

Fig. A.1 **The anatomical position.** From Drake, R et al.: Gray's Anatomy for Students 2e (Churchill Livingstone 2009) with permission.

The axis of the nervous system (or 'neuraxis') and the usage of the terms rostral, caudal, dorsal and ventral has been discussed in Chapter 2 (see Fig. 2.8). Some other key directional terms are illustrated in Figs A.2 and A.3.

A distinction is made between structures that are 'superficial' (meaning closer to the surface) and 'deep'; for instance: the scalp is 'superficial to' the cranial vault, the cerebral cortex is 'deep to' the pia mater.

A number of other terms that are more useful in general anatomy (e.g. words to describe joint movements/positions) will not be discussed here.

Superior
Anterior
Posterior
Inferior

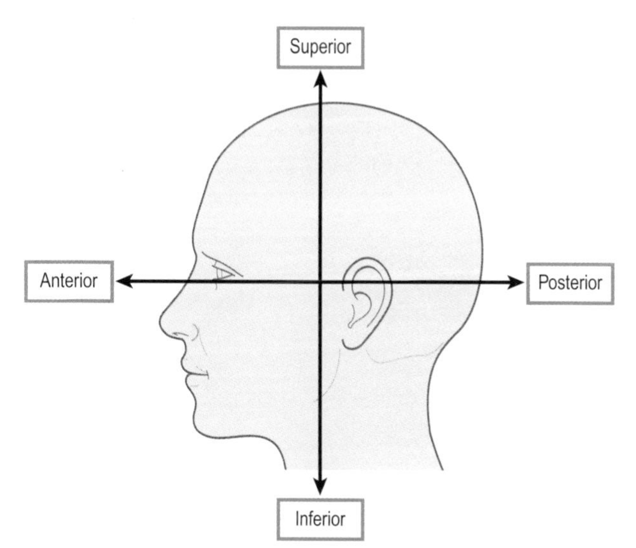

Fig. A.2 **The meaning of the terms anterior, posterior, superior and inferior.**

Lateral
Lateral
Medial

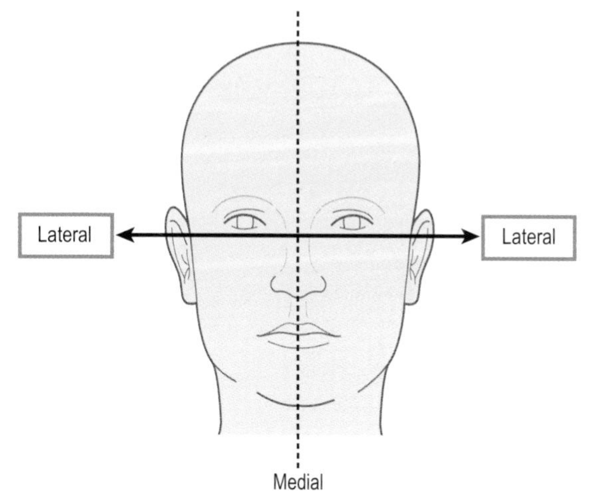

Fig. A.3 **The meaning of the terms medial and lateral.**

Three standard planes of section are described (Fig. A.4). These are used in magnetic resonance imaging (MRI) and computed tomography (CT) scanning of the brain:

- The axial (or horizontal) plane is a transverse section at right angles to the long axis of the nervous system (Fig. A.5)
- The sagittal plane divides the brain into left and right halves, like the path of a well-aimed arrow (Latin: sagitta, arrow) (Fig. A.6)
- The coronal plane is said to encircle the cerebrum like a halo or garland (Latin: corona, halo or crown) (Fig. A.7)

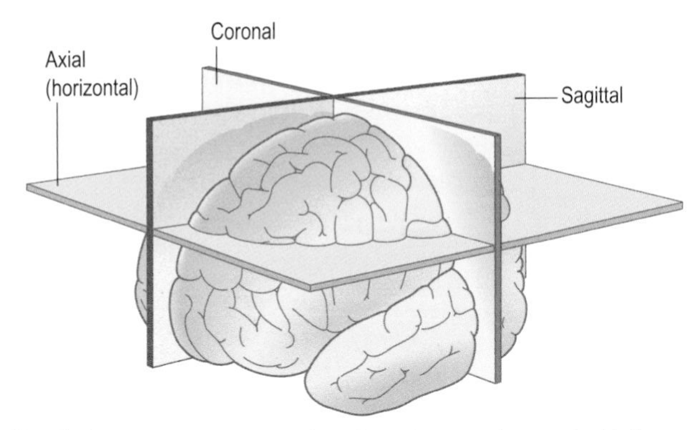

Fig. A.4 **Anatomical planes of section.** These are the standard 'reference planes' used both in cross-sectional anatomy and in medical imaging.

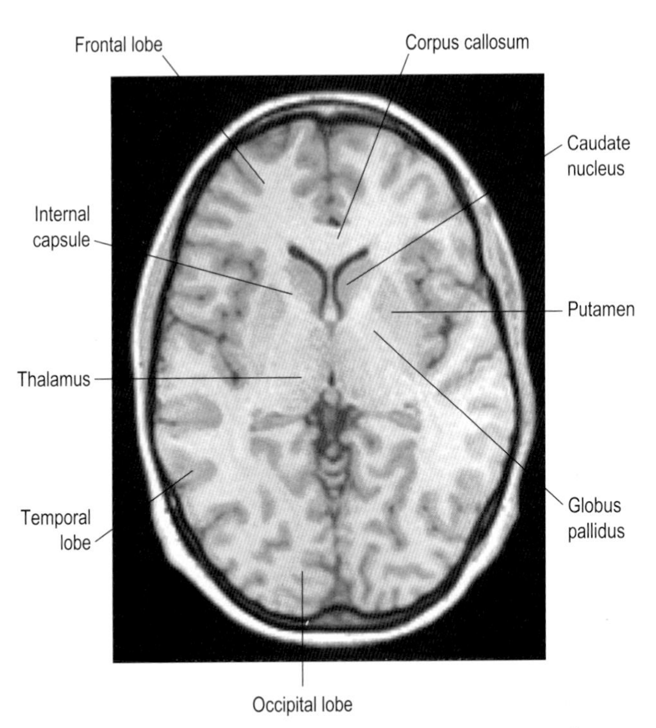

Fig. A.5 **Axial MRI scan of the brain.** Courtesy of Dr Gemma Northam.

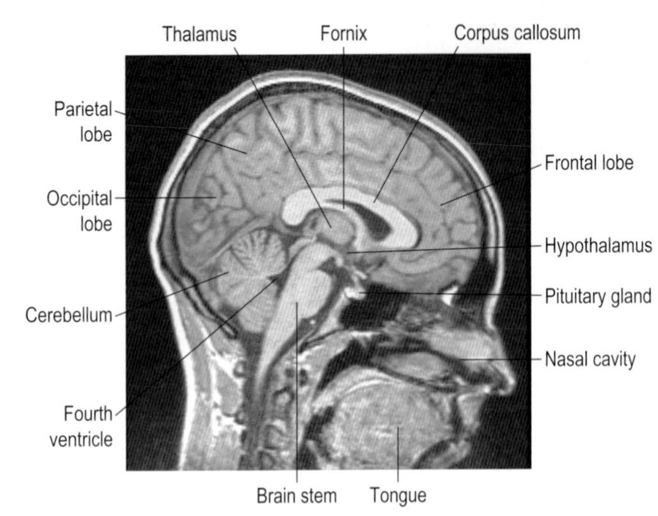

Fig. A.6 **Sagittal MRI scan of the brain.** Courtesy of Dr Gemma Northam.

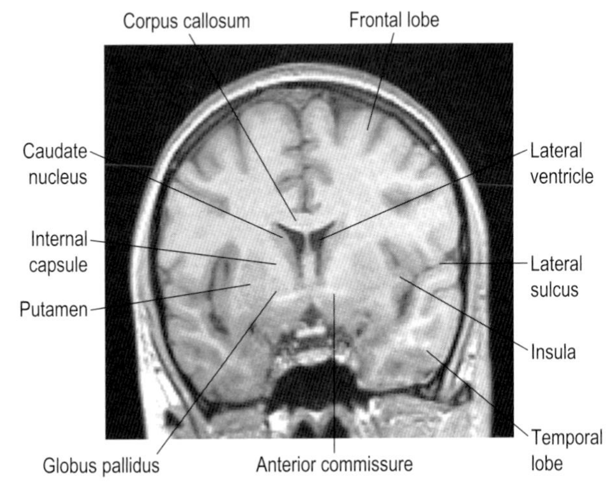

Fig. A.7 **Coronal MRI scan of the brain.** Courtesy of Dr Gemma Northam.

Key Points

- Anatomical descriptions assume that the body is in a standard anatomical position. This means that relationships between body parts do not vary (e.g. the eyes always remain 'superior to' the nose, even when a person is lying down).
- Standard anatomical terms (such as superior, inferior, anterior and posterior) are used to describe the relative positions of structures within the body.
- The terms rostral, caudal, dorsal and ventral (which are less commonly used in clinical medicine) do not mean the same thing in the brain as they do in the spinal cord. This is because the axis of the nervous system changes from horizontal to vertical at the level of the midbrain (see Ch. 2, Fig. 2.8).
- Three standard planes of section (sagittal, axial/horizontal and coronal) are used both in cross-sectional anatomy and medical imaging (e.g. MRI/CT scanning).

Index

Page numbers followed by "f" indicate figures and "b" indicate boxes.

A

B

C

J

K

L

M

N

O